SURGICAL HANDICRAFT
Manual for Surgical Residents and Surgeons

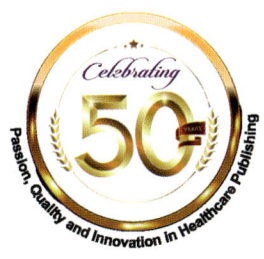

Video Contents

- Insertion of Central Line (Chapter 11)
- Venesection (Chapter 12)
- Tube Thoracostomy (Intercostal Drainage) (Chapter 39)
- Bandaging Techniques (Chapter 43)

SURGICAL HANDICRAFT
Manual for Surgical Residents and Surgeons

Second Edition

R Dayananda Babu MBBS MS MNAMS FIMSA FRCS (Glasgow)
Retired Principal and Professor Emeritus of Surgery
Department of General Surgery
Sree Gokulam Medical College and Research Foundation
Thiruvananthapuram, Kerala, India

Forewords
Santhosh John Abraham
PGR Pillai

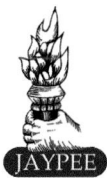

JAYPEE BROTHERS MEDICAL PUBLISHERS
The Health Sciences Publisher
New Delhi | London

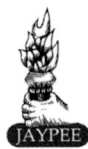 **Jaypee Brothers Medical Publishers (P) Ltd.**

Headquarters
Jaypee Brothers Medical Publishers (P) Ltd
EMCA House, 23/23-B
Ansari Road, Daryaganj
New Delhi 110 002, India
Landline: +91-11-23272143, +91-11-23272703
+91-11-23282021, +91-11-23245672
Email: jaypee@jaypeebrothers.com

Corporate Office
Jaypee Brothers Medical Publishers (P) Ltd
4838/24, Ansari Road, Daryaganj
New Delhi 110 002, India
Phone: +91-11-43574357
Fax: +91-11-43574314
Email: jaypee@jaypeebrothers.com

Overseas Office
JP Medical Ltd
83 Victoria Street, London
SW1H 0HW (UK)
Phone: +44 20 3170 8910
Fax: +44 (0)20 3008 6180
Email: info@jpmedpub.com

Website: www.jaypeebrothers.com
Website: www.jaypeedigital.com

© 2021, Jaypee Brothers Medical Publishers

The views and opinions expressed in this book are solely those of the original contributor(s)/author(s) and do not necessarily represent those of editor(s) of the book.

All rights reserved. No part of this publication may be reproduced, stored or transmitted in any form or by any means, electronic, mechanical, photocopying, recording or otherwise, without the prior permission in writing of the publishers.

All brand names and product names used in this book are trade names, service marks, trademarks or registered trademarks of their respective owners. The publisher is not associated with any product or vendor mentioned in this book.

Medical knowledge and practice change constantly. This book is designed to provide accurate, authoritative information about the subject matter in question. However, readers are advised to check the most current information available on procedures included and check information from the manufacturer of each product to be administered, to verify the recommended dose, formula, method and duration of administration, adverse effects and contraindications. It is the responsibility of the practitioner to take all appropriate safety precautions. Neither the publisher nor the author(s)/editor(s) assume any liability for any injury and/or damage to persons or property arising from or related to use of material in this book.

This book is sold on the understanding that the publisher is not engaged in providing professional medical services. If such advice or services are required, the services of a competent medical professional should be sought.

Every effort has been made where necessary to contact holders of copyright to obtain permission to reproduce copyright material. If any have been inadvertently overlooked, the publisher will be pleased to make the necessary arrangements at the first opportunity. The **CD/DVD-ROM** (if any) provided in the sealed envelope with this book is complimentary and free of cost. **Not meant for sale.**

Inquiries for bulk sales may be solicited at: jaypee@jaypeebrothers.com

Surgical Handicraft: Manual for Surgical Residents and Surgeons

First Edition: 2015
Second Edition: **2021**

ISBN: 978-93-90020-78-2

Printed at: Samrat Offset Pvt. Ltd.

Dedicated to

My teachers and students (both undergraduates and postgraduates in surgery)

My uncle, late Mr N Soman, SILO of Singapore

My parents, late Mr R Raghavan and Mrs N Mallakshy

My sister, late Ms Damayanthi

My wife, Dr Geetha Bhai and son, Deepak D Babu for their love and tolerance of yet another intrusion into the family life as the project took shape.

Great Quotations

"Surgeons believe in practice, not talent. The most important talent may be the talent for practice itself. Practice gives perfection and perfection is the excitement."
Atul Gawande

Halsted principles of surgery "Aseptic technique, gentle handling of tissue, scrupulous haemostasis and tension free, crush free and anatomically proper surgery."
William Stewart Halsted

"To study the phenomenon of disease without books is to sail an unchartered sea, while to study books without patient is not to go to sea at all."
Sir William Osler

"Truth is to be found in simplicity, and not in the multiplicity and confusion of things."
Sir Isaac Newton

"It is tasteless to prolong life, artificially. I have done my share, it is time to go. I will do it elegantly."
Albert Einstein

"The only true wisdom is in knowing, you know nothing."
Socrates

Contributors

Deepak Paul MS
Assistant Professor of Surgery
Department of General Surgery
Sree Gokulam Medical College and Research Foundation
Thiruvananthapuram, Kerala, India

Ganesh Divakar MS MCh (SCTIMST)
Fellow Spine Surgery (AIIMS)
Assistant Professor of Neurosurgery
Department of Neurosurgery
Sree Chitra Institute of Medical Sciences
Thiruvananthapuram, Kerala, India

John S Kurien MS DNB FAIS FICS
Professor of Surgery
Department of General Surgery
Believers Church Medical College
Thiruvalla, Kerala, India

Madhu Muralee
MS DNB (Surgical Oncology)
Professor of Surgical Oncology
Oncology Surgery Division
Regional Cancer Centre
Thiruvananthapuram, Kerala, India

Muhammed Muneer MS
Specialist Surgeon
Department of Surgery
Kerala Government Health Services
Changanassery, Kerala, India

Murali Appukuttan MS DNB MNAMS FAIS FACS FEBS MCh (HPB Surgery ILBS) FEBS (Surgical Oncology) FEBS (Transplant Surgery) DMAS
Gastro, Hepatopancreaticobiliary and Transplant Surgeon
Department of Gestro Surgery
Caritas Hospital
Kottayam, Kerala, India

PG Venugopalan MD
Professor of Anesthesiology
Department of Anesthsia
Sree Gokulam Medical College and Research Foundation
Thiruvananthapuram, Kerala, India

RC Sreekumar MS FRCS (Glasgow)
Postdoctoral Fellowship in Vascular Surgery
Professor of Surgery
Department of General Surgery
Government Medical College
Thiruvananthapuram, Kerala, India

R Dayananda Babu
MBBS MS MNAMS FIMSA FRCS (Glasgow)
Retired Principal and
Professor Emeritus of Surgery
Department of General Surgery
Sree Gokulam Medical College and Research Foundation
Thiruvananthapuram, Kerala, India

Shafeek Shamsudeen MS MCh
Consultant Surgical Oncologist
Department of Surgical Oncology
MVR Cancer Centre
Kozhikode, Kerala, India

Tigy Thomas Jacob D (Ortho) DNB (Ortho)
Professor of Orthopedics
Department of Orthopedics
Government Medical College
Manjeri, Kerala, India

Vinitha V Nair MS FAIS MCh (CTVS) DNB (CTVS) MNAMS FACS (CTVS) FRCS (CTh Eng) FACC MEBCTS (Europe)
Consultant Cardiothoracic and Vascular Surgeon
Department of Cardiothoracic and Vascular Surgery
Caritas Hospital
Kottayam, Kerala, India

Foreword

I was and still is perplexed when Prof R Dayananda Babu asked me to write a foreword to his second edition of the book titled *Surgical Handicraft*. He had the option to select many senior teachers in surgery or senior practicing surgeons to do this and hence my confusion. The only qualification that I can possibly think of is running a popular clinical surgical teaching program across the country.

Prof R Dayananda Babu is one of the most respected Surgical Teacher in this country and had been a recipient of the award of the "Visiting Professorship of the ASI in General Surgery in 2016" for his immense contribution to the clinical teaching of surgery. Prof R Dayananda Babu as known most popularly, had been a mentor to many of the surgeons trained and graduated out of Kerala. Most teaching programs in surgery in India will have the presence of this revered teacher as a lead faculty. As a young entrant into surgery, I had been following his shadow in getting me stuck to the surgical academics.

In the era of an exponential growth of knowledge with availability of many investigative armamentariums, the art of clinical medicine is fading fast. Both patients and clinicians with pretended paucity of time resort to "tests" before even listening to the story of the ailment. By history of illness and thorough physical examination with correct methods of eliciting signs, one can have a definite diagnosis in more than 90% of the situations. The comprehension of symptoms and signs in the diagnostic canvas is as much an art as science is. The ability of the teacher is in initiating this reasonableness in the thoughts of the students in arriving at a clinical diagnosis followed by appropriate investigations and management. Unfortunately the qualified novice in surgery has no exposure to the "skills" in carrying out the procedures involved in managing the patients.

The clinical acumen and profound teaching experience of Prof R Dayananda Babu had been translated into few elegant books which are highly circulated among both undergraduate and postgraduate students in surgery. The book titled the "*Surgical Handicraft*" helps the interns, residents and even the practitioners to adopt the correct methods to perform these procedures.

The book has an elegant style of narration, fine pictorial representation, authentic scientific basis and precise practical steps. The concise package to the learner is of great value during both studentship and well as in actual surgical practice. Contemporary teaching in surgery is facing a huge challenge in moving away from a clinical platform to a physically detached simulator-based teaching. With availability of many institutions for healthcare delivery and medical teaching in the country, most students are not getting enough chances to see and learn the skill and put it into practice.

In the book *"Surgical Handicraft"*, Prof R Dayananda Babu, describes most of the procedures a junior surgical person is asked to carry out in his day-to-day practice. Most of these are not formally taught but are transferred from seniors to juniors and are bound to be learned wrongly without proper supervision. The relevance of this book comes in at this juncture in providing the safe and correct methodology. The second edition is expanded further with inclusion of few additional topics to encompass more areas apart from redrafting the old ones with contemporary scientific tinge. Majority of the chapters are concept driven and if learned well can make a substantial change in the attitude of surgical performance and hence the results. I strongly recommend this book to all surgeons.

Santhosh John Abraham
MS DiPNB (Surg) FRCS (Eng) FRCS (Edin) FRCS (Glas) FACS
Past President, The Association of Surgeons of India

Foreword

Surgery is that branch of medicine in which an operation (handicraft or instrumental intervention) may have a great role to play in the treatment. Hence, different to other medical disciplines, it requires the development of a physical craft with cognitive growth. Accuracy, speed, economy of effort, coordination of actions, efficient and appropriate surgical skill are all important factors in the art and practice of surgery.

There has been a void in Surgical Handicraft Textbooks since Pye's Surgical Handicraft: A Manual of Surgical Manipulations, Minor Surgery (1893). In the preface to the very first edition Pye wrote, "In this book I have endeavored to describe the details of surgical work as it appears from the point of view of house surgeons and dressers in surgical wards".

This book by Dr R Dayananda Babu provides a unique learning environment wherein surgical residents can acquire technical skills, knowledge and confidence; the essentials of the craft of surgery. The contents of the book is appropriately described by its title, *Surgical Handicraft: Manual for Surgical Residents and Surgeons*. This book will help all doctors intending a surgical career or surgically related career as a foundation text and, of course, in day-to-day "general practice" which is fast disappearing.

This book is written with emphasis on standard surgical principles and techniques. It outlines fundamental principles of major and minor surgeries; to ensure the success of procedures, to help to avoid pitfalls and to minimize the risk of complications. The book *Surgical Handicraft: Manual for Surgical Residents and Surgeons* has been written primarily for house surgeons and junior residents, with constant attention to the thought, "Is this something a student should know when he or she finishes undergraduate medical study?" The field of surgical techniques is broad and varied and "Surgical Handicraft" covers the many techniques effectively utilized to perform the training of today's medical graduates, residents and young surgeons with existing evidence-based knowledge.

Dr R Dayananda Babu has been a long-time colleague of mine. His vast knowledge of both theory and the art of surgery is personally known to me. This is his fifth book.

It is an honor to be associated with this book. I recommend this book as a companion and compendium to surgical studies, with full satisfaction.

PGR Pillai
Former Professor and Head, Department of Surgery
Government Medical College, Kottayam
Dean, Faculty of Medicine, Mahatma Gandhi University, Kottayam
Dean of Faculty of Medical Science
Cochin University of Science and Technology
Kochi, Kerala, India

Preface to the Second Edition

This book is meant as a manual for the neophyte interns, postgraduates and all surgical residents, for giving basic surgical skills during their initial surgical career. The emphasis is on standard surgical principles and techniques of major and minor surgeries.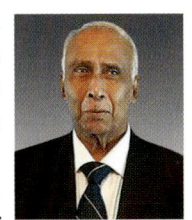

The first edition of surgical handicraft was published in 2015 and it was sold out in 2019. As surgery is a field of everchanging developments and innovations, it was time for a thorough revision of the old chapters of this book. There was also a need for addition of few more important new chapters.

The role of prehabilitation and surgical nutrition is well-known for a successful outcome for a major surgery. New chapters on intestinal anastomosis, vascular anastomosis, feeding jejunostomy, energy sources in surgery, are some of the highlights of this new edition. Chapters on operation theater etiquette, surgical knots, surgical incisions are also included.

The medical profession is facing many challenges in this consumer era and therefore it is important to know the basic concepts of medical ethics in surgical practice, written informed consent for surgery and medical negligence. Effective communication is important for a successful surgical career and therefore a chapter on breaking the bad news is included.

I am sure this revised edition of *Surgical Handicraft* will go a long way in helping the surgical aspirant in acquiring the art and science of basic surgical skills.

R Dayananda Babu

Preface to the First Edition

It is with great pleasure and immense satisfaction I am writing the preface of my second book titled *Surgical Handicraft: Manual for Surgical Residents and Surgeons*.

Medical students who have completed their course and are entering the clinical training, especially in surgery, must be well educated in basics. Most of the time, they are not guided properly during their house surgery. This book is meant for the neophyte intern whose main interest at present is learning multiple choice questions (MCQs) rather than getting hands-on training. The junior residents also get into the surgery departments without proper hands, on exposure during house surgency.

The famous quotation by Virchow is always there in my mind—"Brevity in writing is the best insurance for its perusal." This book is written in a notebook style. The presentation is simple and lucid with liberal use of pictures to facilitate the reading. Basic topics, such as handwashing, gloving, universal precautions, fluid resuscitation, insertion of intravenous cannula, urinary catheter, and nasogastric tube, are discussed. The Interactive DVD provided with this book demonstrates bandaging techniques, central line insertion and tube thoracostomy.

I hope that this book may contribute to improving the training of house surgeons and junior residents. Finally, let me quote Isaac Newton—

"If I have seen a little further it is by standing on the shoulders of giants—My teachers".

R Dayananda Babu

Acknowledgments

This book became a reality because of the constant support and encouragement of Shri Jitendar P Vij (Group Chairman), M/s Jaypee Brothers Medical Publishers (P) Ltd, New Delhi, India.

I am grateful to my esteemed contributors:
- Professor (Dr) John S Kurien MS DNB FAIS FICS (Professor of Surgery, Believers Church Medical College, Thiruvalla)
- Dr Tigy Thomas Jacob D (Ortho) DNB (Ortho) (Professor of Orthopedics, Government Medical College, Manjeri)
- Dr PG Venugopalan MD (Professor of Anesthesiology, Sree Gokulam Medical College, Thiruvananthapuram)
- Dr Ganesh Divakar MS MCh (Associate Professor of Neurosurgery, Sree Chitra Institute of Medical Sciences, Thiruvananthapuram)
- Professor (Dr) RC Sreekumar MS FRCS Post-Doctoral Fellowship in Vascular Surgery (Professor of Vascular Surgery, Government Medial College, Thiruvananthapuram)
- Dr Madhu Muralee MS DNB (Surgical Oncology) (Additional Professor of Regional Cancer Center, Thiruvananthapuram)
- Dr Murali V Appukuttan MS MCh (Consultant, Gastro, Hepatopancreaticobiliary and Liver Transplant Surgeon, Caritas Hospital, Kottayam)
- Dr Vinita MS MCh (Consultant Cardiothoracic and Vascular Surgeon, Caritas Hospital, Kottayam)
- Dr Deepak Paul MS (Assistant Professor of Surgery, Sree Gokulam Medical College, Thiruvananthapuram)
- Dr Shafeeq MS MCh (Consultant Oncosurgeon, MVR Cancer Centre, Kozhikode)
- Dr Muhammed Muneer MS (Specialist Surgeon, Government Health Services, Changanacherry).

I am also thankful to Dr Sagar Sahita, Fobin Varghese, T Saravanam and Nimmy Varghese from Government Medical Collage, Kottayam, Kerala for the interactive DVD. My special thanks to Dr Deepak Paul for spending time out with me in going through the entire proof and correcting it. The medical illustration part of this book was done by Dr Muhammed Muneer and orthopedic chapter by Dr Tigy Thomas Jacob.

My thanks are also due to, my son Deepak D Babu, a final year medical student, who was instrumental in doing the work of 6 new chapters by me for the new edition. My wife, Dr Geetha Bhai, retired Professor of Microbiology, was giving moral support during the entire revision work.

I must thank to Dr Santhosh John Abraham MS FRCS (London) FRCS (Glasgow) FRCS (Edinburgh) FACS (former National President of Association of Surgeons of India, and currently Director of Surgical Educations ASI) for writing the foreword, who is a close friend of mine, a surgeon par excellence.

I would also like to thank, Mr Ankit Vij (Managing Director), Dr Savleen Kaur (Development Editor) of M/s Jaypee Brothers Medical Publishers (P) Ltd, for the editorial help during the entire process of revision of the book. I am also thankful to Arun Kumar C of Jaypee Brothers Medical Publishers, Thiruvananthapuram, Kerala, India.

Contents

1. **Model Conduct for House Surgeons/Residents** 1
   R Dayananda Babu

2. **Duties and Responsibilities of House Surgeons/Interns (Compulsory Rotating Resident Internship—CRRI)** 3
   R Dayananda Babu

3. **9 Tips for House Surgeons/Residents** 6
   R Dayananda Babu

4. **Handwashing Practice** 10
   R Dayananda Babu

5. **Gloving Techniques** 15
   R Dayananda Babu

6. **Ethics and Consent** 19
   R Dayananda Babu

7. **The Operation Theater Etiquette, the Surgical Team, and Assisting at Operations** 25
   R Dayananda Babu

8. **Classification of Surgical Procedures and ASI Classification of Physical Fitness** 33
   R Dayananda Babu

9. **Energy Sources in Surgery** 36
   John S Kurien

10. **Intravenous Cannulation** 54
    PG Venugopalan

11. **Central Venous Catheter** 60
    John S Kurien

12. **Venous Cutdown** 71
    John S Kurien

13. **Local Anesthetics Used for Minor Surgery** 75
    R Dayananda Babu

14. **Digital Nerve Blocks (Finger and Toe Blocks)** 78
    R Dayananda Babu

15. **Surgical Blades, Skin Incisions, and Acute Wound Closure** 81
    R Dayananda Babu

16. **Surgical Incisions** 91
    R Dayananda Babu

17. **Sutures** 101
    John S Kurien

18. **Surgical Knots: Different Types** 106
    Muhammed Muneer

19. **Minor Surgical Procedures of Subcutaneous Swellings** 113
    R Dayananda Babu

20. **Incision and Drainage of Abscess** 119
    R Dayananda Babu

21. **Preoperative Preparation in General for Elective Surgery** 122
    R Dayananda Babu

22. **Preoperative Preparation of Common Operations** 128
    R Dayananda Babu

23. **"Safe Surgery Saves Lives"—A WHO Initiative** 134
    R Dayananda Babu

24. **Prophylactic Antibiotics in Surgery** 137
    R Dayananda Babu

25. **Surgical Site Infection** 142
    R Dayananda Babu

26. **Intravenous Fluids and Postoperative Fluid Management** 147
    R Dayananda Babu

27. **Intestinal Anastomosis** 160
    Madhu Muralee

28. **Vascular Anastomosis** 173
    RC Sreekumar

29. **Nutrition in Surgical Practice** 186
    Murali Appukuttan, Vinitha V Nair

30. **Feeding Jejunostomy** 226
    Shafeek Shamsudeen

31. **Respiratory Complications after Surgery** 233
    Deepak Paul

32. **Prophylaxis and Treatment of Deep Vein Thrombosis and Pulmonary Embolism** 240
    R Dayananda Babu

33. **Burst Abdomen (Wound Dehiscence) and Tension Sutures** 248
    R Dayananda Babu

34. **Methicillin-resistant *Staphylococcus aureus* (MRSA)** 252
    R Dayananda Babu

35. **Ingrowing Toe Nail** 254
    R Dayananda Babu

36. **Nasogastric Intubation (Ryle's Tube)** 257
    R Dayananda Babu

37. **Urethral Catheterization** 262
    R Dayananda Babu

38. **Resuscitation in Trauma** 274
    R Dayananda Babu

39. **Intercostal Drainage Tube** 288
    John S Kurien

40. **Cardiopulmonary Resuscitation** 299
    PG Venugopalan

41. **Head Injury** 307
    Ganesh Divakar

42. **Use of Antiseptics and Ointments for Wound Management** 328
    R Dayananda Babu

43. **Bandaging Techniques** 332
    John S Kurien

44. **Medical Negligence (Professional Negligence/Malpractice)** 344
    R Dayananda Babu

45. **Breaking the Bad News** 349
    R Dayananda Babu

46. **Orthopedics** 353
    Tigy Thomas Jacob

Index.. *421*

Model Conduct for House Surgeons/Residents

R Dayananda Babu

CODE OF CONDUCT

- Character of the physician:
  "An upright man, instructed in the art of healing, Pure in character and diligent in caring for the sick,
  He should be modest, sober, patient, prompt to do his whole duty without anxiety,
  Pious without going so far as superstition."
- Physician's responsibility:
  The objective of the medical profession is to render service to humanity with full respect for the dignity of man.
- Develop the affective domain (heart): "Medicine is an art, not trade.
  A calling, not business,
  A calling in which your heart will be equally used as your head."

  —*William Osler*

"It is with heart one sees rightly,
what is essential is invisible to the eye"
"Where there is a love for humanity, there is love for the art of medicine."

—*Hippocrates*

"To cure occasionally,
To relieve sometimes and To comfort always."

—*Louis Pasteur*

- *Develop soft skills*:
  - Communication (Communicate to the patient and bystanders)
  - *Empathy*: Experiencing the feelings and thoughts of another person
  - *Humility*: State of being humble.
- *Success will depend upon your attitude*:
  - Attitude will decide the altitude
  - "The greatest discovery of my generation is that human beings can alter their lives by altering their attitudes of mind."—*William James* (Harvard University).
- Reliability and punctuality are the two most important qualities of a successful doctor.

- *Dress code*:
    - A clean white coat always looks professional
    - Dirty, polo-necked sweaters are not acceptable.
- *Be well-equipped*:
    - Carry a spiral diary to note down the work, rather than rely on memory
    - Carry stethoscope, pen torch, knee hammer, measuring tape, etc.
- *Never display the arrogance of office*: Arrogance is a sign of ignorance and immaturity.

There is no role for high-handed behavior inside the hospital:
- Never make comments like "This patient should have been sent to hospital much earlier".
- *Primum non-nocere (primarily do no harm)*: In any real doubt or difficulty, consult the senior doctor. Know your limitations.
- A doctor should not run except in dire emergency, such as cardiac arrest or total respiratory obstruction.
- Get along well with seniors, nurses, paramedical staff, technicians, and subordinates. The intelligent resident can learn a lot from the nursing staff.
- Give due respect to senior doctors and doctors coming from other institutions.
- *Be an active listener*: Active listening encourages the patients to tell his or her story of the illness.
- Know how to break bad news (Read tips for house surgeons).
- *Avoid social evils such as smoking, alcohol, and drugs*: Doctor must be a role model for the community.
- Always look confident.

2. Duties and Responsibilities of House Surgeons/Interns (Compulsory Rotating Resident Internship—CRRI)

R Dayananda Babu

1. *Training period*: House surgency is a training period and forms part of the curriculum. Only after successful completion of this training program, you are eligible for permanent registration. You get hands on training of various ward procedures, suturing techniques, minor operations, etc. during this period and you are always supervised by a senior doctor.
2. *Resident doctor (24 × 7)*: The intern is in charge of the life and health of his patient with continuous medical cover. He is on call duty for 24 hours, 7 days a week. He must be staying in the resident's area of the hospital.
3. *Time keeping*: They should report for duty 30 minutes before the consultant is expected. He/she should take preliminary rounds, note down the vital signs, collect the investigation results, write the progress notes and send appropriate investigations, etc. Those who are on casualty duty should relieve the night duty house surgeon at the correct time (8.00 AM).
4. *Inform your whereabouts to the duty nurse and operator*: It is better to display your mobile number in the ward concerned.
5. *Case sheet writing*: Complete the case sheets within 24 hours of admission and this must be written legibly. All documentations in the case sheets must be recorded with date and time. Every day you should write the daily progress in the concerned sheet with date and time. Do not write "repeat 1, 2, 3" when you start a fresh page of doctor's orders (instead write the entire orders). When there is cancellation of an order, cross the order vertically with date and time. It is better to review the entire orders when there are too many cancellations. All laboratory results must be entered in the case sheets. Always use polite language for writing consultations. Use red ink only for writing night instructions. Whenever you attend a call during duty hours, record your clinical findings in the

case sheets and if you prescribe medications, it should be noted in the case sheet with date, time, and your signature. When you discharge a patient, the facing sheet of the case sheet must be filled up. The final diagnosis (if pathology report is there, that will form the final diagnosis) must be written in capital letters, so also the name of the operation. There must be a discharge summary written legibly in the facing sheet. Always mention whether the patient is cured, relieved, dead, or otherwise. If you are discharging a patient Against Medical Advice (DAMA), use the appropriate printed form in the case sheet. *If the patient is sensitive to any drug, it should be noted with block letters in red ink in front of the file/case sheet. This is applicable also for hepatitis B surface antigen (HBsAg) and methicillin-resistant Staphylococcus aureus (MRSA).*

6. *Prescribing drugs*: Always write the prescription legibly (better to write the pharmacological name rather than the brand name) and put your signature along with your full name and designation. If you are not sure about the dose and mode of administration *do not hesitate to ask the senior*. You should also know the contraindications for the drug and the various possible reactions. *Test dose* should be administered for penicillin group of drugs and other drugs which can produce reactions.

7. *Five day rule for antibiotics*: Antibiotics once prescribed should not be continued indefinitely. It is better to ask the consultant whether to continue it or not at the end of 5 days.

8. *Writing a request form for laboratory*: Write the request legibly. Write the name, age, IP No., and unit of the patient. Give a brief clinical history, and mention previous diagnosis and pathology reports, if any. The name of the requesting doctor and designation must be mentioned and should be properly signed.

9. *Getting ready for rounds*: The house surgeon must present the case during rounds. He will be standing on the left side of the patient facing the consultant. He should know the vital signs of the patient, any night events that has happened, drugs given to the patient, and any fresh complaints for the patient.

10. *Attending a call*: While on duty, you will be called to see the patients in the ward. He/she should immediately attend the call, examine the patient after taking brief account of the history and note down the clinical findings in the case sheets with date and time. Ensure that your instructions are executed by the nurse. For a dying patient, institute resuscitative measure and cardiopulmonary resuscitation (CPR), if required. In the event of death of a patient, inform the duty Medical Officer (MO) immediately and act in accordance to his advice.

11. *Preparation of patient for special investigations, invasive procedures, surgical procedures, delivery, etc.*: Carry out the preparations required for a particular procedure. If you do not know the preparation, contact the concerned department/specialist.

12. *Never send unstable patients for scanning and other procedures unattended*: Whenever you send a sick patient to another department, it is your duty to accompany the patient, so that any untoward incident can be tackled.
13. *Consent*: Informed consent must be taken for all procedures, special investigations, and surgical procedures after explaining the procedure. Explain the merits, demerits, benefits expected, and the risks involved in the procedure. Use the language which the patient and relatives can understand. Avoid technical terms. Explain the necessity of the procedure. Discuss also the alternative procedures available. Be realistic, however, do not scare the patient. The consent must be signed by the patient himself if he/she is an adult. It is better to get the signature of a witness.
14. *Arrival of a consultant to see your case*: When another specialist comes to see your case, ensure that you are present there to brief him about the patient and clarify his doubts.
15. *Discharge card and reference letter*: Discharge card is a permanent record which will go to other doctors and hospitals. Therefore, it should be legibly written. The final diagnosis and the name of the operation should be written in capital letters. It is important to enter all significant laboratory values and investigation reports in brief. After writing the card it should be shown to a senior doctor and get it approved before handing over to the patient. Whenever you write a reference letter to another center, it is advisable to prepare it and get it approved by a senior person.
16. *Death certificate and medicolegal formalities are done by the duty medical officer*. Please confirm the death with the help of a senior doctor before declaring it.
17. *Log book*: The log book is permanent record of your day-to-day ward work and it must be completed at the end of your posting. There is a printed assessment sheet for each posting and the book will be evaluated by the concerned unit chief and the appropriate score will be given.
18. *Take leave only after prior sanction*. The house surgeon is eligible for 20 days of leave as noted below:
    - Medicine including psychiatry—3 days
    - Surgery including anesthesia—3 days
    - Specialty [casualty; ear, nose, and throat (ENT); ophthalmology; elective—1 day each]—4 days
    - Obstetrics and gynecology—3 days
    - Pediatrics—2 days
    - Community medicine—3 days
    - Orthopedics—2 days.

9 Tips for House Surgeons/Residents

R Dayananda Babu

Tip 1—Be five star doctors [World Health Organization (WHO)]
The five star qualities of a doctor are:
1. Care provider
2. Leader
3. Manager
4. Decision maker
5. Communicator.

Tip 2—Remember the four pillars of ethics:
1. *Patient autonomy*: The most important norm of medical practice is patient autonomy, which granted the patient the right to get treated or not, the right to accept or reject a certain type of treatment. For instance, certain sections of Christianity called Jehovah Witness do not accept blood transfusion. In such cases, we have to give first preference to the choice of the patient, the second to that of spouse, and third to the view of the relatives.
2. *Beneficence*: All actions of physicians should be aimed at the good of the patient. This is the second norm to be addressed in ethics.
3. *Nonmaleficence*: Nonmaleficence means that doctors should ensure that his approach did not result in a wrong being done to the patient, i.e., *Primum non nocere—primarily do no harm* to the patient.
4. *Spirit of generosity and service*: Spirit of generosity and service is the most ideal for a doctor.

Tip 3—Practice handwashing (Refer to Chapter 4).

Tip 4—Practice universal precautions:
- All hospital staff must adhere rigorously to protective measures which minimize exposure to the diseases transmitted through blood, blood products, and body fluids.
- It is based on the concepts that all persons are potential sources of infection independent of diagnosis or perceived risk.
- The use of universal precautions involves placing barriers between staff and all blood and body fluids.

UNIVERSAL PRECAUTIONS

- Wearing protective gloves (ideally double gloves during surgery—bigger size inside and smaller size outside)
- Wearing protective eyewear (preferably goggles during surgery)
- Wearing mask, protective apron, and gown
- Wearing boots for covering the foot and lower leg during surgery
- Washing hands after removal of the gloves
- Washing hands between patients
- Always use gloves for handling blood, blood products, and body fluids
- Undertaking hepatitis B vaccination
- Covering open wounds
- Staff with infected wounds and active dermatitis must stay off work
- Using safe sharp instrument handling techniques consisting of the following:
  - Never recap a hollow needle after use
  - Sharp instruments should not be passed between surgeon and nurse
  - The sharp instruments are placed into a bowl or tray and which can then be used to transfer
  - Only one sharp instrument be placed in the tray at a time
  - When two surgeons are operating, each surgeon will have their own sharp tray
  - Used needles and other disposable sharp are discarded into an approved sharp container.

Tip 5—Practice evidence-based medicine **(Tables 1 and 2)**.

Tip 6—WHO surgical safety checklist (refer to Chapter 5).

Tip 7—Doctor–patient relationship.

There are several models of doctor–patient relationship. The doctor must be able to shift models as per the clinical situations and needs of the patient.

Table 1: Evidence-based classification of medical literature (Agency for Healthcare Policy and Research).	
Class I evidence	Prospective, randomized controlled trials—the gold standard of clinical trials. Some may be poorly designed, have in adequate numbers, or suffer from other methodological inadequacies and, thus, may not be clinically significant
Class II evidence	• Clinical studies in which the data were collected prospectively and retrospective analyses that were based on clearly reliable data • These types of studies include observational studies, cohort studies, prevalence studies, and case–control studies
Class III evidence	Studies based on retrospectively collected data. Evidence used in this class includes clinical series, databases or registries, case reviews, case reports, and expert opinion

Table 2: Categorization of strengths of recommendations for evidence-based practice.

Level I	This recommendation is convincingly justifiable based on the available scientific information alone. It is usually based on class I data; however, strong class II evidence may form the basis for a level 1 recommendation, especially if the issue does not lend itself to testing in a randomized format. Conversely, weak or contradictory class I data may not be able to support a level 1 recommendation
Level II	This recommendation is reasonably justifiable by available scientific evidence and strongly supported by expert critical care opinion. It is usually supported by class II data or a preponderance of class III evidence
Level III	This recommendation is supported by available data, but adequate scientific evidence is lacking. It is generally supported by class III data. This type of recommendation is useful for educational purposes and in guiding future studies

- *Active-passive model*:
    - The patient is having a passive role and the doctor takes control.
    - The patient takes no responsibility for their care.
    - This model is suitable when the patient is unconscious or bedridden.
- *Teacher-student model*:
    - The doctor is having a paternalistic and controlling role.
    - The patient is having the role of dependence and acceptance.
    - This model is observed during recovery of a patient after surgery.
- *Mutual participation model*:
    - In this situation, there is an equal role between the doctor and the patient and depends upon each other's input.
    - This is applied in treatment of chronic illness such as diabetes and renal failure.
- *Friendship model*: Here, the doctor converts the patient care into a relationship of mutual sharing of personal information and love and hence there is blurring of boundaries of professionalism.

Tip 8—Breaking the bad news [Source—medical records, documentation, and consent by Indian Medical Association (IMA)]:
- No "conspiracy of silence".
- Honesty and openness.
- The question is not whether to tell the patient but when and how.
- Truth is not the enemy of hope.
- The patient is interested in the issue of suffering than the actual diagnosis.
- Let the patient control the flow of information.
- Some relatives insist on not to tell the patient. Explore reasons. Physician's first duty is to the patient. Inform the relatives of the patient's awareness.

- Promise you will go only as far as the patient wants and not take a blunt or confronting approach. Inform them of the outcome of the interview. Offer to see patient and relatives together, if needed.

Tip 9—A nine-point program for better communication
(Better communication is the key to better doctor–patient–nurse relations)
(Source—medical records, documentation and consent by IMA):
- Be clear in your own mind what you want to put across. How and why.
- Make yourself agreeable to the patient. Put the message in the most acceptable form.
- Talk in the language of the patient and relate your message to his own level of intellectual, understanding, prejudice, emotion, and self-interest.
- Aim to arouse the patient's immediate interest and then hold it.
- Choose the right medium.
- Choose the right timing, right intensity, and right length of message.
- Release your hopes and persuasion to what is predictable.
- Use every means to receive and interpret the "feedback". Remember that communication is a hazardous activity prone to mistakes, distortion, and misunderstandings.
- Simply what you want to put over.

4. Handwashing Practice

R Dayananda Babu

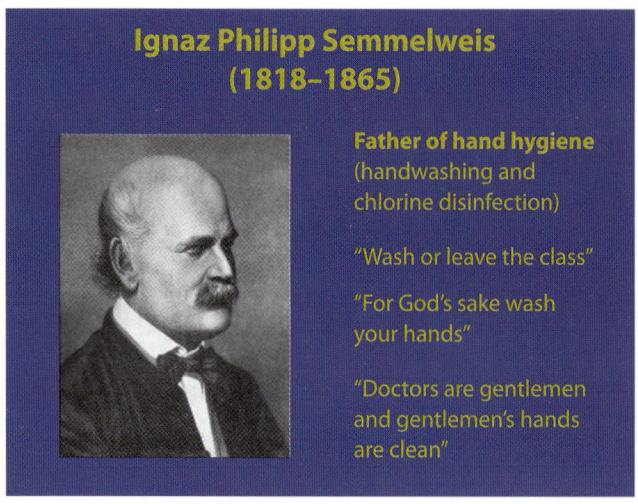

CLEAN HANDS SAVE LIVES WORLD HEALTH ORGANIZATION

"Prevention is better than cure". Nowhere is this saying truer than in the setting of healthcare-associated infections (HAI). Few extra moments of care, some effort, simple precautions, and a little additional investment in hand hygiene practices can translate into shorter hospital stay, reduced costs of care, and avoidance of serious and occasionally life-threatening complications by reducing the HAI.

What to Use for Routine Hand Antisepsis?

Use soap and water (hand washing) for routine hand antisepsis, if hands are visibly dirty or visibly soiled with blood or other body fluids or after using the toilet. Otherwise, use alcohol-based handrubs (handrubbing). At present, alcohol-based hand rubs are the only known means for rapidly and effectively inactivating a wide array or potentially harmful microorganisms on hand.

When to Clean Your Hands?

World Health Organization (WHO) recommends the "My 5 Moments for Hand Hygiene" approach as key to protect the patient, the healthcare worker, and healthcare environment against the spread of pathogens and thus reduced HAI.

Five Moments for Hand Hygiene

- *Moment 1*: Before touching a patient
- *Moment 2*: Before a clean/aseptic procedure
- *Moment 3*: After body fluid exposure risk
- *Moment 4*: After touching a patient
- *Moment 5*: After touching patient surroundings

How to Wash Hand?

Surgical hand preparation should reduce the release of skin bacteria from the hands of the surgical team for the duration of the procedure, in case of unnoticed puncture of the surgical gloves. Medicated soap and alcohol-based preparations are available. Preference should be given for alcohol-based formulations. The initial reduction of the resident flora is rapid and effective with this. Steps before starting hand preparation are:

- Keep nails short and pay attention to them when washing. Most microbes come from beneath fingernails.
- Do not wear artificial nails or nail polish.
- Remove all jewelry (rings, watches, and bracelets) before entering the operation theater.
- Wash hand and arms with a nonmedicated soap before entering the operation theater area or if hands are visibly soiled.
- Clean subungual areas with a nail file.
- Nail brushes should not be used, as they may damage the skin and shedding of cells. If used, nail brushes should be sterile once only use. Reusable autoclavable brushes are on the market.

Procedural Steps

- *Start timing*: Scrub each side of each finger, between the fingers, and the back and front of the hand for *2 minutes*.
- Proceed to scrub the forearms keeping the hand higher than the arm at all times. This helps to avoid recontamination of the hands by water from the elbows and prevents bacteria-laden soap and water from contaminating the hands.
- Wash each side of the forearm from wrist to the elbow for *1 minute*.
- Repeat the process on the other hand and forearm, keeping hands above the elbow at all times. If the hand touches anything at any time, the scrub must be lengthened by 1 minute for the area that has been contaminated.
- Rinse hands and forearms by passing them through the water in one direction only, from fingertips to elbow. Do not move the arm back and forth through the water.

- Proceed to the operating theater holding hands above elbows.
- At all times, during the scrub procedure, care should be taken not to splash water on to surgical attire.
- Once in the operating theater, hands and forearms should be dried using a sterile towel and aseptic technique before donning gown and gloves.

See the pictures for handwashing **(Figs. 1A to I)**.

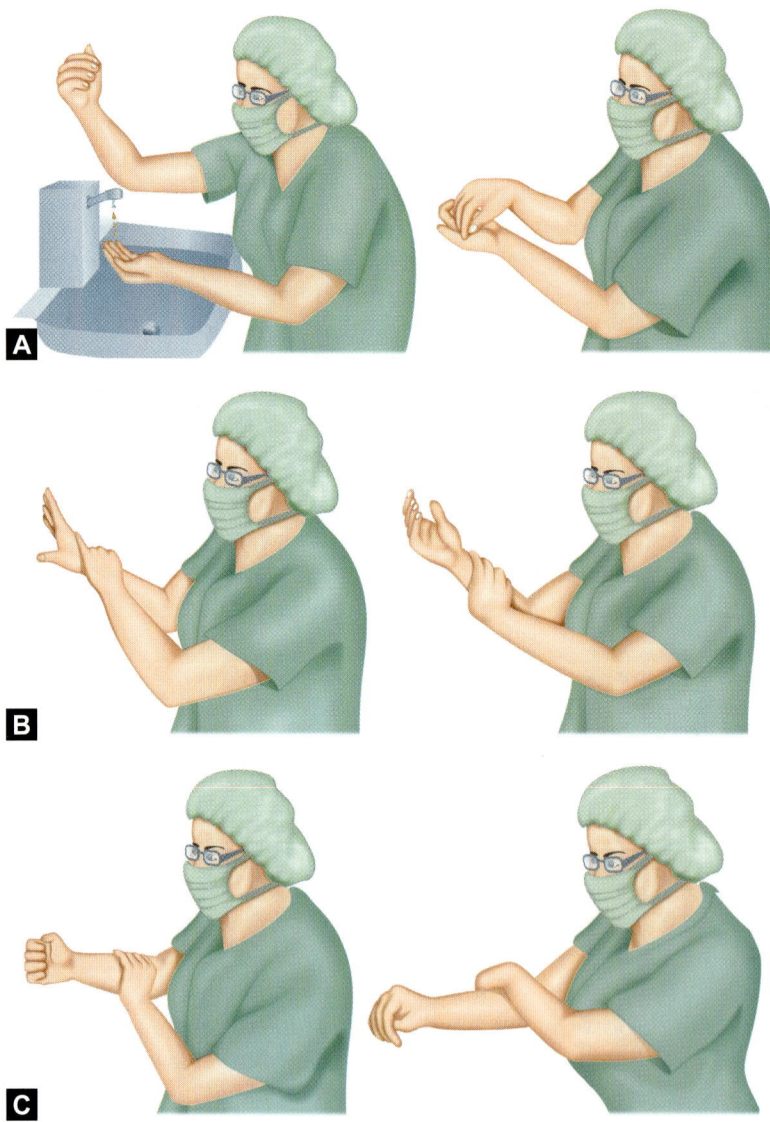

Figs. 1A to C

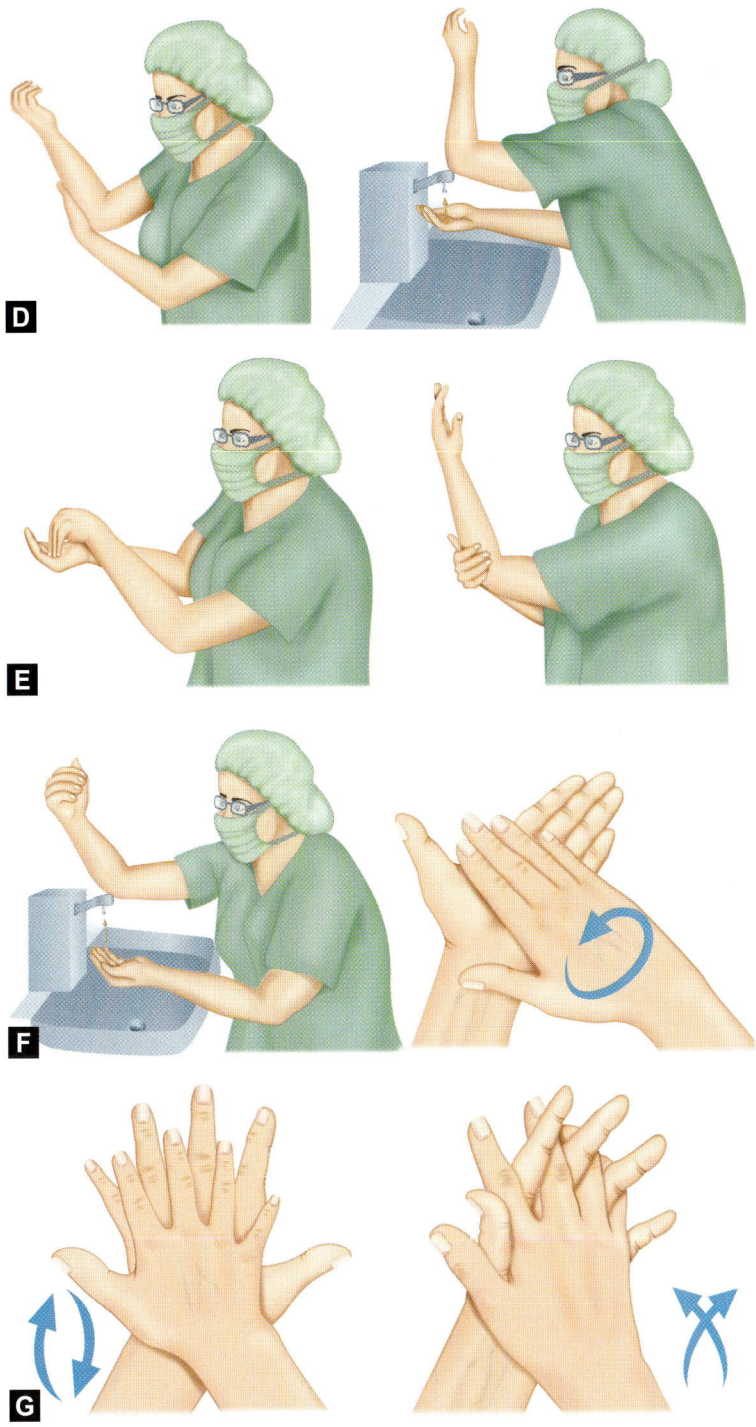

Figs. 1D to G

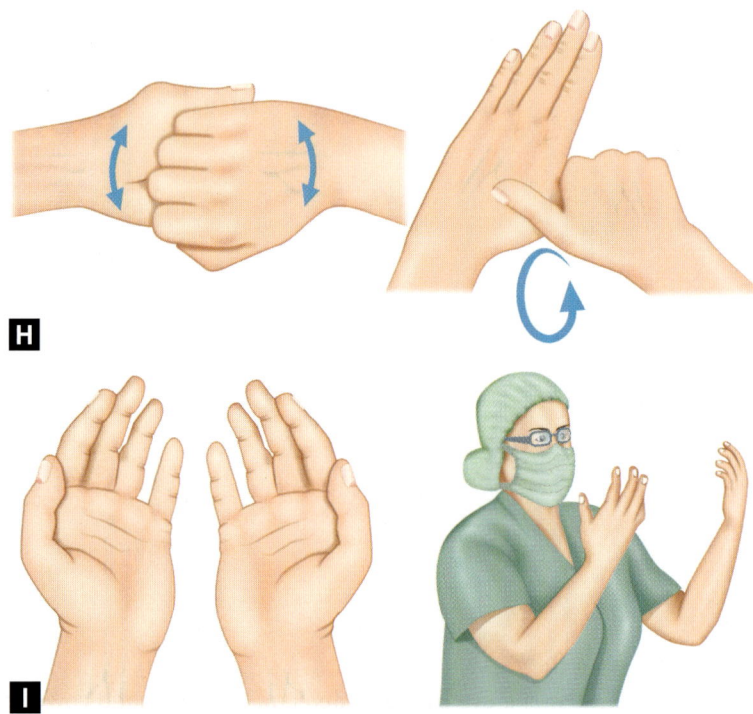

Figs. H and I
Figs. 1A to I: Handwashing steps.

5

Gloving Techniques

R Dayananda Babu

INTRODUCTION

Two methods are used for gloving—(1) the open method and (2) the closed method. The closed method is preferred because there is a less chance for contamination of the outside of the sterile gloves by the hand.

CLOSED METHOD OF GLOVING: STEPS

- The hands are brought only through the cuffs of the gown. See that the cuffs are covering both hands so that the cuff edges have not been touched by the bare hands **(Fig. 1A)**.
- Pick up the sterile first glove by the folded cuff with the hand covered by cuff of the gown **(Fig. 1B)**.
- Place the glove, palm, and thumb down on the forearm of the opposite hand **(Fig. 1C)**.
- Pull the glove cuff over the knitted cuff so that it completely covers the cuff **(Fig. 1D)**.
- Work fingers in to the glove on to the hand using covered hand **(Fig. 1D)**.
- Repeat the procedure on the contralateral side **(Figs. 1E and F; 2A and B)**.

OPEN METHOD OF GLOVING (FIG. 3)

- During gowning, the hands are brought out through the cuff of the gown. After gowning, pick up one glove by its cuff. For this, either hand may be used.
- Pull the glove on to the opposite hand using the cuff and being careful not to touch any other part of the glove.
- With the gloved hand, slide the fingers (excluding the thumb) inside the cuff of the second glove.
- Pull the glove on to the hand and the cuff of the glove over the cuff of the gown (*Caution*: Avoid inward rolling of the glove cuff as it is being brought upon the hand, so that it will not contaminate the outside of the glove from the hand).
- Draw the cuff of the opposite glove over the gown cuff.

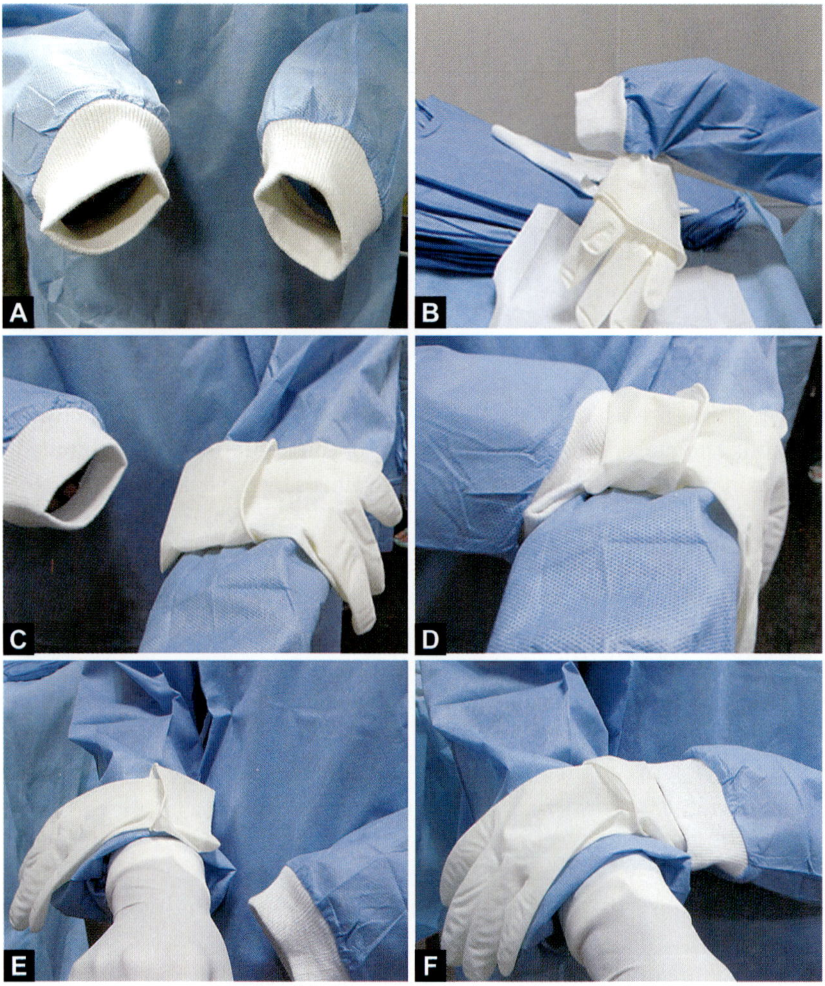

Figs. 1A to F: Steps of closed method of gloving.

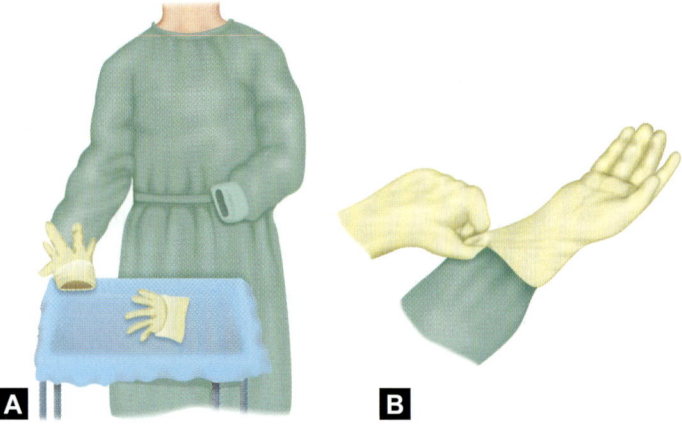

Figs. 2A and B: Closed method of gloving.

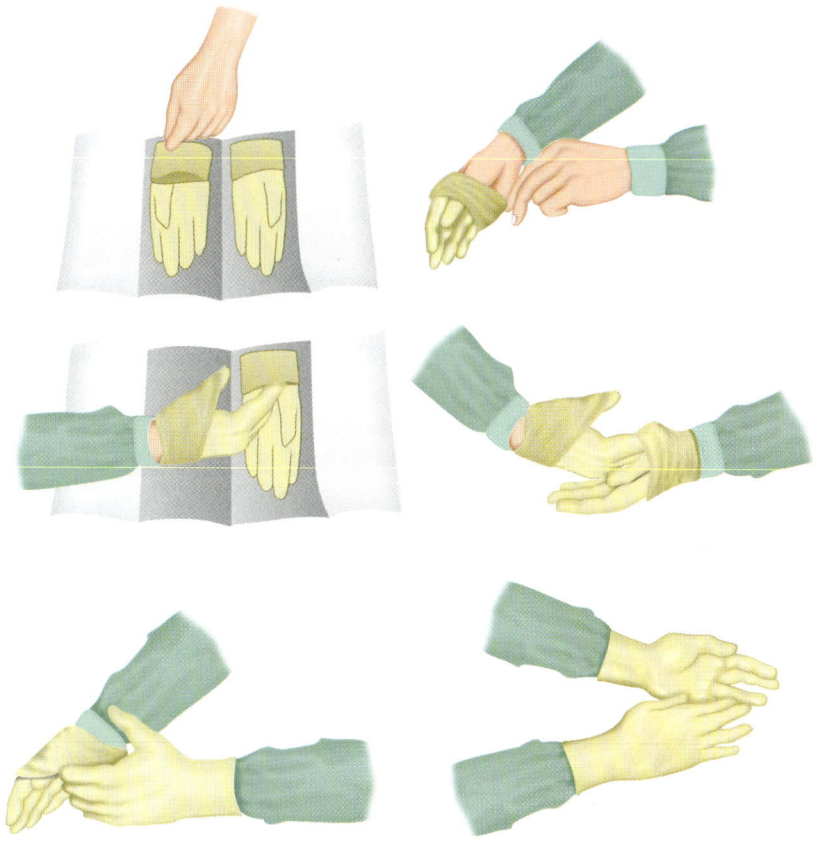

Fig. 3: Open method of gloving.

GLOVING ANOTHER STERILE TEAM MEMBER (FIGS. 4A TO D)

- Pick up the right glove first and turn the glove palm away from you.
- Slide your fingers under the glove cuff and spread the index and middle fingers away from you so that a wide opening is created (*Caution*: The team member's skin must not touch the outside cuff of the glove because it would contaminate the outside of the team members gown).
- After the team member inserts his hand in to the glove, scrub goes up with the glove and the team member pushes his hand down in to the glove.
- Gently release the rim of the glove while unrolling it over the wrist.
- The gown sleeve stockinette cuff must be completely covered.

RULES TO BE OBSERVED WHILE WEARING STERILE GOWN AND GLOVES

- Never drop your hands below the level of the sterile area at which you are working.

Surgical Handicraft

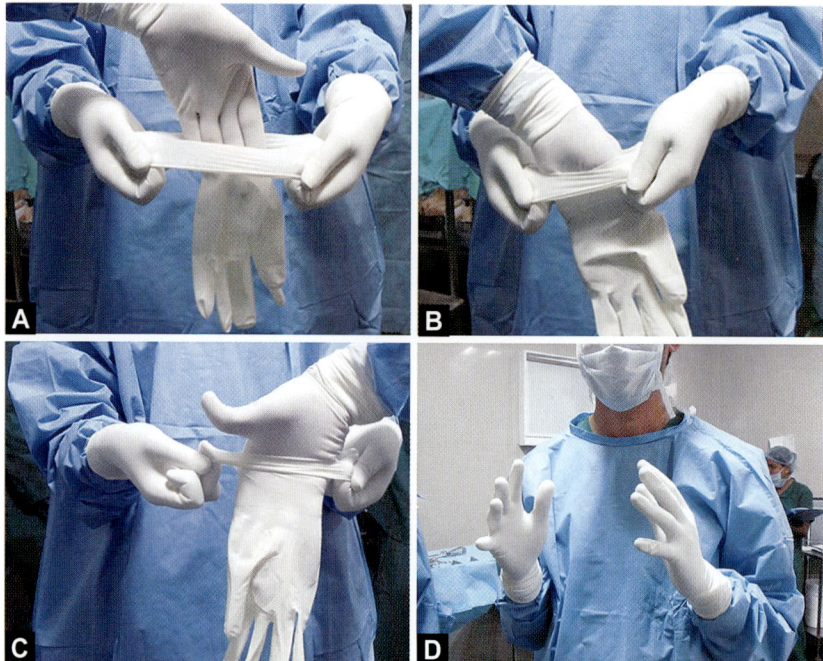

Figs. 4A to D: Steps for gloving another sterile team member.

- Never touch your surgical gown above the level of the axilla or below the level of the sterile area where you are working.
- Never put your hands behind your back. You must keep your hands within your full view all the time.
- Never tuck your gloved hand under your armpits, as axillary region of the gown is contaminated.
- Never reach across an unsterile area for any item.
- Never touch an unsterile object with a gloved hand.

6

Ethics and Consent

R Dayananda Babu

INTRODUCTION

What constitutes good professional practice depends on many factors such as:
- Medical ethics
- Law relating to consent
- Confidentiality
- Personal autonomy
- Trust between patient and doctor.

The doctor may be faced with ethical challenges, especially in matters of life and death to withhold or withdraw life-sustaining treatment is a big challenge. So, also to prolong the life of a patient who is in close to death situation. In the present era, orders like "do not resuscitate" may be an unreasonable demand.

Respecting the privacy of a patient is equally important as patient autonomy, which is called confidentiality. Maintaining the dignity of the patient is very important, especially exposing the private parts in open wards without proper screen. Instead of calling patients name calling him cot no. 9 or case of rectal cancer are dehumanizing. With the explosion of medical technology and knowledge maintaining, standards of excellence is difficult. This needs continuing education throughout a surgeon's life.

Atul Gawande noted that physicians too suffer the emotional reactions of failure when dying patients seek quality rather than quantity of life and often make decisions that worsen the problems by failing to ask the patients their basic wishes. The patient may have a better quality of life by palliative care than invasive treatments.

The four important pillars of medical ethics are:
1. Patient autonomy
2. Beneficence
3. Nonmalfeasance
4. Justice.

For patient autonomy, the most important thing is a prior informed consent.

What is consent?

Informed consent is patient's right and physicians duty. However, broad the consent might be for diagnostic procedure, it cannot be used for therapeutic surgery. It is a practical combination of salesman ship, ethical problem solving, and psychological nurturing. It requires the recruitment of the patient and family as allies in decision-making process. Rather than a legal requirement, informed consent requires an ethical commitment to the patient, your peers, and yourself. In summary, it involves communication, documentation, ethics, and legal issues.

If a medical practitioner attempts to treat a person without valid consent, then he will be liable under both tort and criminal law.

Tort—is a civil wrong for which aggrieved party may seek compensation.

Battery—is an act that either intentionally or negligently directly causes some physical contact with another person without that person's consent.

All medical procedures, examinations, diagnostic procedures, and medical research on patients are potential acts of bodily trespass in the absence of consent. Potential acts of bodily trespass or assault involve Indian Penal Code (IPC) 351. The IPC section dealing with self-defense of the body are Section 96 to 102, 104, and 106.

TYPES OF CONSENT

- Implied or tacit consent—when a patient is coming for consultation, it is implied that patient is willing to undergo inspection, palpation, percussion, and auscultation. Any other examination including intimate examinations requires written consent.
- Written consent—all major diagnostic procedures, anesthesias, surgeries, intimate examinations, age determinations, examination for potency and virginity, and other medicolegal examinations need written consent.
- Proxy consent—the consent given by the relative or guardian (in the case of minor—<18 years).
- Informed refusal—the final decision for any procedure will be taken by the patient based on patient autonomy. The patient has got the right to refuse any form of treatment. In such situations, the informed refusal must be obtained and documented.

When the patient is unconscious and there is nobody to give consent on behalf of the patient and there is imminent danger to the life of the patient, there is no need for formalities including consent. However, it is important to take second opinion from another specialist and document the necessity of the procedure along with signature from a witness.

The consent by the patient for a particular operative procedure cannot be treated as consent for unauthorized additional procedure.

Any additional procedure involving removal of an organ only on the ground that it is beneficial to the patient or is likely to prevent some damages developing in the future is unacceptable. When there is imminent damage to the life or health of the patient and additional procedure is required, in that case, it may be accepted.

SEVEN COMPONENTS OF INFORMED CONSENT

1. Decision-making capacity
2. Voluntariness
3. Disclosure
4. Recommendations
5. Understanding
6. Decision to consent or refuse
7. Autonomous authorization.

The decision is taken by the patient after understanding the treatment options and information disclosed by the doctor. The doctor can recommend treatment options, but the decision is made by the patient voluntarily. The patient will finally intentionally authorize the doctor for a specific procedure. Persons who have attained the age of 18 years are considered to have attained the age of maturity and competent to give consent legally.

For minors (<18 years), parental consent is required for any form of procedure. For physical examination alone, those who are 12 years or above can give consent.

Doctrine of Disclosure

The doctor is bestowed with the final right to decide how much information shall be divulged to the patient. There are no clear parameters laid down by the court regarding the quantum of information. However, it is important to describe the benefits of the operation and the consequences of alternative treatment approaches. In a situation where surgery will produce rapid recovery, what will happen if the operation is not carried out and it is also important to disclose the perioperative complications (such as infection, intestinal leak, hemorrhage, poor healing, and death), disability, and possible recurrence of the condition.

Exceptions to the Obligations to Disclosure

- Patients who choose not to be informed
- Disclosure would cause psychological harm
- Emergencies where valid consent taking is not possible—in such situations, the doctor can exercise *therapeutic privilege*. However, full disclosure will be made to the relatives and it should be documented.

Consent would not be a free consent if it is caused by coercion, undue influence, fraud, misrepresentation, and mistakes.

How consent is taken?

It requires the recruitment of the patient and family as allies in the decision-making process.

"Good communication makes for good medicine and good records are essential for the defense of doctor"—David Bogod.

IDEAL PLACE FOR TAKING CONSENT

Choose a relatively quiet setting away from the chaos of the emergency room, intensive care unit, or operation theater.

Introduce yourself and all members of your team who are present. Conduct the session in sitting position, you sitting at eye level with patient and family. Maintain constant eye contact with each of them. Do not ignore somebody hiding in the corner of the room for she or he may be the one who becomes your enemy. This is not the time to smile or joke around. Just play the serious surgeon committed to the well-being of the patient.

Use simple language preferably in comprehensible nonmedical terms in local language.

Ask questions and assess they are understanding. Be friendly, empathetic but professional, caring, honest, open, and informative. Language must be the one you must use in speaking to one of your own nonmedical relative. Describe the expected benefits of operation, consequences of alternative treatment approaches. Say, e.g. in a case of sigmoid colon carcinoma with obstruction in an elderly patient gives the following options:

- Nonoperative management will result in slow and difficult death
- Surgery will lead onto rapid recovery with long-term cure
- In between, potential difficulties of perioperative complications and death are possible events
- Discuss the general potential for postoperative complications such as infection, leak, hemorrhage, poor healing, must be explained
- Before any major emergency operation, the need for reoperation based on your operative findings must also be revealed and tell them that reoperation represents a continued management effort.

ILLUSTRATE THE PROBLEM AND PLANNED PROCEDURE

Draw schematically the lesion, the segment, or part you want to remove, how you are going to join the ends, need for ostomies, etc. Write the diagnosis the name of the operation and hand over this paper to the family. The members of the family will restudy this piece of paper.

Remember the patient's family is your greatest ally in promoting your plan of action.

Make the family members partners involving them early, confidently, and continuously sitting yourself as a knowledgeable and compassionate advisor.

ETHICAL PROBLEM SOLVING

The operation you offer is ethical if it is expected to save or prolong the patient's life or palliate his symptoms and can achieve this goal with reasonable risk-benefit ratio. You must be convinced that there are nonoperative treatment modalities that are safer or as effective as your proposed operation. The burden of proof is on you.

MEDICOLEGAL CONSIDERATIONS

"Surgery is the most dangerous activity of legal society"—Nyström.

Medicolegal dangers associated with abdominal surgery greatly depend on where you practice. In some places, surgeons can get away with almost anything. Emergency surgery is a legal minefield. Young surgeons tend to be overoptimistic trying to cheer up the family emerging from the operation room assuming a tired hero and announcing—your father is stable, he took the operation very well, and let us hope he will be home next week. It may raise high hope and expectation and subsequent anger and resentment, if complication should develop.

A better script might be—the operation was difficult, however we managed to achieve our goals. The cancer is out. Considering your father's age and other illnesses, he took it well. Let us hope for the best. But you must understand that the road to recovery is long and as I mentioned before, there are still many potential problems ahead.

DOCUMENTATION

What has not been documented in writing did not actually takes place. Your notes can be brief, but must encompass the essentials such as—elderly male patient with diabetes mellitus, chronic obstructive pulmonary disease presented with abdominal pain and distension. The plain X-ray revealed large gut obstruction. Patient is a high-risk patient and the therapeutic options, risks, and potential complications are explained to the patient and family. They understand the need for emergency surgery, need for colostomy, and may need further operation.

AVOID SELLING UNNECESSARY OPERATIONS

Be honest with yourself. Consider the risk-benefit ratio of the procedure. It may be easy to convince a worried family that a futile operation is indeed necessary and then at the time of inevitable mortality, explain that the family forced me to operate. Do not operate on brain dead patients and intubate and ventilate.

"One should advice surgery only if there is reasonable chance of success. To operate without having a chance means to prostitute the beautiful art and science of surgery"—Theodor Billroth (1829-1894).

GOLDEN RULE

"Do unto others as you would have them do unto you". Would you recommend the same treatment to your father, mother, wife, or son. Studies showed that surgeons are much less likely to recommend operations on themselves or their loved ones.

"The patient's family will never forgive a guarantee of cure that failed and the patient will not let the physician forget a pronouncement of incurability if he is so fortunate as to survive"—George T Pack (1898–1969).

SUMMARY

- Informed consent is a patient's right and physicians' duty.
- However, broad the consent might be for a diagnostic procedure, it cannot be used for therapeutic procedures including surgery.
- Consent for a particular operative procedure cannot be treated as consent for an unauthorized additional procedure.
- Separate consent is required for anesthesia and blood transfusion.
- Patient autonomy is one of the most important pillars of ethics and patient's decision to accept or deny a procedure is final.
- Documentation of your consent and discussion with patient is important.

Finally physicians have a moral commitment to place the interest of their patients above their own self-interests. Medical practice cannot be considered as a merely a business. Professionalism in surgery will require firm commitment and willingness to make sacrifices.

The Operation Theater Etiquette, the Surgical Team, and Assisting at Operations

R Dayananda Babu

SURGICAL TEAM

The surgical team consists of the surgeon, anesthetist, theater scrub nurse, and assistants. The responsibilities of the team members vary from institution to institution. However, the overall responsibility always rests with the surgeon. Establishing the identity of the patient, side of the lesion before surgery, and ensuring that the right operation is done for the right patient are important [read the World Health Organization (WHO) Surgical Safety Checklist]. In most of the places, the side for operation is marked with an indelible marker pen. The surgeon himself will finally check and see that the marked site is correct. The ornaments are preferably removed, if required may be taped. The dentures are also removed.

Consent

Read the consent chapter.

Check that the consent form is taken in proper format for that specific operation and signed by the patient.

OPERATING THEATER

Operation theater is a sterile area and it is important to see that the sterile environment is not violated. The risk of contamination should be kept to a minimum. At the entrance of a theater, there will be a changing area, where all the team members will get into the theater attire, consisting of shirt and trousers for all staff. Usually, different color dresses are there for doctors, nurses, and technicians. The dress will be usually cotton because the synthetic material will be associated with generation of electric spark. The outside footwear is changed and shoes/boots specially meant for only theater purpose are worn. In some centers, they use overshoes (shoe cover). Before entering the sterile area, the team will wear disposable caps and masks.

PATIENT

The patient is brought to the theater and transferred to the theater trolley at the entrance of the theater. Usually the patient will be in the preanesthetic area, where the patient will be examined by the anesthesiologist and review the latest laboratory results. The anesthesiologist will put intravenous (IV) cannula and deicide the nature of *premedication* and the type of anesthesia. *Prophylactic antibiotics* if required is administered at this time; it is also important to know the *blood group* and the requirement regarding blood transfusion or requirement for blood products like platelets, fresh frozen plasma, etc. Once they decide that the patient is *fit for surgery*, the patient will be wheeled to the operation theater and transferred to the operating table. It is preferable to have an entry and exit door for each operating room. So that, there will be one-way traffic which will minimize the risk of contamination of equipment. In addition, there should be separate exit for the transfer of contaminated/used instruments, swabs, soiled goods, etc. After surgery, the patient will be transferred to the recovery room through the exit door.

EQUIPMENT

Operation Table

Different types of operation tables are available with automation for changing the level of the table, tilting the table in required positions, kidney bridges, elevation of foot end and head end, etc., with remote control option.

Theater Lighting

The modern operation theaters are fitted with mounted shadowless cold lamps with cameras and monitors. The theater technician should develop some expertise in directing the light to the areas where the surgeon would like to get illuminated properly. For surgical procedures in depth, use of head lamps are recommended.

Surgical Sterile Instruments

The trays with instruments for the particular operation will be arriving from the central sterile department. The sterility of the pack is checked with the change of color of the tape on the instrument pack after the autoclave.

Anesthesia Workstation

This is a Boyles apparatus fitted with a ventilator and its monitor. The modern anesthesia workstation is fitted with all the connections for nitrous oxide, oxygen, and air, in addition to monitors for checking the vitals and pulse oximeter. There will be provisions for monitoring the arterial pressure and central venous pressure. There will be facility for total intravenous anesthesia in a sophisticated workstation.

The Operation Theater Etiquette, the Surgical Team, and Assisting at Operations

Diathermy/Harmonic Scalpel

It is important to have a modern diathermy unit with facility for monopolar and bipolar coagulation. There will be a diathermy plate which will be applied to the patient to provide earthing. It will have both *cut/blend/spray* mode.

Patient warmer and fluid warmer will be available in all the modern operating theaters.

Ultrasonography Machine

Most of the nerve blocks are administered by ultrasonography guidance nowadays for regional anesthesia.

Laparoscopy trolley with carbon dioxide insufflators, the camera, the monitor, and light source is also present.

POSITION OF THE PATIENT

It is the responsibility of the surgeon and his assistants to see that the patient's position in the table is correct. The patient should be properly padded underneath the arms and heels, so as to avoid skin damage. Excessive abduction of the upper limbs should be avoided to prevent neuropraxia. After giving IV muscle relaxant, there is risk for bone and joint injury. Judicious use of sandbags and restraints are used for *lateral position* for kidney exposure and head down position **(Fig. 1)**. For hemorrhoidectomy, the *lithotomy position* is used **(Fig. 2)**. The *Trendelenburg position* (head down) is used for pelvic surgery and varicose vein surgery. Anti-Trendelenburg position (head up) is used for thyroidectomy and upper abdominal surgery. *Lloyd-Davies position* is used for rectal surgery **(Figs. 3A and B)**. *Prone position* or *jackknife position* is used for excision of pilonidal surgery.

URINARY CATHETER

It is preferable to put a urinary catheter in cases of lower abdominal surgery and pelvic surgery which will prevent injury to urinary bladder. This is

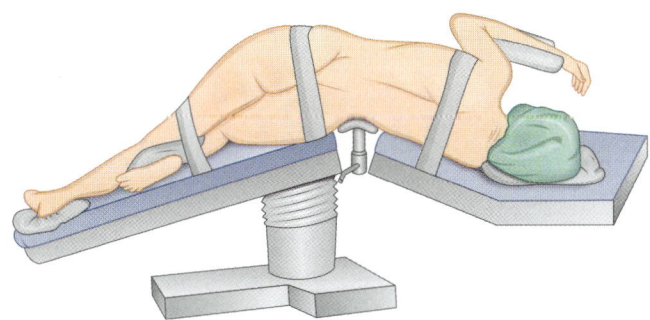

Fig. 1: Lateral position (nephrectomy).

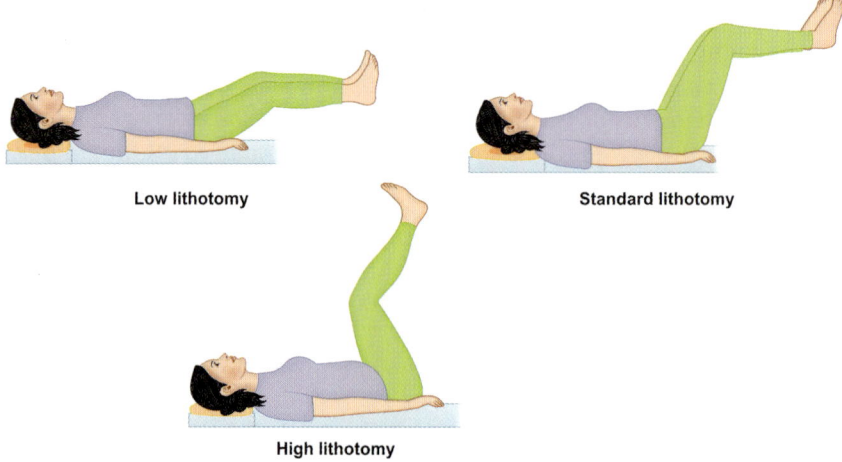

Fig. 2: Different lithotomy positions.

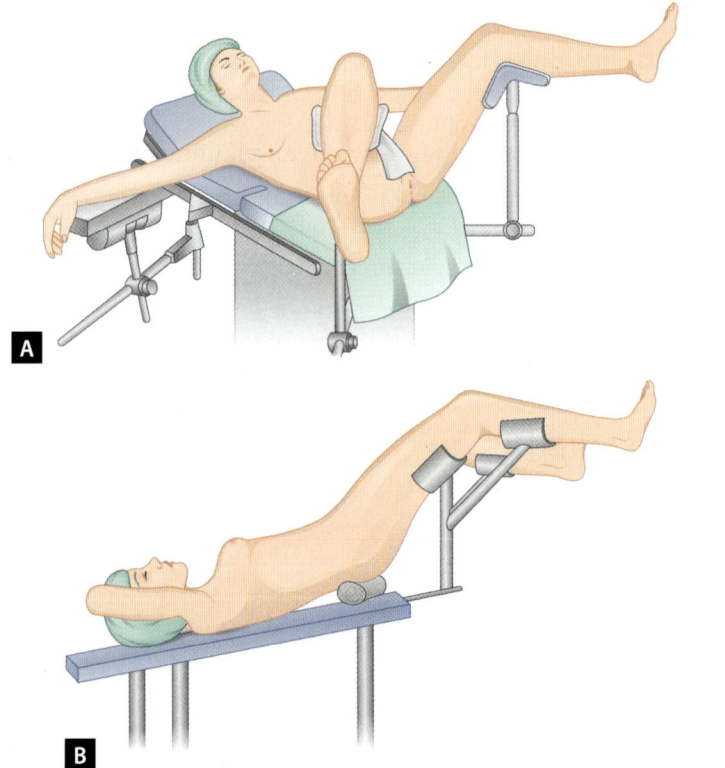

Figs. 3A and B: (A) Lloyd-Davies position; and (B) Head down lithotomy (30°) or legs apart Trendelenburg.

also useful for monitoring the urine output during prolonged surgery. In upper abdominal surgery, a nasogastric tube may be introduced by the anesthesiologist at the beginning of the surgery.

MOVEMENT IN THE OPERATION THEATER

The movement inside the operation room should be kept to a minimum. Those who are not part of the team and observing the surgery should be instructed not to come into physical contact with surgical team or any of the sterile instruments and instrument trolleys in the operating theater. Only minimum numbers of observers are allowed. They should limit their movements during the procedure. They are instructed not to talk during the surgery.

SURGICAL SCRUB TEAM

The surgeon, one or two assistants, and the nurse will now scrub thoroughly at the special washing area designated for this, where adequate warm water is supplied. It is preferable to control the flow of water and antiseptics which can be controlled with either the foot or knee. The antiseptic solution usually used is betadine or Hibiscrub (read the Handwashing Technique). The initial scrub will last for 3 minutes and the subsequent scrubs of 1–2 minutes duration are adequate. After scrubbing, the hands and forearms are rinsed and finally held up above the level of the elbow. At this position, any remaining water will flow downward and fall off at the elbow. Now, the hand and forearms are dried by a sterile towel. Immediately after this, the gown and gloves are put on as mentioned in the Chapter Handwashing Practice.

Draping

Once the patient is anesthetized and positioned, the skin of the operative area is painted with betadine or chlorhexidine (for laparotomy, the skin between the nipple area and upper thigh is painted). The painting will start in the midline and goes laterally. Attention is paid to the umbilicus and groin folds. Sterile drapes are then placed to cover all the areas, except the part to be incised. The towels are clipped in place using towel clips passing through the drapes only.

Positioning of the Surgical Team

The surgeon will usually stand on the side of the organ to be operated and the first assistant stands opposite to the surgeon. The scrub nurse will also be standing on the opposite side. Additional assistants or nurses may position on both sides depending on the requirement of the surgeon.

Table Height

The table height will be decided by the operating surgeon, usually at the elbow level of the surgeon. The assistants and nurses will elevate themselves, if required on footstools.

Instruments and Swabs

Surgeon will now check the instruments and swabs with the scrub nurse which will be documented and displayed on the mounted board.

The surgeon will now proceed to start the operation after taking permission from the anesthetist. See that the diathermy is connected and working.

ASSISTING AN OPERATION

- The responsibility of the first assistant is to ensure adequate exposure of the operation field.
- Assist the surgeon to secure hemostasis.
- Anticipate the surgeon's requirements and act accordingly.
- "Assisting is not resisting"—avoid interference of surgeon's movements and in no way, the assistants hand should come in the way of the surgeon.
- Maintain vigilance throughout the procedure and see that errors are avoided.
- The retractor should be handled judiciously and gently as instructed by the surgeon. Excessive retraction may tear tissues, e.g., liver tear by Kelly retractor.
- The assistant should not lean on body of the patient.
- The assistant should keep the operating field dry and free of blood. Careful use of a surgical suction device will be useful, especially with multiple orifices.
- Do not rub the field rather does dab. Excessive rubbing will dislodge the clot.
- Bleeding is dealt by applying pressure on pack.

HEMOSTASIS

The bleeding may be arterial, venous, or capillary oozing. The bleeding may be from named vessels or unnamed branch. Nearly all cut arteries will contract after a few minutes and the bleeding will stop. In case of atherosclerosis and hardened arteries, this will not happen.

Options for Controlling the Bleeding

- Catch the bleeding vessel with an artery forceps (not the surrounding tissue). This may be dealt with either by *coagulation with a diathermy*.
- Ligation—for ligating the vessel, the hemostat is applied in such a way that it is facing upward. A ligature is passed around the vessel and ligated with a square knot. The knot can be tied either by instrument or by hand tying.
- When a vessel cannot be identified, it is recommended to undersew the bleeding point using absorbable suture material like polyglactin.
- The capillary oozing can be controlled with gentle pressure or by hot wet gauze packs. One can also use hemostatic agents like *Surgicel* as a last resort.

- *Bone wax*—this is used for controlling oozing from the cut edge of the bone.
- *Temporalis muscle pieces* are used by neurosurgeons for controlling bleeding. The muscles are rich sources of thromboplastin.
- *Calamitous bleeding*—this is massive bleeding in cavities like abdomen following trauma. In such a situation, packing the abdomen with largest packs available is an option. Pack each quadrant of the abdomen followed by the central part. This is a damage control procedure and once the patient is stable, formal exploration for the identification of the bleeding vessel may be carried out. At this stage, the individual vessel can be safely clamped and repaired.

GLOVE CHANGING

During the procedure, there is likely chance of a tear/puncture in the glove with resultant contamination. This is a very common problem and should be identified as early as possible and should be changed. It is also preferable to change the gloves after handling infected material and malignant tumor. It is preferable to use fresh gloves for the final closure in such cases.

END OF THE OPERATION BEFORE CLOSURE

The surgeon and scrub nurse will make sure that the swab and instrument counts are correct. Always ensure adequate hemostasis. If required, a *tube drain* may be put (corrugated drains are not recommended because they act as two-way traffic for infection). For closed spaces like neck and for thyroid, a closed suction drain is put. In the abdomen, it is preferable to keep one drain in the subhepatic position in the right paracolic gutter and another one in the pelvis. The drain must be stitched in position to avoid dislodgement.

OPERATION NOTE

The detailed operation note should be written by the surgeon himself or may be dictated by the surgeon to the assistant, containing the details such as the incision, findings with pictures drawn, the steps of the procedure, and closure including the suture materials used for it. It should also contain the names of the surgeon, anesthesiologist, scrub nurse, and assistants. The nature of anesthesia, the time of beginning, and end of the procedure along with the date and time should be documented.

PATHOLOGY SPECIMEN SENDING

At the end of the procedure, the specimen should be properly marked and put it in a bottle containing adequate formalin (10%). The specimen should be adequately oriented in cases of malignancy for reporting of the margins. In cases of nodal dissection, it is important to label it separately. The requisition forms must contain the necessary clinical details, the investigation findings, and the previous pathology reports if any, which will guide the pathologist for their final reporting. If specimens are there for microbiological examination, that should be signed in another bottle containing saline.

FROZEN SECTION

If frozen section study is required, the surgical team should inform the pathology department before hand so that they will be ready in the operation theater at the time of surgery for collecting the specimen for pathological study.

HIGH-RISK PATIENTS

Take *universal precautions* for all suspected high-risk patients including wearing a plastic apron, double gloving, use of goggles, etc. (read Chapter 9: Tips for House Surgeons/Residents). The main high-risk groups are human immunodeficiency virus (HIV) and hepatitis B. The hepatitis B is more infective than HIV. Suspect hepatitis B when there is history of *jaundice, blood transfusion, and tattoos*. Suspect HIV in drug addicts, male homosexuals, hemophiliacs, and anorectal pathology. Take precaution during ward procedure also. The use of sharp instruments like scalpel should be minimized. It is preferable to use diathermy or scissors for cutting. Use of stapling devices will go a long way in preventing injuries during intestinal anastomosis. The sharp instruments should not be transferred from hand to hand, instead use a tray or dish for this purpose. After the procedure, all the disposable items are properly disposed. The theater should be cleaned with 1% hypochlorite solution.

8. Classification of Surgical Procedures and ASI Classification of Physical Fitness

R Dayananda Babu

INTRODUCTION

They are classified into emergency, urgent, scheduled, and elective.

Emergency

Immediate operation—operation required within 2-3 hours, for example, ruptured aneurysm, abdominal injuries, chest trauma, etc. Here, resuscitation is carried out simultaneously with surgical treatment.

Urgent

The surgery is carried out after resuscitation as early as possible, usually *within 24 hours*. The typical examples are visceral perforations, intestinal obstructions, peritonitis, strangulated hernia, perforated appendix, embolism, etc.

Scheduled

Here the operation is required *within 3 weeks*. The examples are surgery for malignancies—breast carcinoma, colon carcinoma without obstruction, soft tissue malignancies, cardiac surgeries, etc.

Elective Procedures

Here the date for surgery will be decided by the surgeon and patient after optimization and to the convenience of the patient and the surgical department. The examples are surgery for uncomplicated hernia, elective cholecystectomy, thyroidectomy, excision of benign swellings, hemorrhoids, fistula-in-ano, hydrocele, etc.

ANOTHER CLASSIFICATION

The operations are classified into minor, intermediate, major, extra major, and complex.

Minor

This is a surgical procedure lasting <30 minutes. It may be done as a daycare procedure and the anesthetic of choice will be local/short general anesthesia.

Intermediate

Here the surgical procedure will last from 30 minutes to 1 hour.

Major

The procedure will last 1–2 hours.

Extra Major

The procedure will last 2–4 hours.

Complex

The procedure will last >4 hours.

AMERICAN SOCIETY OF ANESTHESIOLOGISTS PHYSICAL STATUS CLASSIFICATION SYSTEM

- *American Society of Anesthesiologists 1 (ASA 1)*: A normal healthy patient, e.g., fit, nonobese [body mass index (BMI) < 30 kg/m^2], and a nonsmoking patient with good exercise tolerance.
- *American Society of Anesthesiologists 2 (ASA 2)*: A patient with mild systemic disease, e.g., patient with no functional limitations and a well-controlled disease (e.g., treated hypertension, obesity with BMI < 35 kg/m^2, frequent social drinker, or a cigarette smoker).
- *American Society of Anesthesiologists 3 (ASA 3)*: Patient with severe systemic disease that is not life-threatening, e.g., patient with some functional limitation as a result of disease (poorly treated hypertension or diabetes, morbid obesity, chronic renal failure, a bronchospastic disease with intermittent exacerbation, stable angina, and implanted pacemaker).
- *American Society of Anesthesiologists 4 (ASA 4)*: A patient with severe systemic disease that is a constant threat to life, e.g., patient with functional limitation from severe life-threatening disease [unstable angina, poorly controlled chronic obstructive pulmonary disease, symptomatic congestive heart failure, recent (<3 months ago) myocardial infarction, or stroke].
- *American Society of Anesthesiologists 5 (ASA 5)*: A moribund patient who is not expected to survive without the operation. The patient is

not expected to survive beyond the next 24 hours without surgery, e.g., ruptured abdominal aortic aneurysm, massive trauma, and extensive intracranial hemorrhage with mass effect.

- *American Society of Anesthesiologists 6 (ASA 6)*: A brain dead patient whose organs are being removed with intention of transplanting them into another patient.

The addition of "E" to the ASAP (ASA 2E) denotes an emergency procedure.

Note: There is no specific classification assigned to patients with moderate systemic disease.

9

Energy Sources in Surgery

John S Kurien

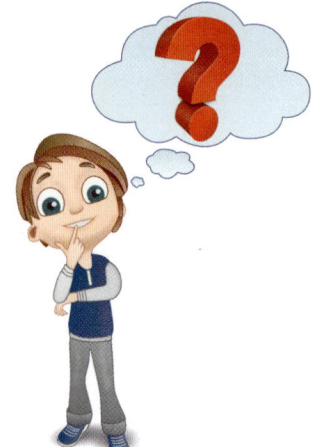

Cautery!! What strikes in your mind on hearing the word "cautery"?

In Latin, *cauterize* means "to burn or brand with a hot iron".

Actual cautery refers to the metal device, generally heated to a dull red glow, to use as an identification mark in cattles in barns. So, it is electrocautery and not just cautery **(Figs. 1 and 2)**.

Electrocauterization is the process of destroying tissue (or cutting through soft tissue) using heat conduction from a metal probe heated by electric current. The procedure stops bleeding from small vessels (larger vessels being ligated). Electrocautery applies high frequency alternating current by a *unipolar* or *bipolar* method. It can be a continuous waveform to cut tissue or intermittent to coagulate tissue.

The electrically produced heat in this process inherently can do numerous things to the tissue, depending on the waveform and power level, including cauterize, coagulate, cut, and dry (desiccate). Thus, electrocautery, electrocoagulation, electrodesiccation, and fulguration are closely related and can co-occur in the same procedure when desired.

HISTORY

William T Bovie (September 11, 1882 to January 1, 1958) **(Fig. 3)** was an American scientist who is credited inventing the Bovie electrosurgical generator **(Fig. 4)**. He said that electric current above certain frequencies could cut tissue without inducing muscular contraction. He used such knowledge to create his electrosurgical device and he first employed it in neurosurgical cases with Harvey Cushing, known as the father of neurosurgery **(Fig. 5)**. Bleeding had been the significant obstacle in neurosurgery until Bovie and Cushing began to employ the device in 1926.

Bovie's device allowed Cushing to reexplore operations in patients with brain masses that had been declared inoperable. While the device

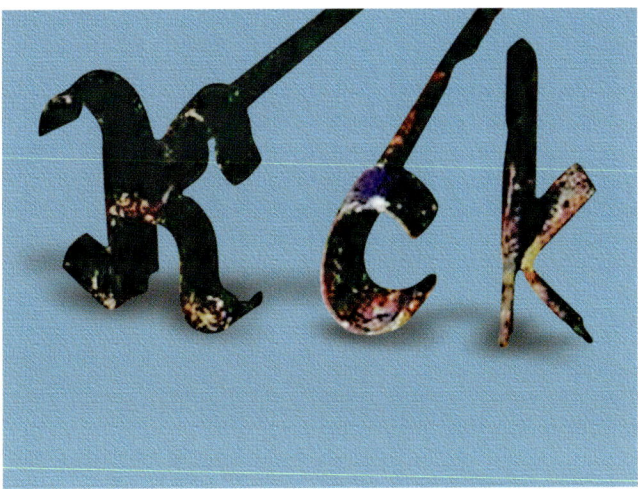

Fig. 1: Cautery iron used for branding cattle in olden days by heating in fire. The word cautery should be used only for this.

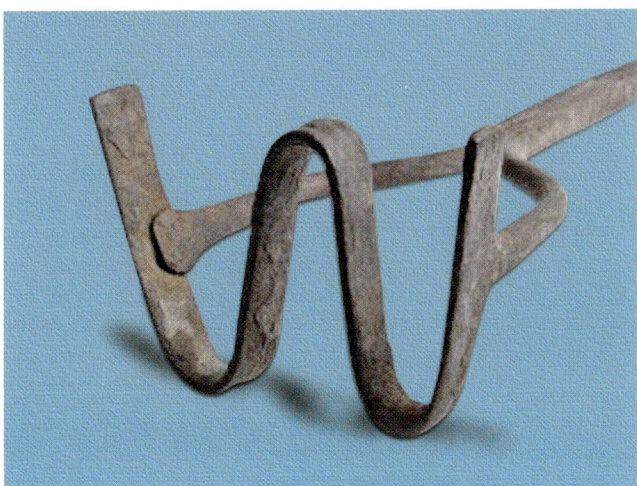

Fig. 2: A type of cautery branding iron in the shape of a letter used to brand cattle by heating directly in fire.

revolutionized surgery, there were occasional technical problems. Cushing recalled an instance in which the current from Bovie's device short circuited through a retractor. Electricity traveled up to Cushing's arm and to his headlight, an experience that Cushing described as "unpleasant to say the least". In another case, the Bovie's device briefly ignited ether gas that was being given to a patient during surgery.

ELECTROSURGICAL UNIT

Electrosurgical units (diathermy machines) were first introduced during the early 20th century to facilitate hemostasis and/or the cutting of tissue during

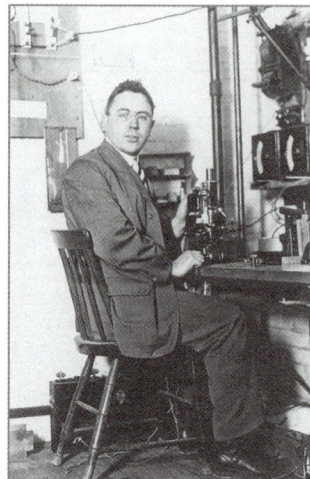

Fig. 3: Dr William T Bovie.

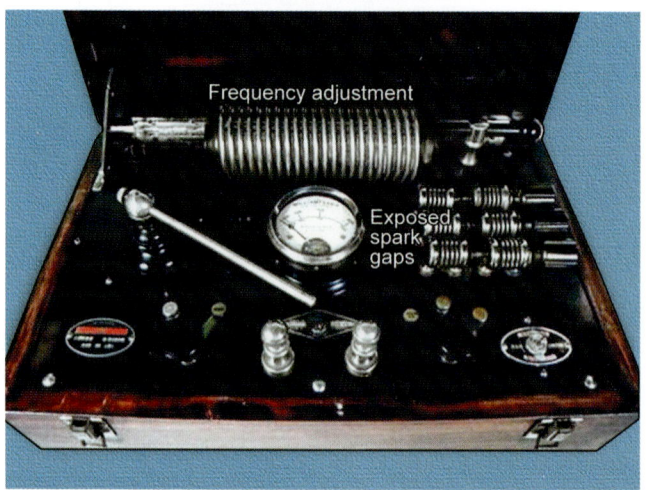

Fig. 4: Bovie electrosurgical generator.

surgical procedures **(Fig. 6)**. This is achieved by passing normal electrical current via the diathermy machine and converting it into a high-frequency alternating current (HFAC). The HFAC produces heat within body tissues to coagulate bleeding vessels and cut through tissue. At this high frequency of over 300,000 Hz, the nervous system and muscles are not affected when the current passes through the body and hence electrocution does not occur.

Due to the high risks of injury to both patients and staff which could lead to permanent disfigurement or death, guidance is required for staff using electrosurgical machines.

There are two different types of electrosurgery: (1) monopolar and (2) bipolar. Monopolar electrosurgery is the emittance of the HFAC from the

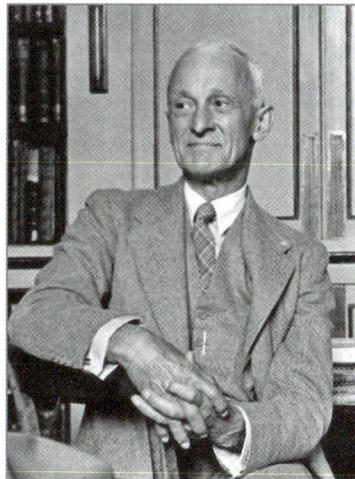

Fig. 5: Dr Harvey Cushing.

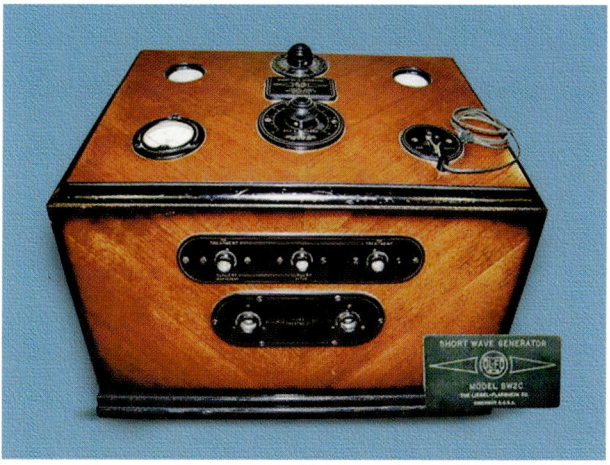

Fig. 6: First electrosurgical diathermy machine.

diathermy via an active electrode through the patient's body tissues and returned back to the diathermy machine via a return electrode or patient return pad or dispersive electrode.

Bipolar electrosurgery is the passage of the HFAC from the diathermy machine using only the patient's tissue grasped between a pair of bipolar forceps, to form a complete electrical circuit within the patient. Bipolar diathermy does not require a patient return pad as both active and return electrodes are combined within the forceps **(Figs. 7A and B)**.

Electrosurgery has three effects on body tissue:
1. Cut (linear vaporization)—generation of heat destroys tissue cell.
2. Coagulation (desiccate)—tissue cells contract to increase normal clotting.
3. Fulguration—cell walls destroyed through dehydration **(Fig. 8)**.

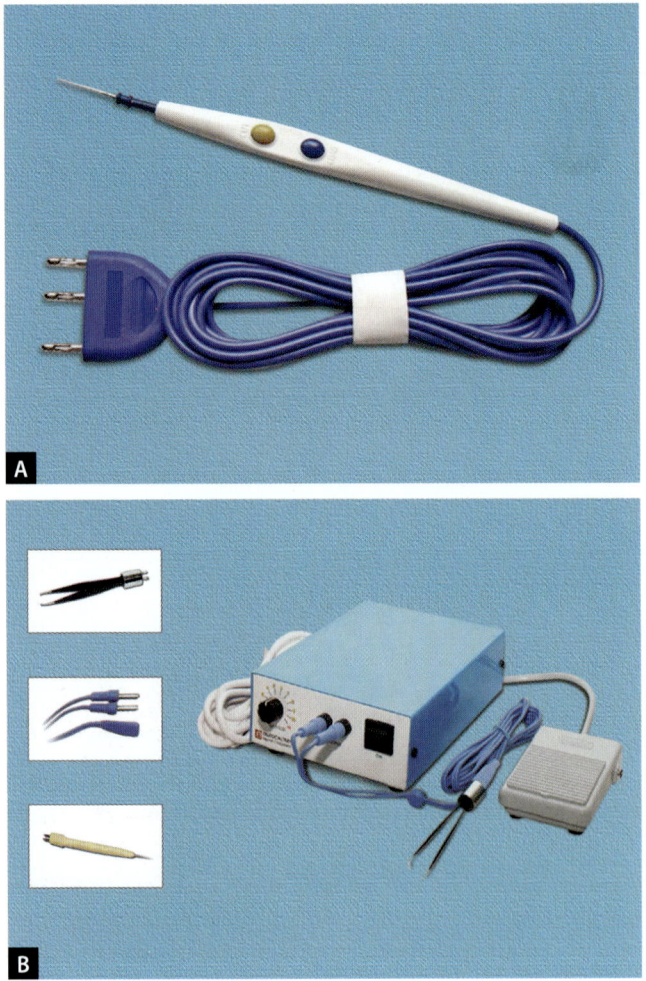

Figs. 7A and B: (A) Monopolar diathermy lead; and (B) Bipolar diathermy unit with lead and footswitch.

Each of these processes generates smoke plume which contains chemical byproducts (e.g., acrylonitrile and hydrogen cyanide) which can be absorbed by the skin and lungs, carbonized tissue, blood particles, and viral deoxyribonucleic acid particles; infectious viruses and bacteria have also been noted. Hence, it is ideal to use a suction tip to suck off these gases while using diathermy.

Monopolar instrument is a pencil type, the active electrode is placed in the entry site, and can be used to cut tissue and coagulate bleeding. The return electrode pad is attached to the patient, so the electrical current flows from the generator to the electrode through the target tissue to the patient return pad and back to generator. The dispersive electrode can be used in the split manner, so that partial detachment of the dispersive electrode plate cuts off the current **(Figs. 9 and 10)**.

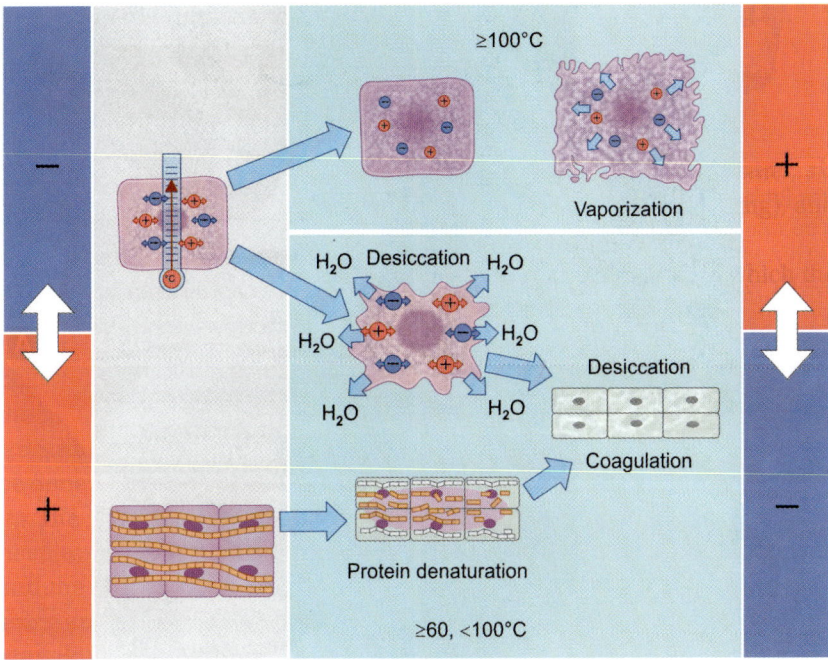

Fig. 8: Coagulation, desiccation, and vaporization are the processes happening during diathermy depending on the temperature at the tip of the electrode.

In bipolar instrument, the electrons flow between two adjacent electrodes. The tissue between the two electrodes is heated and desiccated. It is usually used for coagulation of vessels without thermal injury. It uses lower voltages, so less energy is required. But because it has limited ability to cut and coagulate large bleeding areas, it is more ideally used for those procedures where tissue can be easily grabbed on both sides by the forceps electrode.

Cutting can also coagulate, but it takes 6 minutes to do it and desiccation is homogeneous. With coagulation, desiccation is faster but it is nonhomogeneous **(Fig. 11)**.

There are lots of thermal injury mechanisms with these instruments. If not taken proper care of, it includes dispersive electrode—if there is partial detachment of the patient plate and if it is not placed obliquely touching the skin and it should not be over any bony prominence in the body.

According to the Association of Perioperative Registered Nurses journal, around 40,000 patients are burned by faulty electrosurgical unit every year. Mechanical injuries due to dispersive electrode include application site issue and partial detachment and due to active electrode injury is direct extension, inadvertent activation and current diversion due to direct coupling, and insulation failure.

Direct coupling: It occurs when one conductive element of the circuit touches or arcs to an instrument outside the intended circuit.

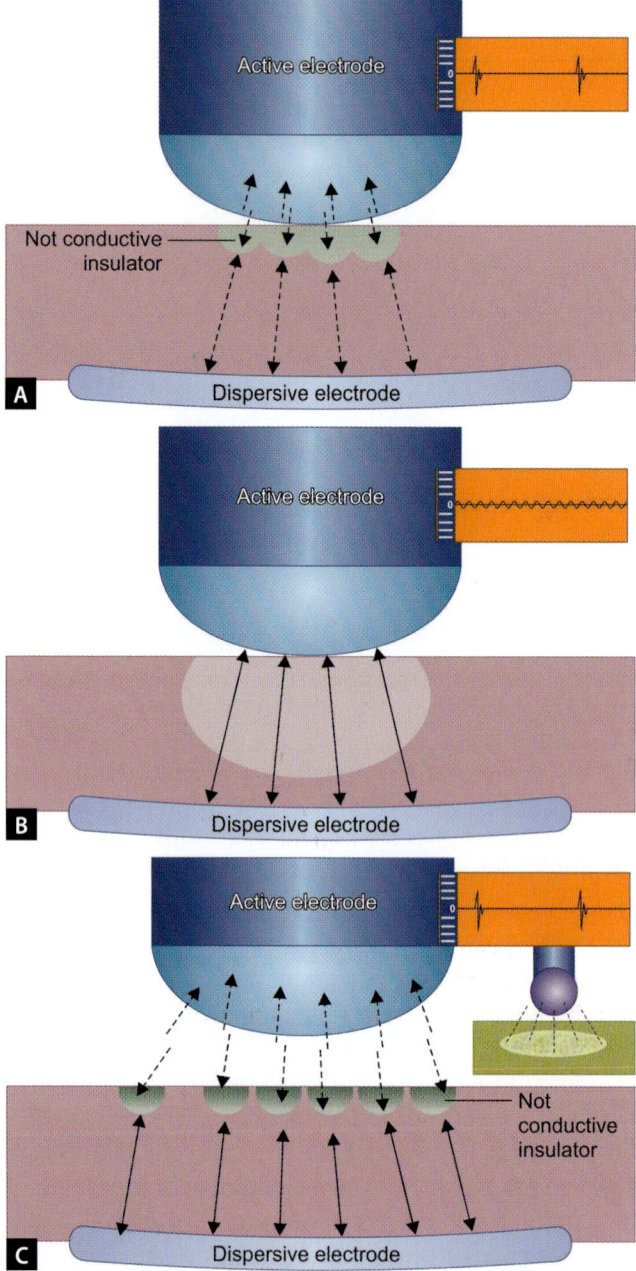

Figs. 9A to C: (A) 60–100°C → Desiccation; (B) 100°C → Vaporization; and (C) Temperature goes up to 400°C and individual cells are carbonized.

It always activate the monopolar only after touching the forceps held by the surgeon.

If the monopolar is touched on the forceps above the surgeon's hand and not at the tip of the forceps, the current may pass from the instrument

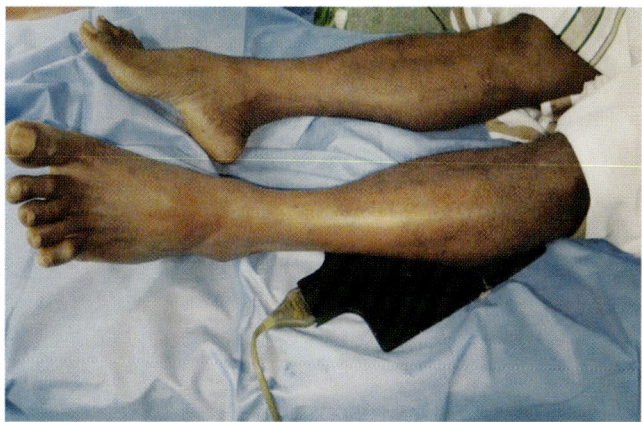

Fig. 10: Dispersive electrode only partially in contact with patient.

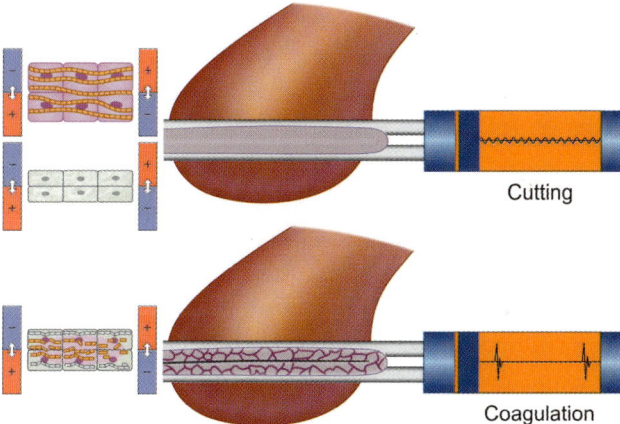

Fig. 11: Cutting occurs with the diathermy tip moving within a water vapor envelope. Coagulation occurs directly.

to the surgeon and so he may get an electric shock. So, always activate the monopolar pencil by touching the instrument close to the tissue.

Capacitance is defined as stored electrical charge when two conductors are separated by an insulator. Capacitive coupling occurs when the circuit is completed by the insulator. It occurs only with the use of monopolar instrumentation mainly in laparoscopy. So, avoid crossing of graspers while using monopolar cautery to prevent the electric current crossing to the other grasper and causing injury elsewhere. Use bipolar coagulation, if possible, to avoid this complication.

As the tissue is being treated, the tissue impedance changes. When the tissue impedance increases on the gallbladder side, after the tissue is charred, then the current starts to flow toward the duodenum and the duodenum may get burned **(Fig. 12)**. Effect may manifest only on the third day by a duodenal perforation.

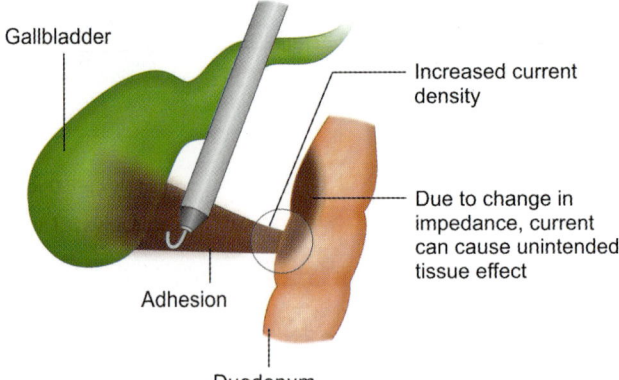

Fig. 12: Monopolar current spread to bowel, after charring of the intended tissue is over, because the generator continues to increase the tip voltage.

If the sensitivity of the monitor is increased, it interferes with the electrocardiogram, but varying the sensitivity decreases the chance of detecting arrhythmias.

ULTRASONIC DEVICES

Harmonic scalpels, unlike radiofrequency (RF) energy devices, have oscillating jaw which oscillates at a frequency of 55,000 Hz. As a result, this mechanical energy is converted to thermal energy which produces the same effects of vaporization, desiccation, and protein coagulation, without the inherent risk associated with an electrical circuit.

The ultrasonically activated scalpel (UAS) is characterized by its ability to cut and coagulate tissues simultaneously with relatively low heat and limited lateral thermal injury. The UAS has been used routinely in a number of general surgeries, including laparoscopic surgeries and open surgeries of the lung and liver **(Fig. 13)**.

The basic mechanism for coagulating bleeding vessels by UAS is similar to that of electrosurgery or lasers, in that vessels are sealed and occluded with denatured protein. However, the manner in which protein is denatured is different for each modality. Electrosurgery and lasers denature protein by heating the tissues with electric current in the former and light in the latter at a very high temperature. The UAS denatures protein by transferring mechanical energy to ultrasonic high frequency vibration (25 kHz/s–55 kHz/s). The vibration breaks hydrogen bonds and produces frictional heat. This frictional heat produces lower maximum temperature and slower increase in tissue temperature than the heat from electrocautery. The cutting mechanism for the UAS is also different from that observed with electrosurgery or laser surgery. UAS cuts tissues by a relatively sharp blade vibrating at 25 kHz–55 kHz over a distance of up to 100 μm.

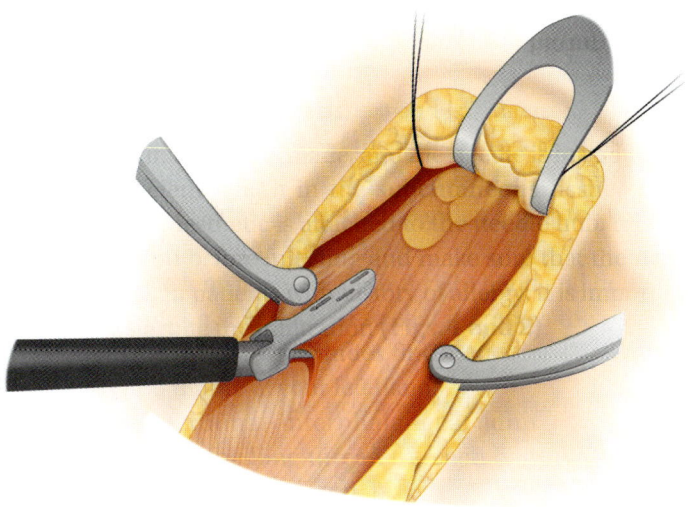

Fig. 13: Harmonic scalpel (ultrasonic activated scalpel).

Advantages

- Minimal lateral thermal tissue damage
- Minimal charring and desiccation
- Ultrasonic technology can reduce the need for ligatures with simultaneous cutting and coagulation
- Fewer instrument exchanges simplify procedure steps
- No electricity to or through the patient
- Greater precision near vital structures
- Minimal smoke for improved visibility in the surgical field.

The ultrasonic shear handles contain piezoelectric ceramic disks which convert electrical energy to mechanical energy which is transferred to the shaft and amplified by silicon nodes. Excursion of the oscillating jaw can be adjusted between 50 and 100 µ, which leads to more effective cutting and coagulation, respectively **(Fig. 14)**. Increasing the power setting increases the excursion of the fixed blade and enhances cutting.

Harmonic Focus

The harmonic focus is described in **Figure 15**.

Harmonic Wave

The harmonic wave is described in **Figure 16**.

Harmonic Ace

The harmonic ace is described in **Figure 17**.

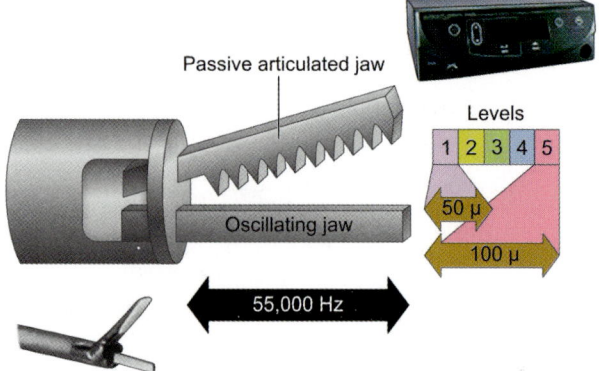

Fig. 14: Fixed jaw of the ultrasonic shears moves to and fro.

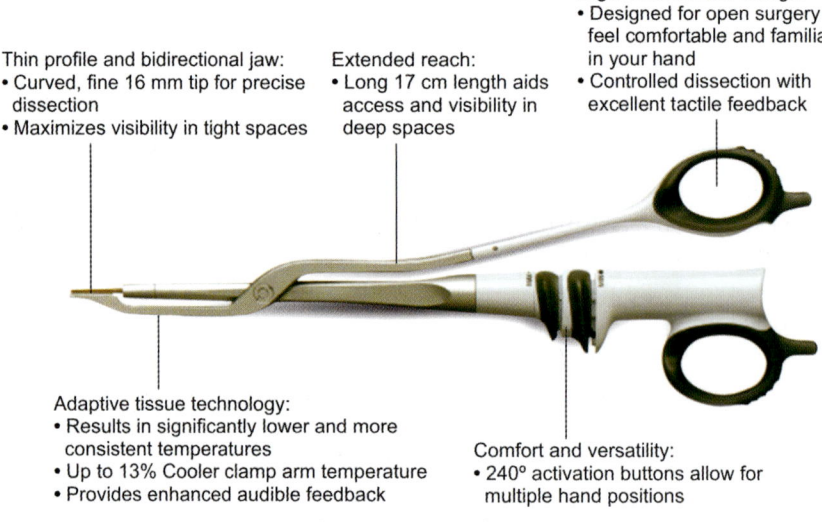

Thin profile and bidirectional jaw:
- Curved, fine 16 mm tip for precise dissection
- Maximizes visibility in tight spaces

Extended reach:
- Long 17 cm length aids access and visibility in deep spaces

Ergonomic scissor design:
- Designed for open surgery to feel comfortable and familiar in your hand
- Controlled dissection with excellent tactile feedback

Adaptive tissue technology:
- Results in significantly lower and more consistent temperatures
- Up to 13% Cooler clamp arm temperature
- Provides enhanced audible feedback

Comfort and versatility:
- 240° activation buttons allow for multiple hand positions

Fig. 15: Harmonic focus.

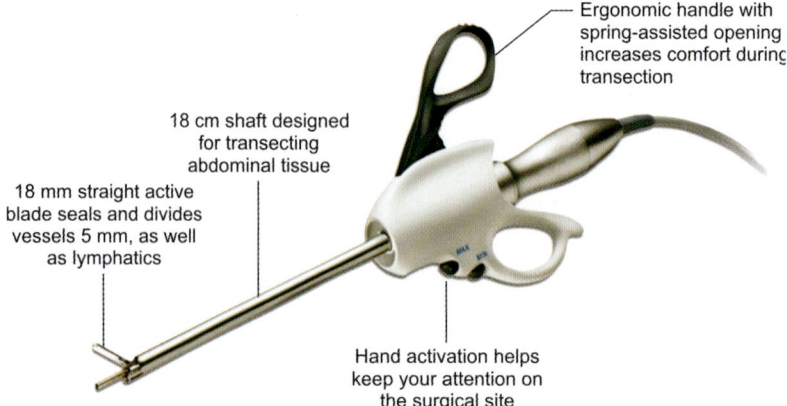

18 mm straight active blade seals and divides vessels 5 mm, as well as lymphatics

18 cm shaft designed for transecting abdominal tissue

Ergonomic handle with spring-assisted opening increases comfort during transection

Hand activation helps keep your attention on the surgical site

Fig. 16: Harmonic wave.

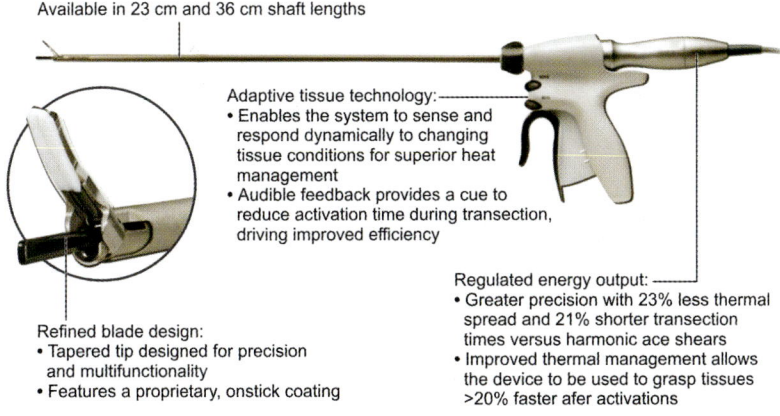

Fig. 17: Harmonic ace.

CAVITRON ULTRASONIC SURGICAL ASPIRATOR (FIG. 18)

The cavitron ultrasonic surgical aspirator (CUSA) is an innovative tool for dissecting through the liver parenchyma, which can potentially reduce intraoperative blood loss and perioperative morbidity. The CUSA system is a powerful ultrasonic aspirator and dissector with a wide application not only in liver surgery, but also in other surgical specialties like neurosurgery as well. CUSA Excel is an ultrasonic surgical aspirator, where fragmentation, suction, and irrigation occur simultaneously, allowing the surgeon to remove tissue with accurate control. In liver surgery, it is an invaluable tool, particularly in a situation where the tumor is closely adjacent to a vital structure that needs to be saved. CUSA will enable dissection around any structure that needs to be preserved.

The CUSA console provides an alternating current of 23,000–36,000 Hz to the handpiece where the current passes through a coil inducing a magnetic field. This in turn excites a transducer of nickel alloy laminations which produces vibrations along its long axis to an attached surgical tip. Tissues with weak intracellular bonds like liver are easiest to get fragmented.

The handpiece of the CUSA contains a hollow titanium tip which vibrates longitudinally along its axis, driven by a transducer **(Figs. 19A and B)**. The vibration occurs with a frequency of 23 kHz and with an adjustable stroke of 0–300 μ. The tip of the device, placed in contact with the target tissues, destroys and emulsifies the cell membranes, which are irrigated and removed through a built-in suction tube. Since vessels >0.5 mm in diameter, nerves and fibrous tissue capsules contain much collagen, they rebound with the ultrasonic vibration waves emitted by the CUSA and consequently they are left unimpaired by the procedure. The larger the degree of tip excursion of the CUSA, the greater is the power added to fragment the target tissues **(Fig. 20)**. The effectiveness also depended upon the amount of water contained in the tissues.

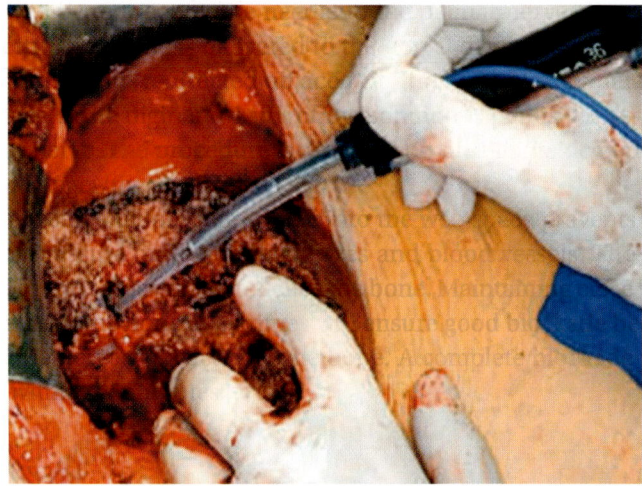

Fig. 18: Cavitron ultrasonic surgical aspirator for dissecting liver parenchyma.

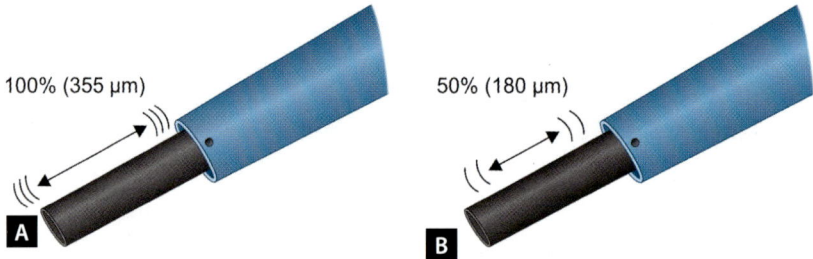

Figs. 19A and B: Hollow titanium tip in handpiece of cavitron ultrasonic surgical aspirator.

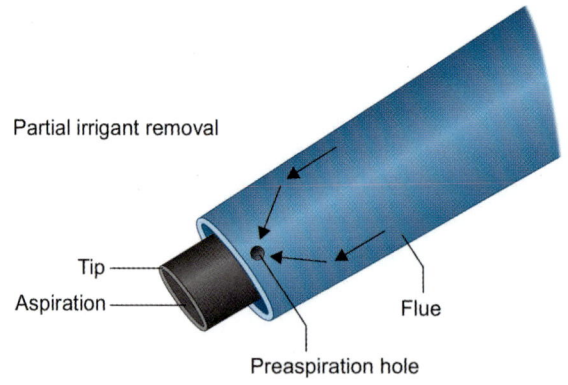

Fig. 20: CUSA tip.

RADIOFREQUENCY ABLATION

Radiofrequency ablation (RFA) is a medical procedure in which part of the electrical conduction system of the heart, tumor, or other dysfunctional tissue is ablated using the heat generated from medium frequency alternating current (in the range of 350–500 kHz). RFA is generally conducted in the outpatient setting, using either local anesthetics or conscious sedation anesthesia. When it is delivered via catheter, it is called radiofrequency catheter ablation.

Two important advantages of RF current (over previously used low frequency alternating current or pulses of direct current) are that it does not directly stimulate nerves or heart muscle and therefore can often be used without the need for general anesthetic and that it is very specific for treating the desired tissue without significant collateral damage **(Fig. 21)**.

The main applications in surgery are:
- Ablation of varicose veins
- Palliative ablation of liver secondaries.

It uses the same principles of RF electrosurgery. But when it comes in contact with a blood vessel in the zone of ablation, the heat is transferred from the target tissue to the flowing blood. This result in ablation zone distortion—"heat sink effect". Hence, secondaries near a vessel need other modes of ablation **(Figs. 22A and B)**.

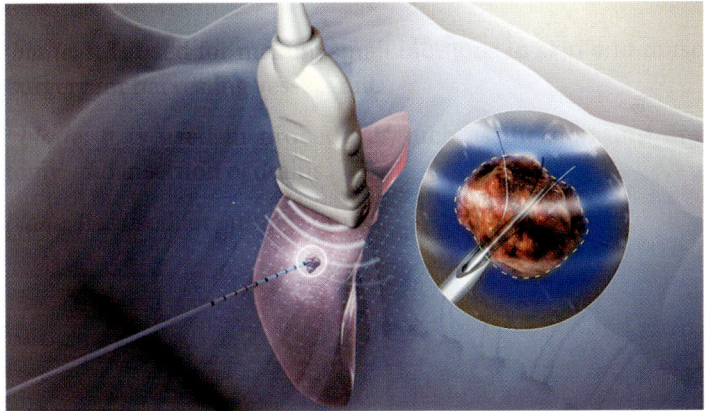

Fig. 21: Tissue ablation using radiofrequency.

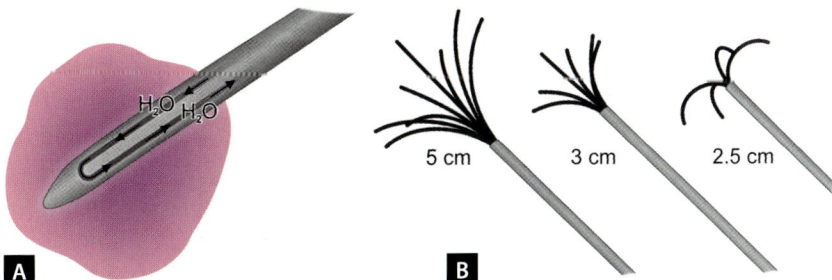

Figs. 22A and B: Probe with detachable radiofrequency ablation types called TINES.

CRYOABLATION

It is a mirror of RFA, except that tissue is destroyed through freezing with the use of liquid nitrogen, cryoprobes. The mechanism of action includes cell membrane disruption due to ice crystals, induction of apoptosis, and blood coagulation in capillaries. The objective of cryoablation (*kryo* = "cold" in Greek and *ablatus* = "to carry away" in Latin) is to reduce the temperature of the target tissue to below the lethal −20°C. This requires a continuous removal of energy from the entire target tissue **(Fig. 23)**.

There are three ways that thermal energy may be transferred from one volume to another: (1) by conduction, the transfer of energy (or heat) from an object to a another at a lower temperature by virtue of physical conduct (direct molecular kinetic energy exchanges); (2) by convection, the transfer of energy (or heat) from an object to another at a lower temperature, with one of the objects being a flowing fluid (thus providing a continuously refreshed heat sink or heat source); and (3) by radiation, which removes radiant energy from all bodies above absolute zero temperature. The chance for secondary

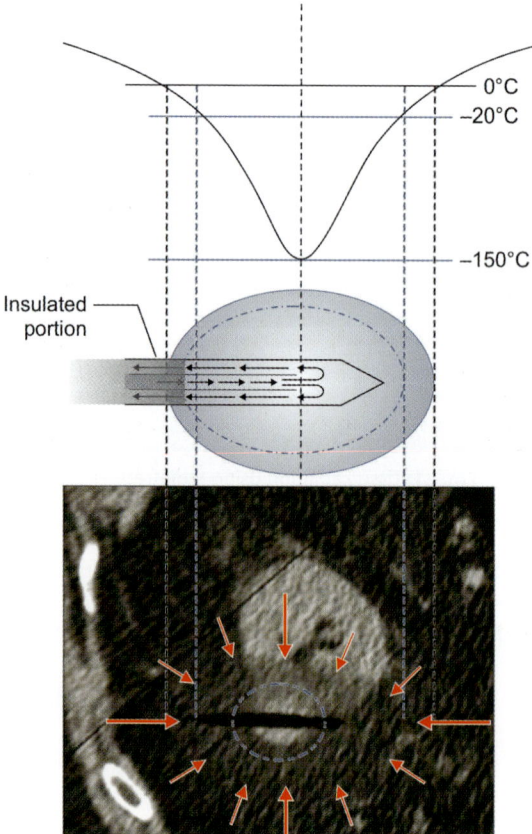

Fig. 23: Cryoablation.

hemorrhage is more with cryoablation. Multiple cryoprobes can be used simultaneously.

"Cryoshock" refers to cardiopulmonary collapse after a seemingly uneventful cryoablation. It is a diagnosis of exclusion and the risk increases with increasing patient age, increasing size of ice ball, and preexisting cardiac or pulmonary disease. The risk is mitigated by staging the procedure and avoiding large-diameter ice balls.

It is better to err on the side of using more cryoprobes than have to retreat a residual tumor. Two probes placed at the margins of the target mass are far better than one probe going right through the mass's center, even if the single probe's ice ball theoretically covers the mass.

Even though the temperature reading of the probe can reach –150° to –160°C, the distance between the tumor margin (dashed blue circle) and the edge of the ice ball (red arrows) is the crucial factor that determines the efficacy of ablation. The temperature rises quickly as a function of the distance from the probe and reaches 0°C at the edge of the ice ball. The lethal temperature for mammalian tissue is –20°C or colder. Therefore, an ablation margin is required between the target tumor and the edge of the visible ice ball to ensure complete ablation. A 5 mm margin is thought to be adequate to ensure that the target tumor reaches the lethal temperature of –20°C. The solid black line piercing the target lesion (dashed blue circle) is the "ghost" of the removed probe, which remains filled with air as the surrounding ice ball prevents it from collapsing.

OTHER BIPOLAR CUTTING AND COAGULATING DEVICES FOR LARGER VESSELS UP TO 7 mm

LigaSure

A new electrothermal bipolar tissue sealing system recently has been applied in abdominal and pelvic surgery, mostly through laparoscopy. The use of this sealing system allows the surgeon to improve vessel sealing with minimal thermal spread to the surrounding tissue **(Figs. 24 to 26)**.

The LigaSure vessel sealing system allows hemostasis by vessel compression and obliteration through the emission of bipolar energy. It includes:
- An electrosurgical generator able to detect the characteristics of the tissue closed between the instrument jaws; it delivers the exact amount of energy needed to seal it permanently.
- Several types of instruments that seal and, in some cases, divide the tissue:
  - LigaSure Atlas is a surgical endoscopic device (diameter: 10 mm, length: 37 cm) that seals and divides vessels up to 7 mm in diameter.
  - LigaSure V is a single-use endoscopic instrument (diameter: 5 mm, length: 37 cm) able to seal and divide.
  - LigaSure Lap is a single-use endoscopic instrument (diameter: 5 mm, length: 32 cm).

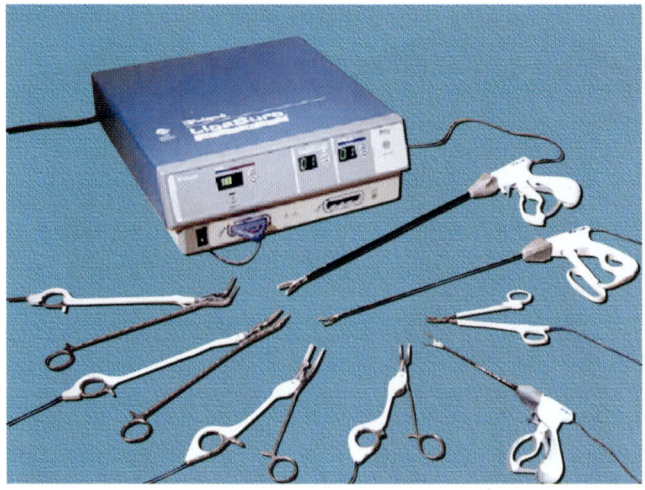

Fig. 24: LigaSure unit with probes.

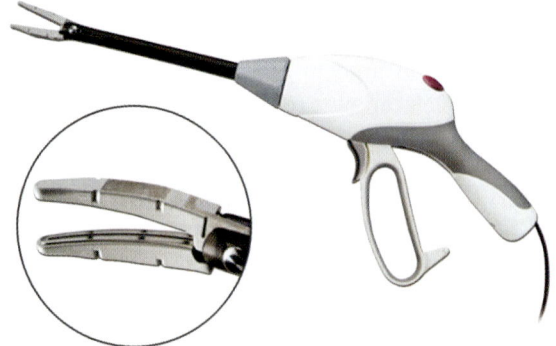

Fig. 25: LigaSure tip.

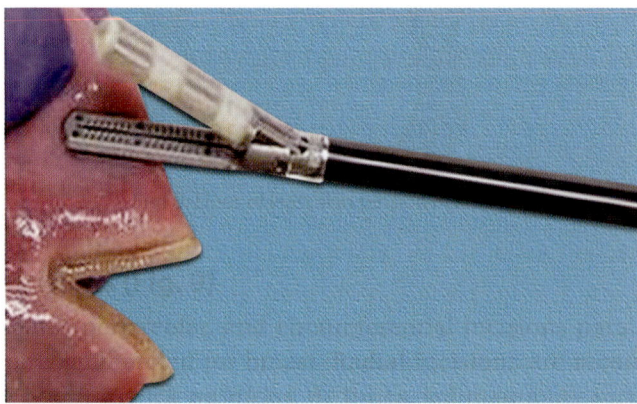

Fig. 26: LigaSure tip effect.

- LigaSure Precise is a single-use instrument (length: 16.5 cm) for open procedures specifically designed to provide permanent vessel occlusion to structures that require fine grasping.
- LigaSure Std is a reusable instrument.

This technique is different from the conventional coagulating methods that achieve vessel sealing by tissue carbonization. In fact, the heat generated from the bipolar energy determines the fusion of collagen and elastin in the walls of the vessel with the creation of a permanent sealed zone. The system detects the thickness of tissue to be coagulated and automatically defines the amount of energy required and the delivering time. An acoustic signal informs the surgeon when the vessel obliteration is complete and its division is possible. The seal zone shows a translucent appearance that is easy to recognize. Furthermore, this sealing system has a minimal thermal effect on the tissues surrounding the sealing line.

10 Intravenous Cannulation

PG Venugopalan

HISTORY

Sir Christopher Wren used a quill and bladder and injected opium into drops in 1656. Two English physicians published continuous method of transfusion in 1935. Metal needles were already in use prior to World War II. First reported use of plastic cannula dates back to July 5, 1950 by David Massa. The original manufacturer of this cannula with stylet was available through the Rochester Products Company, MN. The advances of Rochester needle have truly revolutionized the safe practice of intravenous (IV) therapy worldwide.

INDICATIONS

- Administration of IV medicines
- Transfusion of blood or blood components
- Maintenance or correction of hydration levels, if unable to tolerate oral fluids
- Potential venous access.

CONTRAINDICATIONS

- The presence of injury or damage
- The presence of infection as suggested by inflammation, phlebitis, and cellulitis
- Veins which are mobile or tortuous or sited near a bony prominence
- If IV therapy is predicted to be long-term
- Continuous infusions or therapies which are vesicant or have a pH of <5 or >9.

SITE SELECTION FOR CANNULATION

Preference should be given to a site where:
- Veins are accessible, unused
- Easily detected by palpation and/or visual inspection and appear healthy and patent
- Vein should feel soft and bouncy to the touch and refill quickly following compression
- Long straight veins with a large lumen are ideal.

Intravenous Cannulation

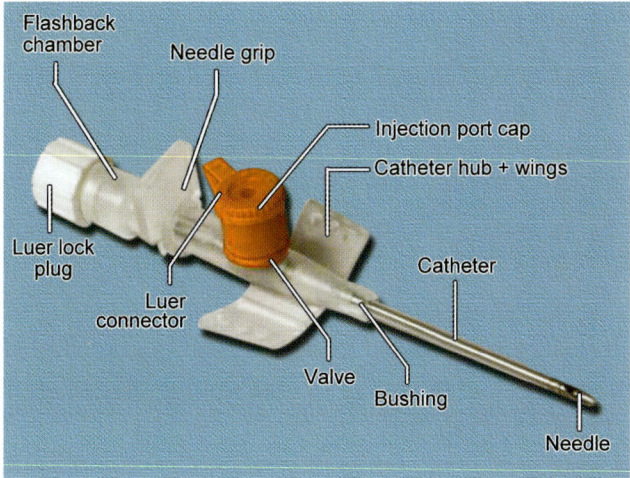

Fig. 1: Parts of intravenous cannula.

Most common veins used are basilica or cephalic veins of the forearm. This allows the placement of a variety of different sized cannulae in an area which is easily immobilized and does not cause too much restriction in patient activity. The antecubital fossa should only be used as a last resort as the effects of extravasation are more devastating, difficult to immobilize, uncomfortable to the patient, and may hamper other procedures such as venepuncture and blood pressure recording. The use of patient's dominant arm should be avoided, whenever possible.

DEVICE INFORMATION AND CHOICE OF CANNULA

A number of different types of peripheral cannulae are available. Incidence of vascular complications increases as the ratio of cannula external diameter to vascular lumen increases. Therefore, the smallest gauge cannula should be used in any given situation. Each cannula has a volume of fluid that can be infused on the external package. This will also inform the practitioner of an appropriate size. For the administration of viscous fluids/drugs, larger gauge needles may be required. In addition, larger gauge needles are used routinely in emergency situations **(Fig. 1 and Table 1)**.

Factors Influencing Choice of Cannula
- The purpose of cannulation
- Proposed drug administration
- Expected duration of cannula placement
- Size of vein to be cannulated.

EQUIPMENT LIST
- Sharps container
- Procedure tray

Table 1: Specifications for cannula.

Gauge	Color code	External diameter (mm)	Length (mm)	Flow rate (mL/min)
14 G	Orange	2.1	45	240
16 G	Gray	1.8	45	180
18 G	Green	1.3	32/45	90
20 G	Pink	1.1	32	60
22 G	Blue	0.9	25	36
24 G	yellow	0.7	19	20
26 G	Violet	0.6	19	13

- Cannulation pack which includes:
    - 1 small drape
    - 2 dry swabs
    - 1 IV cannula dressing
    - 1 customized cannulation label
    - 1 needle-free extension set
    - Gloves
    - Appropriate cannula for the purpose and length of infusion
    - 5 mL sterile saline and syringe
    - Disposable tourniquet
    - Prepared infusion
    - Alcohol handrub.

TECHNIQUE

Explain and discuss the procedure to the patient and get a verbal consent. Select cannulation site as described previously. Ensure that the patient is seated on a bed/chair with a back support. The use of local anesthetic injection (needs to be administered a few minutes before cannulation) or anesthetic cream (Emla cream, Ametop gel, cryogesic spray) should be considered. Hands should be cleaned as per Hand Hygiene policy. Collect equipment identified in equipment list. Where possible establish if the patient is at risk due to prolonged bleeding time. Ascertain if the patient has any known allergies to the dressing which is to be used. Use an alternative dressing, if necessary.

Clean hands before and after palpating the skin. Extend the limb and support on a pillow. Apply tourniquet to the chosen limb **(Figs. 2 to 11)**.

Steps of TV Cannulation

Use the following methods to encourage venous access:
- Ask the patient to clench and unclench his/her fist.
- Lower the extremity below the level of heart.
- Stroke veins with fingertip.

Intravenous Cannulation

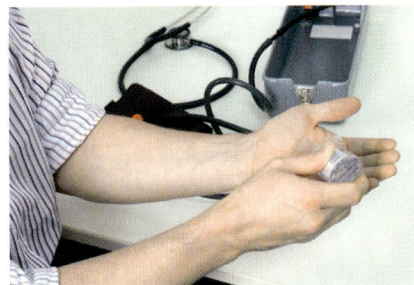

Fig. 2: Sanitization of hands (preferably to wear gloves).

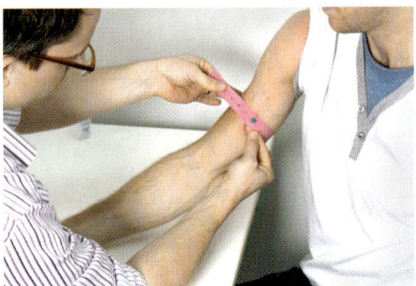

Fig. 3: Applying tourniquet.

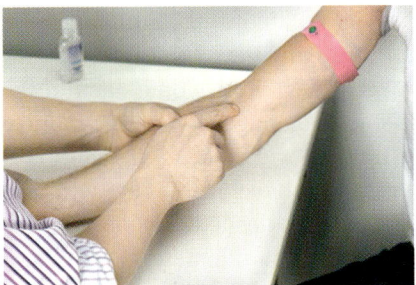

Fig. 4: Rechecking the vein.

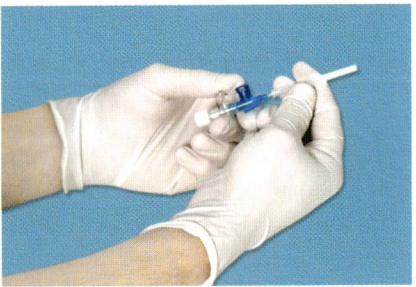

Fig. 5: Removal of needle from the cap.

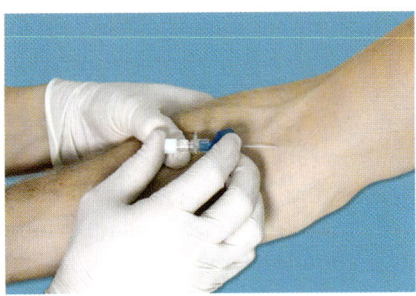

Fig. 6: Insertion of needle at 30°.

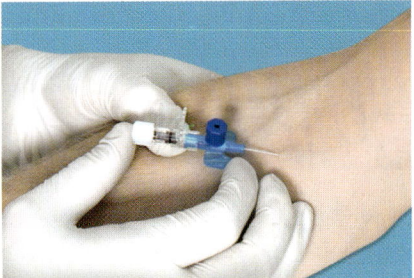

Fig. 7: Flashback of blood seen in hub of cannula.

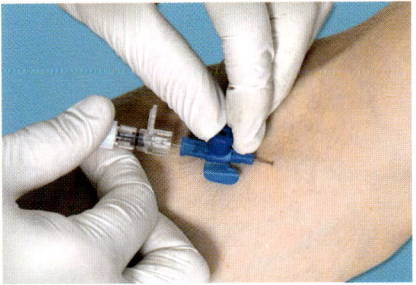

Fig. 8: Advance rest of the cannula into the vein.

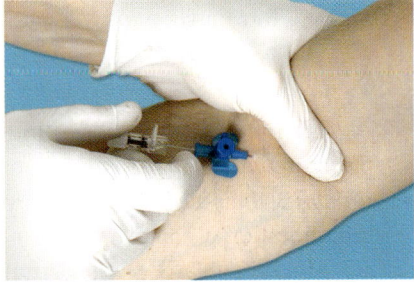

Fig. 9: Applying pressure to the vein at the tip of the cannula and removing the needle.

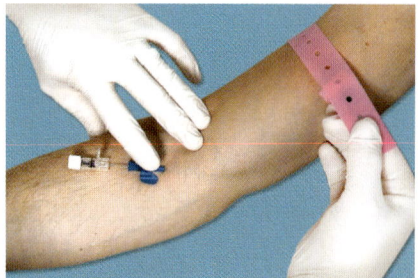
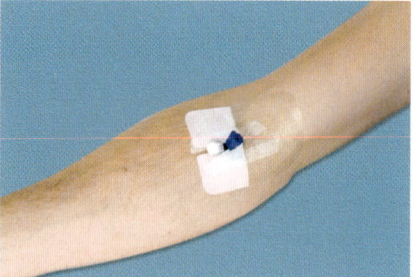

Fig. 10: Release of tourniquet.

Fig. 11: Plaster applied to cannula to fix it in place.

- Apply heat pad or immerse hand in warm water (under supervision). Lightly palpate selected vein and assess its suitability for cannulation.

Thoroughly clean the site with alcohol swab and then allow to air dry for at least 1 minute. Put on disposable gloves. Check expiry date of cannula. Remove cannula cover and inspect for signs of damage. Do not completely remove introducer. Anchor the vein by holding the surrounding skin taut using your nondominant hand. Insert cannula, bevel up, in line with the vein and at an angle of between 5 and 10°. Observe flashback of blood in the cannula chamber. Level off the cannula advance a few millimeters further into the vein. Withdraw introducer approximately 5 mm. Advance the cannula further into the vein observing for continued flashback of blood along the cannula. Release tourniquet. Apply gentle but firm pressure over the vein at distal end of cannula and then withdraw the introducer and place it directly into sharps container. Attach an extension set, either a needle-free extension set or prepared infusion set to the end of the cannula. Flush the cannula with 5 mL of 0.9% sodium chloride. Observe for signs of swelling or discomfort. Apply a sterile transparent dressing using an aseptic technique, ensuring that the entry site is visible and the date label is completed and attached to the dressing. If an infusion set is being used, ensure this is secured in double loop on the patient's arm using hypoallergenic adhesive tape. Document date, time, position, and size of the cannula. Ensure the insertion site is inspected regularly for signs of infection/phlebitis. Sites must be inspected prior to administration of medication 4 hourly, if an infusion is in progress or if the patient complaints of pain or discomfort around the site. When the cannula is removed, this must be recorded in the relevant documentation.

COMPLICATIONS

- *Accidental damage*: Nerve, tendon, or artery may be inadvertently punctured causing pain and damage.
- *Phlebitis*: It is characterized by pain and discomfort resulting from inflammation of the intima of the vein. The three main types are:
  1. Mechanical—damage/irritation by a cannula that is too large for the vein or inadequate securement of the cannula which allows for movement.

Table 2: Visual infusion phlebitis score.

Signs	Score	Stage / Action
IV site appears healthy	0	No signs of phlebitis **Observe cannula**
One of the following is evident: • Slight pain at IV site • Redness near IV site	1	Possible first sign of phlebitis **Observe cannula**
Two of the following are evident: • Pain • Erythema • Swelling	2	Early stage of phlebitis **Resite the cannula**
All of the following signs are evident: • Pain along the path of the cannula • Erythema • Induration	3	Medium stage of phlebitis **Resite the cannula** **Consider treatment**
All of the following signs evident and extensive: • Pain along the path of the cannula • Erythema • Induration • Palpable venous cord	4	Advanced stage of phlebitis or start of thrombophlebitis **Resite the cannula** **Consider treatment**
All of the following signs evident and extensive: • Pain along the path of the cannula • Erythema • Induration • Palpable venous cord • Pyrexia	5	Advanced stage of thrombophlebitis **Initiate treatment** **Resite the cannula**

(IV: intravenous)

2. Chemical—drugs which cause irritation (pH <5 or >9 or extreme osmolarity or vesicant). Vesicant drugs can cause blistering and necrosis, if they leak into the surrounding tissues.
3. Bacterial—poor hygiene or aseptic techniques leading to infection. Assessed by VIP score (Visual Infusion Phlebitis Score) **(Table 2)**.

- *Hematoma*: Hematoma may form if the cannula pierces the front and/or back wall of a vein. This can occur during insertion or removal of the cannula and may render the vein unsuitable for further cannulation. Treated by firm pressure applied for 3–5 minutes.
- *Extravasation*: This is the leakage of vesicant fluids or drugs into surrounding tissues which can cause local necrosis.
- *Prolonged bleeding time*: This may be due to a medical condition or drug therapy. It increases the risk of bruising or hematoma formation and worsens the consequences of inadvertent arterial puncture.
- Blood spillage.
- Needle or blood phobia.
- *Vasovagal faint/syncope*: This is due to innervation of the autonomic nervous system. Ensure that the patient is sitting/lying in a chair/bed whilst undertaking the procedure. However, if the patient begins to feel faint or appears pale and sweaty, the procedure should be stopped immediately. The cannula should be resited at the first signs of inflammation or discomfort.

11 Central Venous Catheter

John S Kurien

INTRODUCTION

"Two roads diverged in a wood and I, I took the one less traveled by, and that has made all the difference." No one was perhaps more inspired by this Robert Frost quote than Werner Forssmann, who in 1929, while still a surgical resident, inserted by himself, a ureteric catheter into his basilic vein, and then not only advanced it into the right atrium of his heart, but also walked up a flight of stairs to the X-ray department to confirm this most dramatic of self-experimentations of our time. Forssmann ended up being suspended from residency, but he received the Nobel Prize in Medicine in 1956, and we ended up being gifted with the vast world of central venous access devices (CVADs).

CATHETER MATERIAL

Polyurethane and silicone are usually used since they are inert, hence, biocompatible and resistant to chemical and thermal degradation. They possess sufficient tensile strength to pass through skin and subcutaneous tissue, but once inside the body, they soften, thereby reducing mechanical trauma to the vein walls.

CATHETER SIZE

The outside diameter (OD) decides the catheter size, which is measured by the following two systems:
1. The Gauge system developed in England which varies inversely with the OD.
2. The French system developed in France which varies directly with the OD and is very simple to understand (French size × 0.33 = OD in mm) and the commonly used system in India.

CATHETER FLOW

The flow within these vascular tubes can be explained by the Hagen-Poiseuille equation:

$$Q = \frac{\Delta P \pi r^4}{8 \eta l}$$

Central Venous Catheter

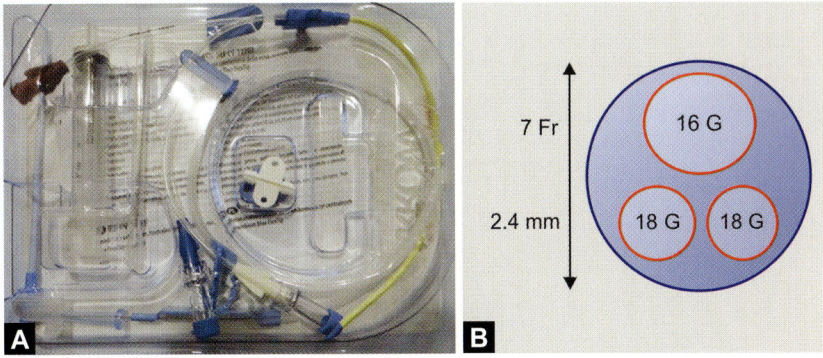

Figs. 1A and B: (A) A 7 Fr central venous catheter; (B) Cross-section of a 7 French central venous catheter shows three lumens. A 16 G distal lumen and two 18 G—medial and proximal lumens.

The equation indicates that the flow (Q) through a catheter will increase as the pressure gradient (ΔP) across the catheter and the radius (r) of the catheter increase, whereas to increase the flow, its length (l) as well as the viscosity (η) of the fluid passing through it has to decrease.

This explains why the flow through a 16 G venous cannula, only 1.2 inches in length, will be much greater than that in a 16 G central venous catheter (CVC) measuring 8–12 inches in length. When rapid volume insertion is necessary, the shortest available large bore catheter is the optimal choice.

The flow through a 16 G peripheral venous cannula of 1.2 inches length is approximately 13 L/hr, whereas the flow through a 7 Fr CVAD of 6 inches length is 3.4 L/hr via the distal lumen of size 16 G, and 1.8 L/hr through the medial and proximal lumens of size 18 G each.

A 7 Fr CVC is the usual choice in adults **(Figs. 1A and B)**.

CENTRAL VENOUS CATHETERS (FIGS. 2A TO D)

They are usually 15–30 cm long with 2–4 infusion channels. Multiple channels increase the diameter of a CVC, which thereby increases the chance of a catheter-induced thrombosis. Avoid CVC longer than 20 cm.

To ensure that there is no mixing of the contents in each lumen, the opening ports are arranged separately at the end—the proximal, middle, and distal opening.

Triple lumen CVCs are of two sizes. The length varies. The 16 cm one is shorter and used for right-sided procedures while the longer CVCs (20 cm or more) are preferred for left-sided central venous cannulations, due to the longer path taken from the left side to reach the superior vena cava (SVC).

Antibiotic-coated catheters are available (e.g., minocycline, rifampin, chlorhexidine, and silver sulfadiazine).

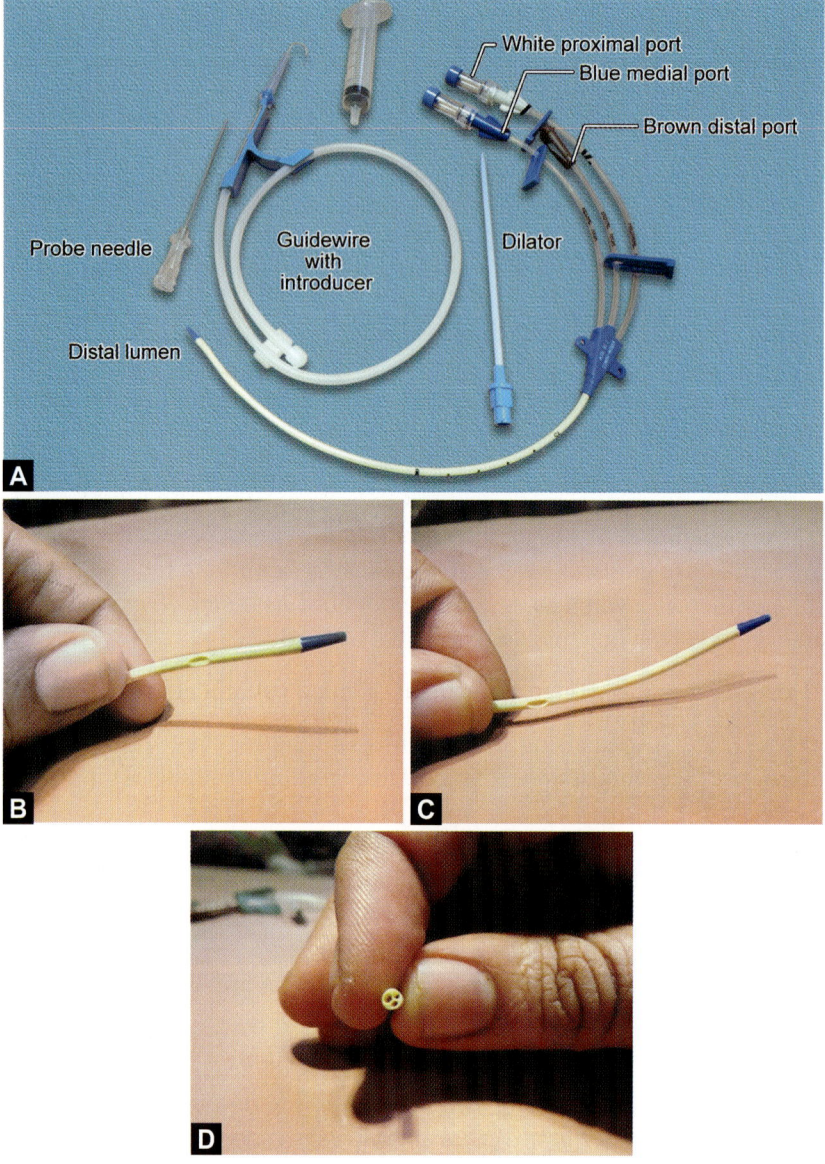

Figs. 2A to D: (A) Parts of central venous catheter (CVC); (B) Medial lumen; (C) Proximal lumen; (D) Cross-section showing three lumens.

Insertion Technique

The modified Seldinger technique was developed in the 1950s. Simply put, it consists of five easy steps to ensure safe venous access. The following images are of a right subclavian vein cannulation:

- Insert a needle into the vein. One can identify venous blood by its dark color, absence of spurting, and absence of platelet clumps. When one

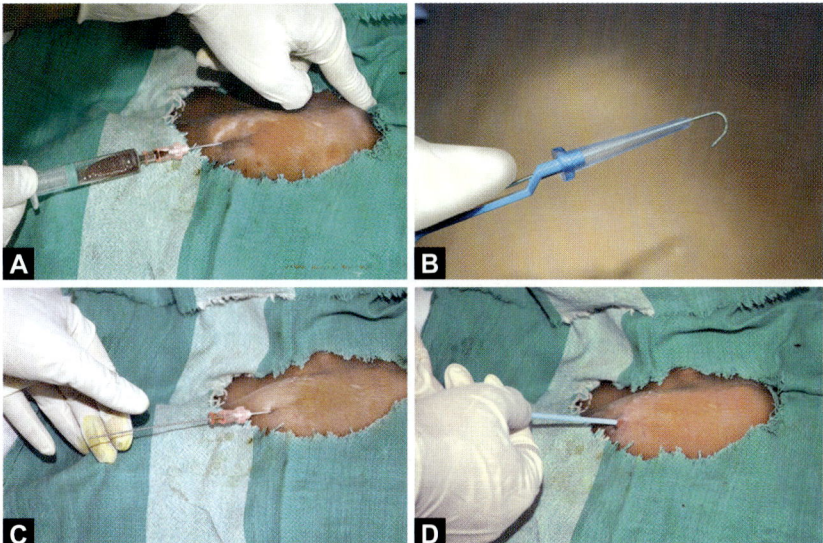

Figs. 3A to D: Inserting the needle into the vein.

disconnects the syringe, movement of blood column at the open end of the needle (in a vein) moves to and fro with each breath **(Figs. 3A to D)**.
- Keep aspirating throughout the procedure till the vein is entered.
- Pass a guidewire through the needle once it is in the vein. Hold the introducer between the thumb and index finger and retract the curved "J-Tip" of the guidewire into the introducer so that the tip becomes straight. Now push it into the probe needle, few centimeters at a time, gently with the thumb. No need to force it in as it may cause rupture of vessel walls.
- Remove the needle. While doing so, expose the tip of the needle a little and catch hold of the part of guidewire just beyond the tip. Only then pull out the needle, otherwise there is a chance that the guidewire comes out along with the needle.
- Insert the dilator over the guidewire to dilate the skin and subcutaneous tissue so as to allow the consecutive smooth passage of the catheter along the guidewire into the vein. This should also be gentle. Do not force the dilator through a vessel wall or other vital structures **(Figs. 4A and B)**.
- Now remove the dilator, being careful not to lose grip on the guidewire at all times. It is now time to guide the CVC over the guidewire. Hold the part of the guidewire still visible distal to the tip of the central catheter, and retract it till a portion of the guidewire comes out proximally, through the distal (brown) port of the catheter. Once this portion of the guidewire is gripped, we can be sure that we will not lose the guidewire into the vein while inserting the catheter, over the guidewire.

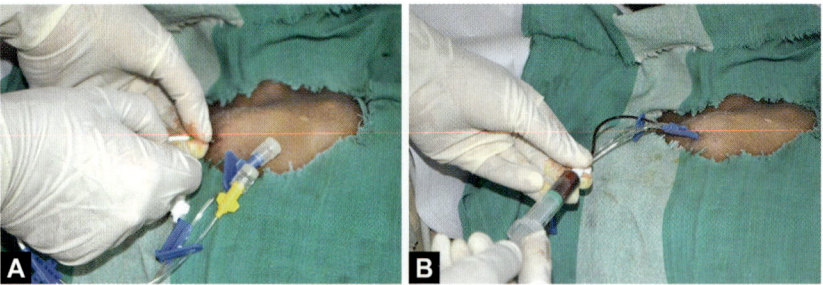

Figs. 4A and B: Inserting the catheter along the guidewire in the vein.

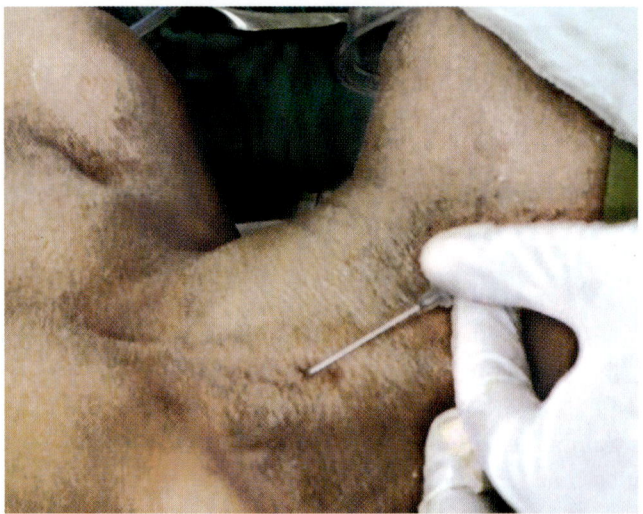

Fig. 5: Internal jugular vein cannulation.

- Once the CVC is in, remove the guidewire. Keep all parts of the catheter set sterile till the procedure is complete (just in case we have to reinsert). Now flush all the three ports with heparin saline and check for backflow of blood. If a CVC has backflow, only then is the central venous pressure (CVP) measured from that port accurate **(Fig. 5)**.

Peripherally Inserted Central Catheters

They are smaller in diameter because they are inserted into smaller peripheral veins. They are twice the length (50–70 cm) of the triple lumen catheters as they have to travel a longer distance to reach the right atrium. A chest X-ray is always taken to locate the position of catheter tip. Peripherally inserted central catheters (PICCs) have only a minimal risk of infection; therefore, these are easier to introduce than CVCs and can be left in place for several weeks. Plus we can avoid the grave complications of CVC such as pneumothorax and carotid rupture. The only problem is catheter-induced axillary and subclavian thrombosis.

Hemodialysis Catheters

These are large bore catheters usually of size 12 Fr having flow rates of around 200–300 mL/min required for effective hemodialysis. These catheters are usually inserted into the internal jugular vein (IJV) and left in place till an arteriovenous shunt is created by the vascular surgeon for long-term use. Never insert a hemodialysis catheter into the subclavian veins. There is a significant risk of subclavian vein stenosis that will affect venous outflow of the ipsilateral arm, thereby rendering the arm unsuitable for creation of an arteriovenous shunt later on.

CENTRAL VEIN CANNULATION

General Principles

Whenever a vein is cannulated, injury to the vessel wall causes inflammation. This incites thrombosis which is propagated by the sluggish flow in a small vein. Hence, larger the vein diameter, better are the flow rates and lesser are chances of local thrombosis.

The three most commonly accessed central veins have the following flow rates **(Table 1)**.

Nine veins are commonly cannulated for percutaneous central venous access. More commonly used veins include:

- Subclavian
- Internal jugular
- Femoral
- Basilic (antecubital fossa approach).

Veins used less commonly include:
- Axillary (anterior or lateral approaches)
- External jugular
- Brachial (mid-upper arm approach)
- Cephalic (antecubital fossa approach)
- Brachiocephalic (supraclavicular approach).

If ultrasound facility is available, puncture under ultrasound guidance is ideal:
- *Long-axis view*: The beam is aligned with the long-axis of the blood vessel. Since both the needle and the vessel are in the plane of the ultrasound

Table 1: Flow rates of most commonly accessed central veins.		
Vein	Maximum diameter	Maximum flow rate
• Internal jugular • Subclavian • Femoral	• 22 mm • 12 mm • 16 mm	• 2,000 mL/min • 800 mL/min • 1,100 mL/min

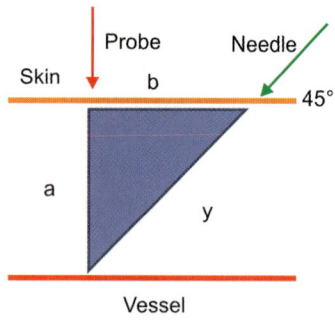

Fig. 6: Calculating the distance of probe from the vessel lumen using Pythagoras Theorem.

beam, we can visualize the path which the probe needle takes to reach the vessel lumen.
- *Short-axis view*: The beam runs perpendicular to the long-axis of the blood vessel (red arrow). Since we get only a cross-section of the vessel in this view, we can visualize the probe needle (green arrow) only after it enters the vessel lumen. Still, this is the preferred technique since we can actually calculate the distance of skin the needle has to pierce so as to reach the vessel wall (y).

For example, if we hold the probe at 90° to the vessel wall in this view, and pierce the skin holding the needle at a 45° angle, we can calculate the distance it has to pierce the skin using Pythagorean Theorem, as this arrangement forms a right-angled triangle **(Fig. 6)**. Plus if we ensure that the distance of the probe from the vessel (a) is equal to the distance of probe from needle (b), our triangle becomes an isosceles triangle, where:

$$a^2 + b^2 = y^2$$
$$\text{if } a = b$$
$$\sqrt{2a^2} = y = 1.4a$$

Hence, suppose we know that the distance of probe from the vessel is 4 cm and we keep the needle 4 cm away from the probe, and pierce the skin at a 45° angle, we have to pierce for a distance of 1.4 × 4 = 5.6 cm to reach the vessel lumen.

Indications
- Peripheral venous access is difficult [obesity, intravenous (IV) drug abusers, agitated patient]
- Delivery of hemodynamic drugs straight to the heart
- Multiple IV medications
- Total parenteral nutrition
- Long duration IV therapy
- Hemodialysis
- Transvenous cardiac pacing

- Hemodynamic monitoring (central venous pressure and pulmonary artery catheters).

Contraindications: Even a severe coagulation disorder is not a contraindication for CVCs in those who need them.

Sterile precautions: Always maintain strict aseptic precautions during a CVC insertion. Applying chlorhexidine-based solution to the insertion site and allowing it to air dry for 2 minutes, maximizes its antimicrobial activity, and it lasts beyond 6 hours after a single application.

Positioning

A head low Trendelenburg position of 15° below horizontal fills up the IJV and subclavian system of veins, making venous cannulation much easier. But avoid the head low position in cardiac failure patients (already have venous congestion) and head injury patients (already have raised intracranial pressures). These patients may symptomatically worsen if positioned this way.

LANDMARK METHODS

Internal jugular vein: There are two approaches to the IJV using surface landmarks—
- *Anterior approach*: For the anterior approach, the operator first identifies the triangular area at the base of the neck created by the separation of the two heads of the sternocleidomastoid (SCM) muscle. The IJV and carotid artery run through this triangle. The operator first locates the carotid artery pulse in this triangle; once the artery is located by palpation, it is gently retracted toward the midline and away from the internal jugular vein. The probe needle is then inserted at the apex of the triangle (with bevel facing anteriorly) and the needle is advanced toward the ipsilateral nipple at a 45° angle from the skin. If the vein is not entered by a depth of 5 cm, the needle should be drawn back and advanced again in a more lateral direction **(Fig. 7)**.
- *Posterior approach*: For the posterior approach, the insertion point for the probe needle is 1 cm above the point where the external jugular vein crosses over the lateral edge of the SCM muscle. The probe needle is inserted at this point (with the bevel facing anteriorly and directed horizontally to the opposite side) and then advanced along the underbelly of the muscle in a direction pointing to the suprasternal notch. The IJV should be encountered 5–6 cm from the insertion point.
 Carotid artery puncture is the most feared complication while doing this technique. If the needle is pierced into the carotid, remove it and apply firm compression for 5–10 minutes. However, if the catheter has already been inserted into the carotid artery, removing it could be life-threatening,

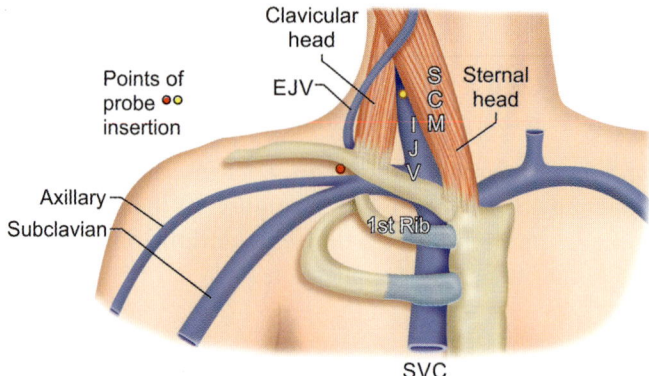

Fig. 7: Anatomy of neck veins and axillary veins reaching the superior vena cava (SVC). (EJV: external jugular vein; IJV: internal jugular vein; SCM: sternocleidomastoid)

due to uncontrolled bleeding. It is better to leave the CVC in its place and call the vascular surgeon.

Subclavian vein: The subclavian vein can be located by identifying the portion of the SCM muscle that inserts on the clavicle. The subclavian vein lies just underneath the clavicle at this point, and the vein can be entered from above or below the clavicle. This portion of the clavicle can be marked with a small rectangle at the base of the clavicular head of the ipsilateral SCM muscle, to guide insertion of the probe needle.

- *Infraclavicular approach*: The subclavian vein is typically entered from below the clavicle. The probe needle is inserted at the lateral border of the rectangle marked on the clavicle, and the needle is advanced (with the bevel facing anteriorly) along the underside of the clavicle in a direction that would bisect the rectangle into two triangles. The needle should enter the subclavian vein within a few centimeters from the surface. It is important to keep the needle on the underside of the clavicle, and to literally "walk on the clavicle" to reach its inferior most border, to avoid puncturing of the subclavian artery, which lies deep to the subclavian vein. When the needle enters the subclavian vein, the needle should be directed toward the ipsilateral sternoclavicular joint so the guidewire will advance in the direction of the SVC.
- *Supraclavicular approach*: Identify the angle formed by the lateral margin of the SCM muscle and the clavicle. The probe needle is inserted so that it bisects this angle. Keep the bevel of the needle facing anteriorly and obliquely advance the needle along the underside of the clavicle in the direction of the opposite nipple. The vein should be entered at a distance of 1–2 cm from the skin surface (the subclavian vein is more superficial in the supraclavicular approach). When the vein is entered, direct the needle horizontally to ipsilateral sternoclavicular joint so the guidewire will advance in the direction of the SVC.

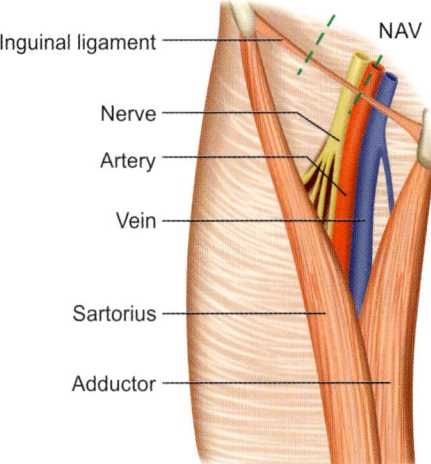

Fig. 8: Femoral vein.

Femoral vein (Fig. 8): It begins by locating the femoral artery pulse and insert the probe needle vertically, 1–2 cm medial to the pulse; the vein should be entered at a depth of 2–4 cm from the skin. If the femoral artery pulse is not palpable, draw an imaginary line from the anterior superior iliac crest to the pubic tubercle, and divide the line into three equal segments. The femoral artery should be just underneath the junction between the middle and medial segments and the femoral vein should be 1–2 cm medial to this point.

Complications

- *Venous air embolism*: If during CVC insertion, the patient develops sudden onset dyspnea, either it is a pneumothorax or a massive air embolism. Venous air embolism may be clinically silent or lead to cardiogenic shock or acute embolic stroke. The Trendelenburg position during catheter insertion helps prevent this complication. The consequences are fatal, if 200–300 mL air enters the system within a few seconds.
  Best investigation to detect air in the heart chambers is transesophageal echocardiography (TEE). But the best noninvasive method is Doppler ultrasound which converts flow velocities to sound. Air in the cardiac chambers produces a characteristic high-pitched sound.
  Pure oxygen breathing, left lateral decubitus position, and chest compressions may help.
- *Pneumothorax*: Pneumothorax is more related to subclavian vein cannulation than IJV cannulation. The operator aspirates air into his syringe while trying to enter the vein using Seldinger approach, by accidentally piercing the lung apices. An immediate X-ray should be taken, preferably in an upright position with patient at the end of

forced expiration. Sometimes, the immediate X-ray may be normal as pneumothorax from central venous cannulation is generally not detectable for up to 48 hours postprocedure. Hence, serial X-rays should be considered. Also, sometimes sick patients cannot sit upright for an X-ray and we accept the supine X-ray film, because something is after all better than nothing. Bear in mind that up to 50% of pneumothoraces are missed on a supine film. Brightness mode (B-mode) ultrasonography (USG) should be used in these cases.

- *Catheter tip position*: A postprocedure X-ray tell us the location of the CVC tip. Ideally, it should be at or just above the level of carina, since carina marks the junction of SVC and the right atrium where pericardium attaches. If a CVC enters the SVC from the left IJV or subclavian, it has to take an acute turn at the junction of left innominate vein and SVC. Sometimes, it abuts against the wall at this junction and a sudden shoulder movement may cause the tip to perforate through the wall. Blood leaks into the thorax. Massive hemothoraces may need emergency thoracotomy. If the tip is below the level of carina, and the tip perforates through the vein wall, blood will leak into the pericardial space instead of the thorax. Cardiac tamponade can be rapidly fatal.

Keep flushing the central line from time-to-time with heparin saline to prevent thrombotic blockage of the CVC. Sometimes, the CVC is not completely blocked but there is enough thrombosis to prevent backflow of venous blood. This will overestimate the CVP measurement. Hence, it is advisable to flush the CVC 2–4 hourly taking sterile precautions (dilute 1 mL = 5,000 units of heparin in 500 mL of normal saline to make heparin saline).

Venous Cutdown

John S Kurien

INTRODUCTION

With the advent of central venous access devices (CVADs) and intraosseous infusions, the popularity of the venous cutdown procedure has come down. Recently, the Advanced Trauma and Life Support Textbook made the venous cutdown procedure as an optional skill for its trainees. But one should not forget that for the occasional trauma patient in shock, who has a feeble femoral pulse or a burn victim with burns in almost every part of the body amenable to access via a CVAD, the venous cutdown procedure could be life-saving.

Venous cutdown is usually done in the great saphenous vein (GSV), median cubital vein, cephalic vein, and basilic vein, but any large subcutaneous superficial vein can be accessed.

ANATOMY

The GSV originates from where the dorsal vein of the first digit (the large toe) merges with the dorsal venous arch of the foot. After passing anterior to the medial malleolus (where it often can be visualized and palpated), it runs up the medial side of the leg. Usual landmark for the GSV is 1 cm anterior and superior to the medial malleolus **(Fig. 1)**.

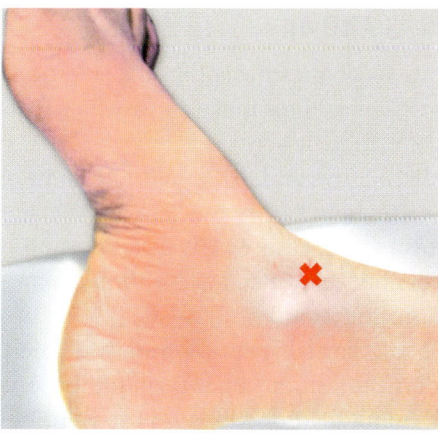

Fig. 1: Site of incision just above and in front of medial malleolus.

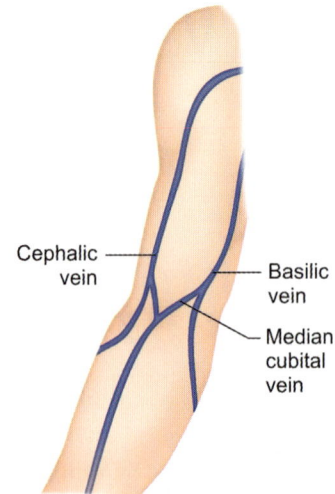

Fig. 2: Venous anatomy of upper limb showing medial cubital vein.

Basilic Vein

Basilic vein originates on the medial (ulnar) side of the dorsal venous network of the hand and travels up the base of the forearm, where its course is generally visible through the skin. It is more commonly used by vascular surgeons for creating arteriovenous (AV) fistulas for patients on long-term hemodialysis.

The median cubital vein lies in the cubital fossa superficial to the bicipital aponeurosis **(Fig. 2)**. It usually forms an H-pattern with the cephalic and basilic veins making up the sides, sometimes an M-pattern, where the vein branches to the cephalic and basilic veins, making this site a good candidate for venous access, thereby called "house surgeon's friend."

APPROACH (FIGS. 3 AND 4)

Prepare and infiltrate local anesthesia into the skin over the landmark and after ensuring aseptic precautions make a transverse incision perpendicular to the long axis of the vein to be accessed.

Now close the skin sutures and fix the cannula to the skin using sutures.

By using blunt dissection, isolate the vein, taking care not to damage its walls. Tie the vein using a 1-0 suture at its distalmost portion. Insert another thread under the vein but do not tie it. This thread allows us to manipulate the vein without damaging its walls.

Using a No. 11 blade partially, cut the vein wall and using a small sized artery forceps widen the lumen. Insert a large bore venous cannula or appropriately sized infant feeding tube into the vein. While inserting, keep the cannula/infant feeding tube on flow to allow smooth insertion with

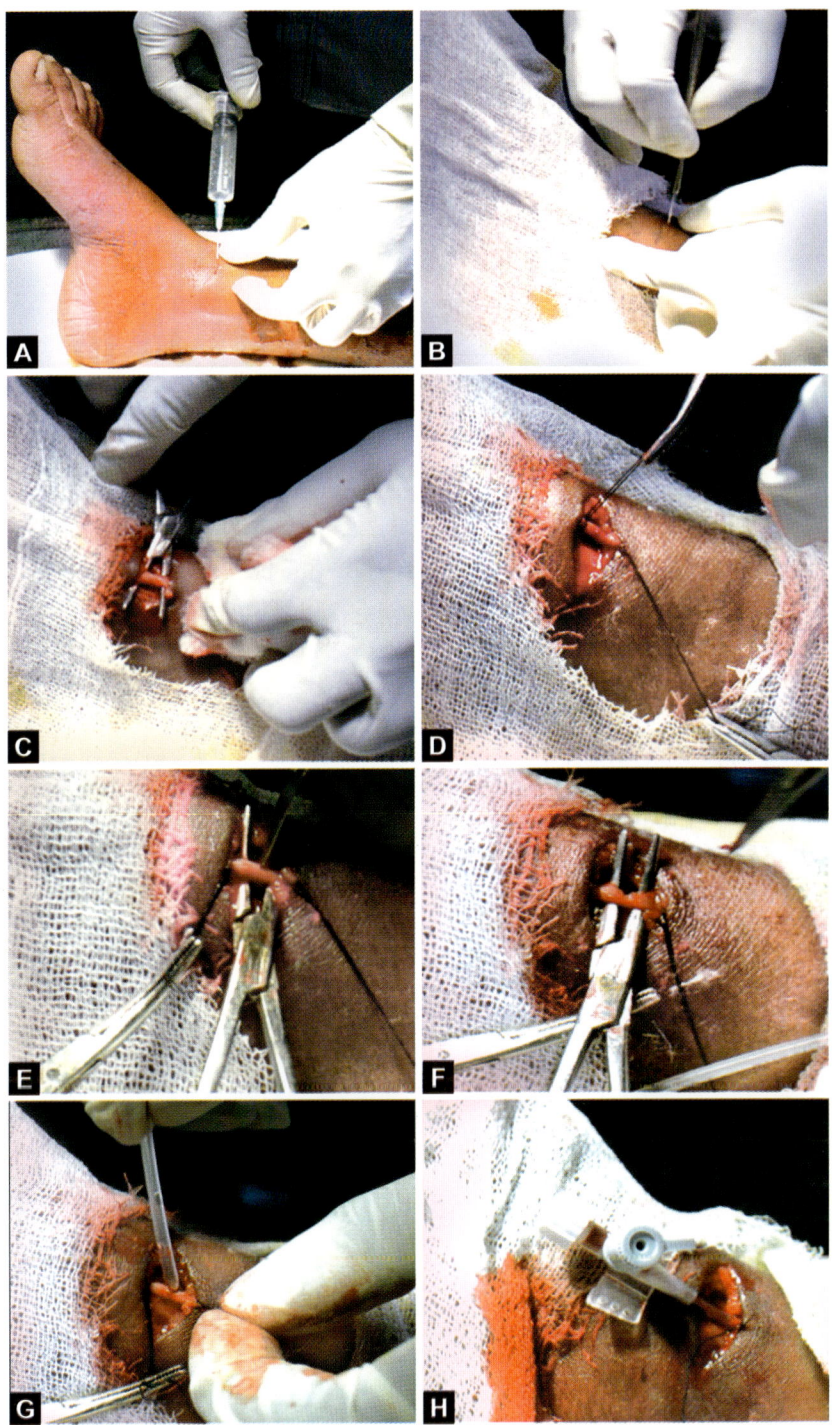

Figs. 3A to H: Infiltration of local anesthesia.

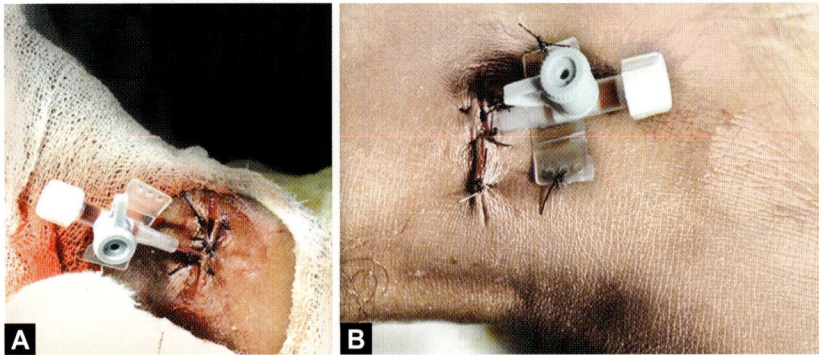

Figs. 4A and B: Cannula insertion after the procedure and the wound sutured.

minimal damage. Alternatively, a large bore venous cannula can be inserted (gray or green) if the appropriate sized infant feeding tube is not available (No. 6 or 8).

Once the vein has been accessed, check for the flow and then securely fix the cannula to the vein just accessed, by tying the suture we had introduced proximally to manipulate the vein.

Now close the skin sutures and fix the cannula to the skin using sutures.

COMPLICATIONS

The complications of venous cutdown insertion are cellulitis, hematoma, phlebitis, perforation of the posterior wall of the vein, venous thrombosis, and nerve and arterial transection. The great saphenous venous cutdown can result in damage to the saphenous nerve due to its intimate path with the GSV, resulting in loss of cutaneous sensation in the medial leg.

13. Local Anesthetics Used for Minor Surgery

R Dayananda Babu

INTRODUCTION

A large number of procedures can be performed under local anesthetic techniques. It produces initial pain while injecting (field block), later on, analgesia will occur in the infiltrated operative site.

Small diameter pain fibers are blocked first and larger ones carrying touch sensation are retained or blocked later. The largest motor fibers will be spared.

Action depends mainly on the rate of blood perfusion in the tissue. Reabsorption of local anesthetic will be faster in areas such as face, and it is better to add vasoconstrictors such as adrenaline to prolong the duration of action.

Adrenaline should be avoided in areas such as digits (for ring block), tip of nose, ear lobes, and shaft of the penis. These areas are supplied by end arteries and adrenaline will result in gangrene of the related areas.

It takes 5 minutes to get action, and if there is inflammation, it takes more time.

Using lignocaine warmed to 37°C results in less pain on injection than does at room temperature and a faster neural blockade. Counter irritant such as pinching nearby skin can increase the comfort of the patient.

LOCAL ANESTHETICS

Lignocaine is a fast-acting local anesthetic. It easily diffuses through the tissues. The duration of action lasts between 20 and 90 minutes. Use of adrenaline will reduce the bleeding and increase both the duration of action and the maximum safe dosage. Commonly used local anesthetic is 0.5% and 1% for skin infiltration. Two percent is used for decreasing the volume in areas such as digits for nerve block. **Table 1** illustrates the maximum dosage of local anesthetics for adults.

In children and old age patients with hepatic disease, renal impairment, epilepsy, or heart block, etc., lower dose must be used.

Prilocaine and bupivacaine are safest for intravenous (IV) anesthesia as it slows reabsorption from the circulation. It has a slow onset of action

Surgical Handicraft

Table 1: Maximum doses of local anesthetic advised in adults.

Drug	Maximum dose without epinephrine (adrenaline)	Maximum dose with epinephrine
Xylocaine	4 mg/kg	7 mg/kg
Bupivacaine	3 mg/kg	
Safe volume for 0.5% xylocaine	40 cc	100 cc
Safe volume for 1% xylocaine	20 cc	50 cc
Safe volume for 2% xylocaine	10 cc	25 cc

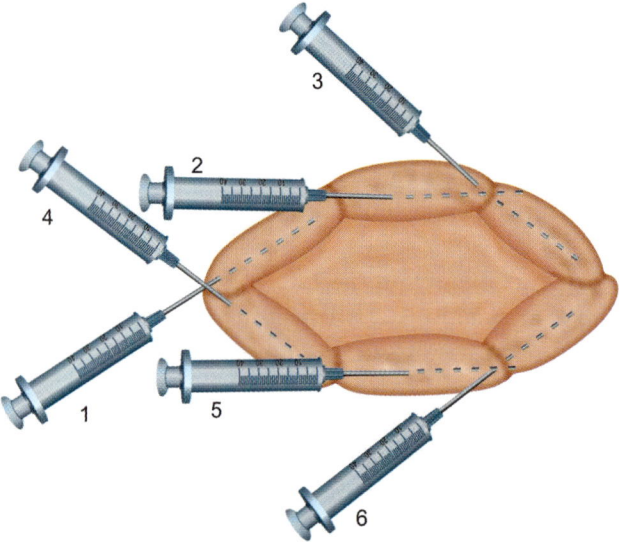

Fig. 1: Local anesthetic infiltration.

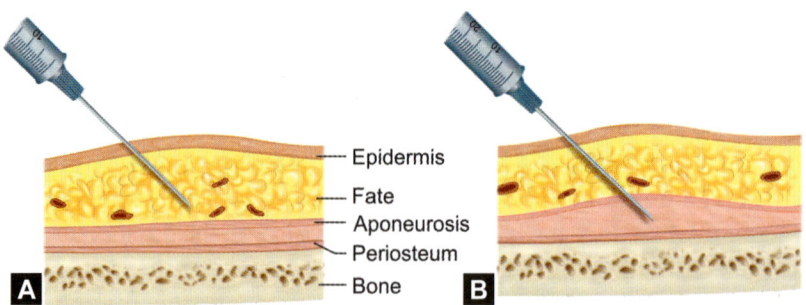

Figs. 2A and B: Method of infiltration of scalp. (A) Correct; (B) Incorrect.

than lignocaine and has no added benefit for its use as an agent for local infiltration. It has long duration of action (4–6 hours).

Use of adrenaline which acts mainly on small intradermal vessels will minimize the bleeding. Bleeding can still be expected to appear from larger and deep vessels. It is helpful in vascular areas such as face and scalp. It is combined with lignocaine in a strength of 1:200,000 (5 µg/mL).

Infiltration of Local Anesthetic

Initially, a small dermal wheal is made, and the needle is introduced through the wheal for sufficient length in the subcutaneous tissue. The syringe containing the local anesthetic is attached to the needle hub. It is important to withdraw the piston before injecting and make sure that the needle tip is not inside the vessel. In patients with history of allergy, it is important to give a test dose before starting the infiltration **(Figs. 1 and 2)**.

14 Digital Nerve Blocks (Finger and Toe Blocks)

R Dayananda Babu

ANATOMY

There are four digital nerves for each finger/toe including the thumb and great toe **(Fig. 1)**. The palmar digital nerves have the most extensive sensory distribution **(Fig. 2)**. They are responsible for the distal finger and fingertips sensation including the nail bed. Although the dorsal nerves have a lesser distribution, there is sufficient overlap with the palmar nerves. All four branches on each finger/toe must be blocked to achieve complete digital anesthesia. The digital nerves are immediately adjacent to the phalanges and these structures act as landmarks for locating the nerves.

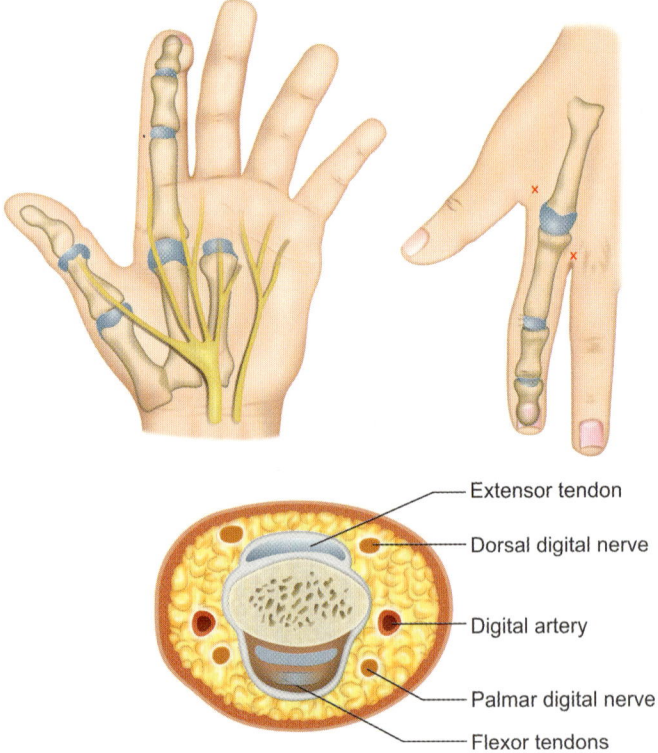

Fig. 1: Section of digit showing the dorsal and palmar digital nerves.

Digital Nerve Blocks (Finger and Toe Blocks)

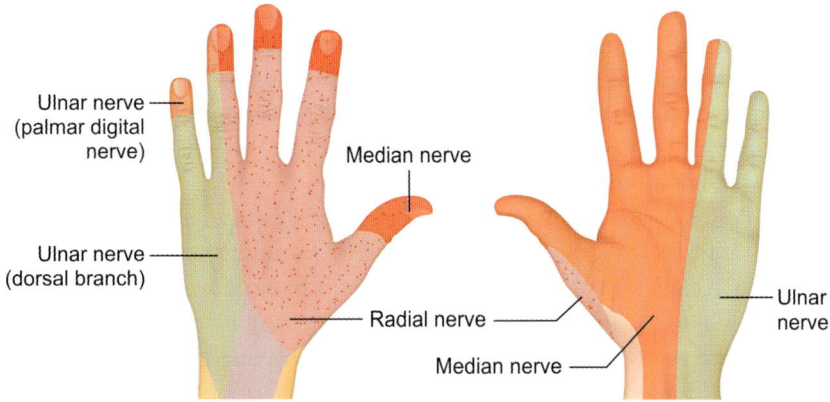

Fig. 2: Sensory innervations of the dorsal and palmar view.

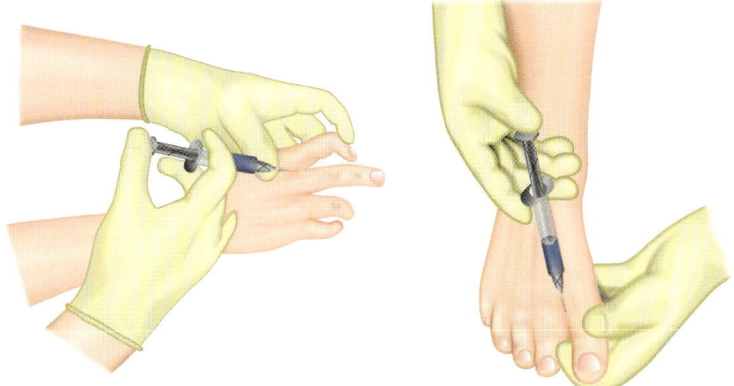

Fig. 3: Performing digital nerve block in hand and toe.

Indications

- For suturing of the wounds distal to the level of the mid proximal phalanx/toe
- For removal of nail
- For paronychia drainage
- For pulp abscess drainage
- For repair of lacerations of the digits.

TECHNIQUES FOR DIGITAL NERVE BLOCK

For the procedure, 1% lignocaine without adrenaline is recommended. Usually 4 mL of the solution is used.

Small needle of sizes 24–28 gauge are used for injection. Two needle pricks are used to block the nerves on either side. The needle is introduced into the dorsolateral aspect of the proximal phalanx in the web space just distal to the metacarpophalangeal joint. The dorsal digital nerve is approached first followed by redirecting the needle to the palmar nerve. Approximately 0.5 mL of the anesthetic is delivered to the dorsal digital now. The needle is then withdrawn and redirected adjacent to the bone of the phalanx to the volar surface of the digit and 1 mL of the solution is deposited at the site of the palmar nerve. The procedure is repeated on the other side of the digit to achieve full finger/toe anesthesia **(Fig. 3)**.

The deposition of local anesthetic into the web space prevents excessive buildup of pressure on the digital nerves and blood vessels. The needle is advanced in such a way that it touches the bone. Maintaining close proximity of the needle to the bone at all times will ensure good blockade because the course of the nerve is adjacent to the bone. A complete blockade is usually achieved within 4–5 minutes.

Surgical Blades, Skin Incisions, and Acute Wound Closure

R Dayananda Babu

SURGICAL BLADES

Skin incisions are usually made with surgical blades.

Surgical blades are pressed firmly at right angles to the skin and then pressed down gently across the skin in the desired direction to create a clean incision.

Surgical blades with scalpel should never be passed by direct hand-to-hand process but always be passed in a kidney dish to avoid injury.

Types of Blades Generally Used (Fig. 1)

No. 10 blade: It is used for making small incisions in skin and muscles, in plastic surgery for harvesting vessel graft.

No. 11 blade: It is used in procedures such as incision and drainage, arteriotomy, and insertion of drains.

No. 12 blade: It is used for cutting sutures.

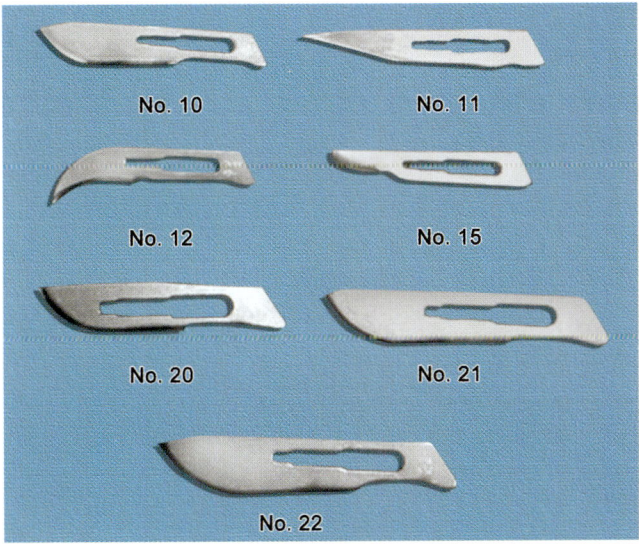

Fig. 1: Types of surgical blades.

No. 15 blade: It is used in minor surgeries such as excision of small swelling.

No. 20 blade: It is used for making big incisions.

No. 21 blade: It is used for abdominal incisions.

No. 22 blade: It is used for abdominal incisions.

SKIN INCISIONS

The incision site, extent, and direction should be planned before making an incision **(Figs. 2 and 3)**.

The incision should be placed parallel to the skin tension lines (Langer's lines) to achieve a better scar. These are the lines of preferred orientation

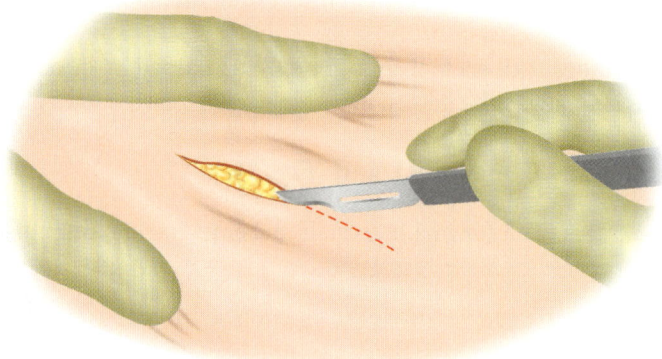

Fig. 2: Method of holding the knife for incision.

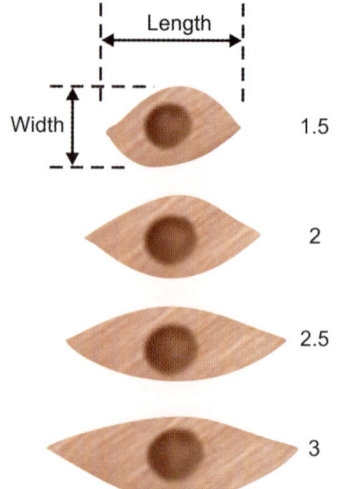

Fig. 3: Length of ellipse should be approximately 2.5–3 times the width to prevent dog ear.

of wounds and take into account lines of least skin tension and skin folds. **Figure 4** shows the preferred incision lines in the face and neck (trunk and limbs). Incisions should be avoided in bony prominences and crossing skin creases.

A wound made at 90° to the lines of maximum tension will tend to spring open. An incision along the line of maximum skin tension will tend to have the least tension across the wound. **Figures 5 to 8** show the lines of least skin tension in different parts of the body.

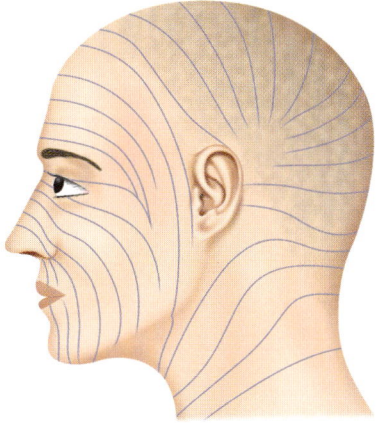

Fig. 4: Preferred incision lines for least skin tension.

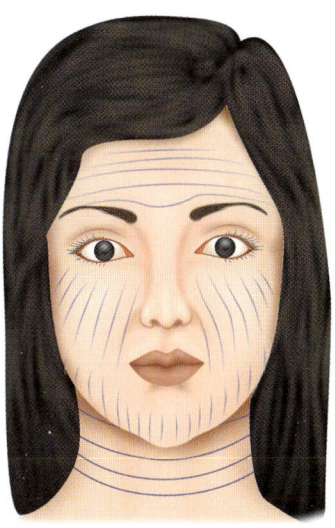

Fig. 5: Lines of least skin tension on face.

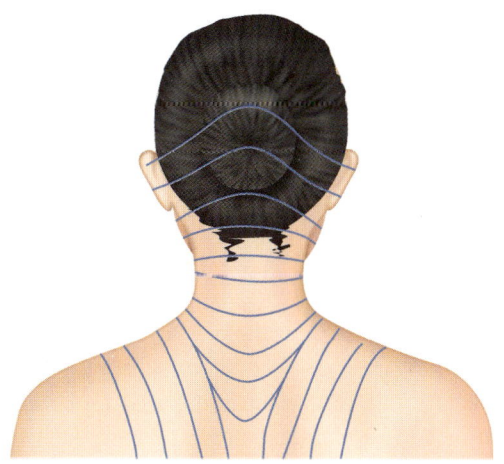

Fig. 6: Lines of least skin tension on back.

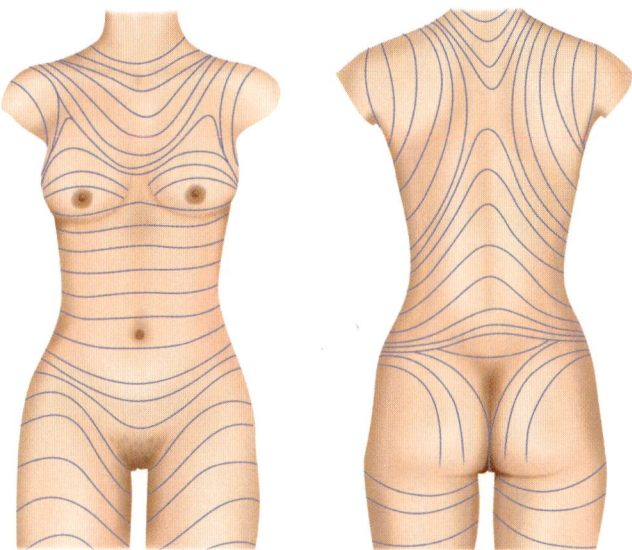

Fig. 7: Lines of least skin tension of trunk.

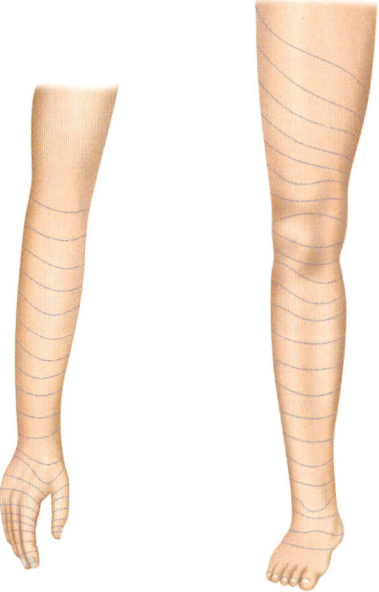

Fig. 8: Lines of least skin tension in limbs.

Breast Incisions (Fig. 9)

Circumareolar, periareolar, and circumferential incisions parallel to the areola are recommended for breast. Radial incisions are recommended only for 3 and 9 o'clock positions. At times, submammary incisions are recommended.

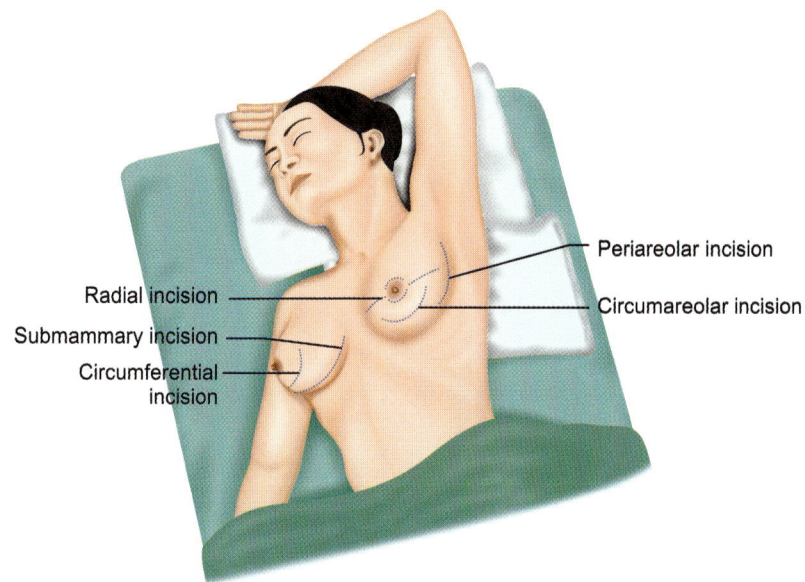

Fig. 9: Recommended breast incisions.

Identifying Skin Tension Lines

If the area is compressed in the direction of planned surgery, the skin will wrinkle easily across the lines of maximum tension. Minimum wrinkling occurs and skin movement is less along the tension lines.

WOUND CLOSURE

There is no ideal wound closure technique that is applicable to all situations. The site and the tissues involved should be taken into consideration before planning closure.

For any wound closure to heal well, there should be a good blood supply and no tension on the closure.

Suture Techniques

The edges of any wound should be treated as gently as possible. Trauma can be minimized by toothed forceps. Adequate hemostasis is critical **(Figs. 10 and 11)**.

Simple Interrupted Suture (Figs. 12A and B)

Needle is positioned with its middle third within the jaws of needle holder.

One wound edge is gripped and slightly everted; needle is pushed into skin at 90° and using the curve of the needle, it is advanced into the center of the wound.

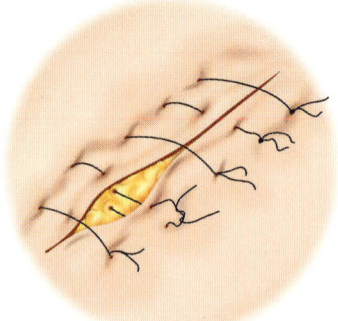

Fig. 10: Combination of simple and mattress.

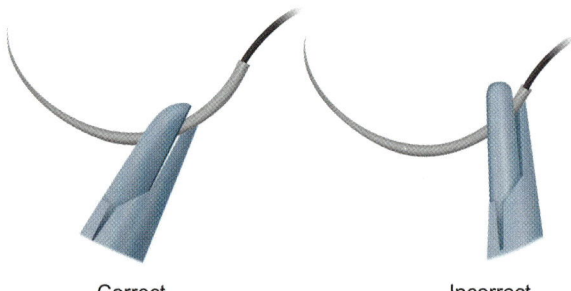

Correct   Incorrect
Fig. 11: Method of holding needle.

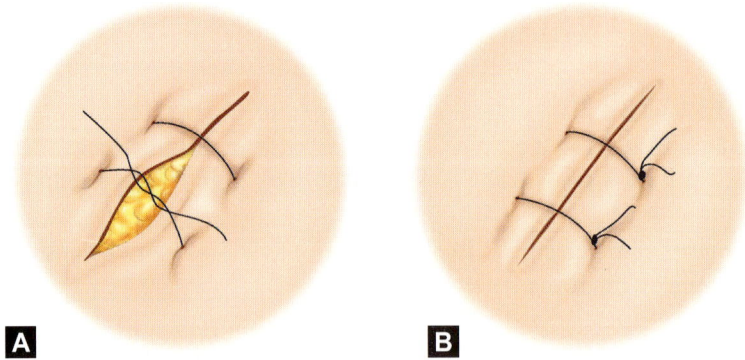

Figs. 12A and B: Simple suture knots pulled to one side.

The opposite edge of the wound should be slightly everted and the needle is advanced in an equal and opposite action using the curve of the needle.

The tip of the needle is retrieved using tissue forceps and not fingers; the thread is pulled leaving 2–3 cm at its tail end.

The initial throw of the suture is double and is pulled firmly but not tightly.

The second throw is single and should be opposite to the initial throw forming a reef knot which is stable.

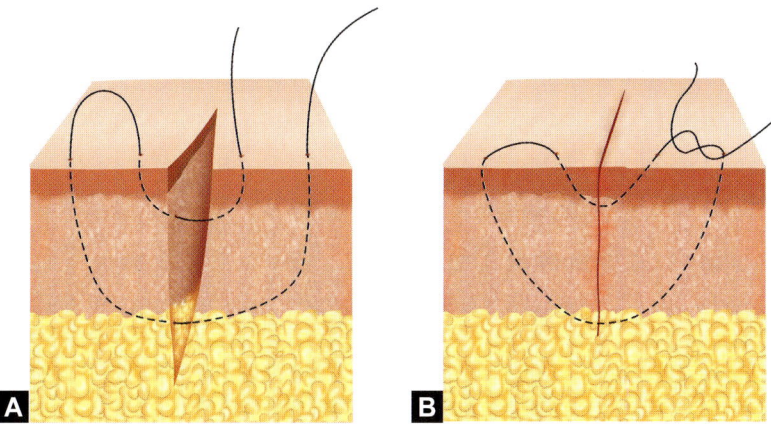

Figs. 13A and B: Vertical mattress suture.

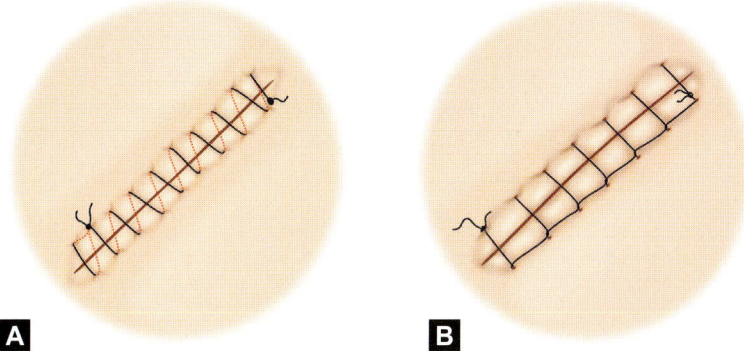

Figs. 14A and B: Continuous suture. (A) Simple running suture; (B) Locking running (blanket) suture.

Interrupted sutures should be spaced evenly and should draw wound together without leaving redundant tissue at either end of the wound (a dog ear).

The knots should not lie directly over the wound.

Vertical Mattress Suture (Figs. 13A and B)

This is an alternative to simple interrupted sutures in wounds that are in tension. The skin is punctured twice on each side of the wound. A deep, wide bite is taken first, then a smaller reverse bite is taken in the same plane traversing the edges of the wound once again. A square knot is tied as before.

These sutures are very useful in producing accurate approximation of the wound edges.

Continuous Sutures (Figs. 14A and B)

The first suture is inserted as an interrupted suture but rest of the sutures are inserted in a continuous manner until the far end of wound is reached. The suture is pulled until the edges appose, but not too tight to allow for tissue edema postoperatively. The end is tied to the final loop. It is quick and easy to insert.

The running sutures are locked by hooking the needle under the previous loop on taking each bite, this is called *"locked running sutures" or "blanket sutures"* (*see* **Fig. 14B**).

Running Subcuticular Suture (Fig. 15)

This technique is used where a cosmetic appearance is important and where the skin edges may be approximated easily. It is a dermal suture that removes risk of suture marks. The needle is introduced approximately 3 mm away from the tip of the wound advanced into the center of the incision.

A small bite is taken in the dermis on one side of the wound with needle held in the same plane as the skin surface. An equal but opposite bite is taken from the other edges lightly further down the wound. The suture is advanced down the length of the wound 3–5 mm at a time. When the far end of the wound is reached the needle is advanced from the center of the wound to the skin surface some 3 mm outside the wound. Both ends may be tied with knots back on themselves. Suture material used can either be absorbable or nonabsorbable. The ends may be secured using a buried knot when absorbable sutures are used.

Alternatives to Sutures

Skin Adhesive Strips

These are used where there is no skin tension and minimal moisture present around the wound.

It is useful for suturing the hernia wound where each needle track is likely to be a potential source of infection.

It is also used to minimize spreading of the scar.

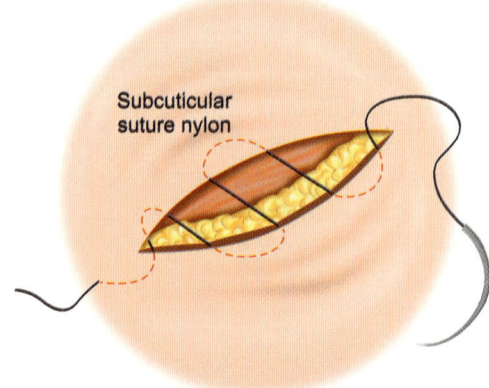

Fig. 15: Running subcuticular suture using nylon.

Tissue Glue

The glue is based upon a solution of N-butyl-2-cyanoacrylate monomer. The wound must be clean, dry with no skin tension and perfect hemostasis. Glue, when applied to a wound, polymerizes to form a firm adhesive bond.

Skin Clips

They can be placed faster than suture insertion and will produce a very neat scar. They are responsible for lowering predisposition to infection. A special instrument is required to remove them.

SUTURE REMOVAL

Simple interrupted sutures are removed using sharp, thin bladed scissors. The sutures are cut close to the skin surface as possible, and with gentle traction at 90° to the wound edge, the suture is removed parallel to the skin surface.

Vertical mattress sutures should be cut next to the knot near the skin surface.

The deep loop is then pulled through and cut near the skin surface on the opposite side of the wound. The remaining superficial loop may be removed by traction on the knot.

The continuous or running sutures should be removed in small sections to minimize wound contamination.

Subcuticular sutures are removed by trimming at one end as it emerges from the skin and pulling on the other end while applying gentle countertraction on the wound **(Fig. 16)**.

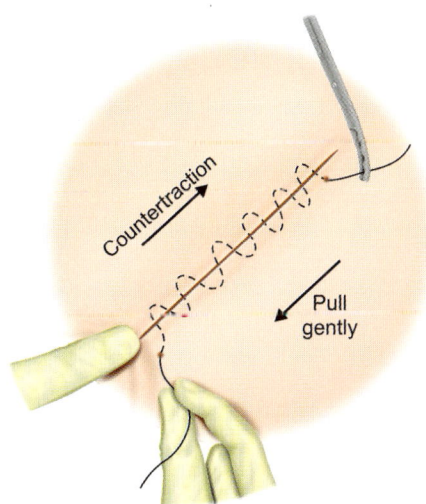

Fig. 16: Suture removal.

When to Remove Suture

- Sutures on the scalp, face, and neck can be removed on the 4th day.
- Open hernia sutures are removed on 6–7 days.
- Mastectomy wound sutures can be removed on the 7th day.
- Open cholecystectomy wound sutures are removed on the 7th day.
- Midline laparotomy wounds are removed on the 10th day.
- Amputation stump above knee and below knee can be removed on the 12th day.

16. Surgical Incisions

R Dayananda Babu

ABDOMINAL INCISIONS

Abdominal incisions may be *vertical*, *horizontal*, and *oblique*. Vertical may be midline or *paramedian* or *lateral paramedian*. Midline incisions may be upper midline or lower midline or full length midline. The horizontal incisions are *Pfannenstiel* or *Lanz* incision. In addition, *oblique incisions* are there. For example, McBurney's gridiron incision for appendicectomy, loin incision for kidney exposure, and Kocher's subcostal incision for cholecystectomy **(Fig. 1)**.

UPPER MIDLINE INCISION

The patient will be in supine position and under general anesthesia. It is used for accessing the stomach, duodenum, gallbladder, colon, liver, and

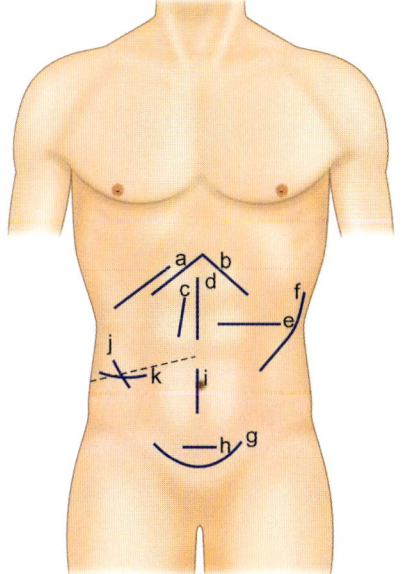

a: Kocher's subcostal
b: Bilateral subcostal/Rooftop (chevron)
c: Right paramedian
d: Upper midline
e: Transverse abdomen incision
f: Rutherford–Morrison
g: Pfannenstiel incision
h: Suprapubic
i: Lower midline
j: Gridiron
k: Lanz

Fig. 1: Abdominal incisions.

spleen. The incision extends from the xiphisternum to the umbilicus. The layers are:
- Skin and subcutaneous tissue
- Linea alba
- Extraperitoneal fat and peritoneum.

The peritoneum is held between artery forceps/Kocher's forceps and held away from the abdominal contents. It is incised with a scalpel. Two fingers are then inserted into the abdomen for protecting the viscera and safe division of the peritoneum upward and downward. The peritoneal cavity and the viscera are inspected systematically (the stomach, duodenum, jejunum, ileum, cecum, ascending colon, transverse colon, descending colon, sigmoid colon, etc.). The jejunum is identified by putting the hand into the left side of the vertebrae and identifying the fixed end of the jejunum at the ligament of Treitz. In addition, the gastrocolic omentum is incised and the posterior surface of the stomach and the pancreas is palpated. Both kidneys are also palpated. In the upper abdomen, the liver and spleen are palpated. The gallbladder is palpated for stones and growths. The lower end of esophagus and the hiatus is inspected.

Closure of the Abdomen

This can be done either in a layered manner by closing the peritoneum with absorbable sutures and the linea alba with nonabsorbable or delayed absorbable continued suture (read the "Closure Technique" in Burst Abdomen Chapter). Another option is mass closure, where all layers of the wound except skin are sutured with nonabsorbable or delayed absorbable continuous suture. The skin may be closed with subcuticular sutures or simple or mattress sutures or skin clip.

Advantages of Midline Incision

- Ease of performance and quick access
- Least vascular
- Easy to close.

Note:
- Linea alba is the strongest fascial layer of the abdomen. Previously, it was thought that it was a weak structure and therefore paramedian incisions were favored.
- There is no deep fascia for the abdomen.
- The hematoma and wound infections are negligible as compared to paramedian incision.

LOWER MIDLINE INCISION

This is done for access to the pelvic organs and sometimes for appendicectomy. The incision extends from the umbilicus to the pubic symphysis. It is preferable to put a urinary catheter to empty the bladder preoperatively to prevent injury to the urinary bladder during the incision. The layers are similar to the upper midline incision. In the lower part of the incision, because of the lack of posterior rectus sheath, the two rectus abdominis muscles will be seen lying closely in the midline. Complete pelvic examination (uterus, ovaries, bladder, rectum, and prostate can be examined in addition to a pelvic appendix) is possible by this incision.

Full Length Midline Incision

Sometimes after putting an upper midline incision, a wider access may be required, where the pathology may be in the pelvis. In such situations, the incision may be extended down by skirting the incision at the umbilical region.

PARAMEDIAN INCISION

The paramedian incision may be upper paramedian or lower paramedian. They are usually put 2 cm lateral to the midline and parallel to it. The layers are:
- Skin and subcutaneous tissue.
- Anterior rectus sheath is opened vertically.
- The rectus muscle will be seen. There are three tendinous intersections in the upper part above the umbilicus. The tendinous intersections should be carefully dissected and the rectus muscle is retracted laterally to expose the posterior rectus sheath. There are no tendinous intersections in the lower half and, therefore, retracting the muscle laterally is easier. The muscle should never be retracted medially because the nerve supply for the muscle is coming from the lateral aspect and the muscle will atrophy.
- The posterior rectus sheath is incised vertically along with the peritoneum after holding it between two Kocher's forceps. Hold and feel and make sure that no viscera are held in the forceps. Sometimes, it may be required to release the forceps and reapply. Now the peritoneal cavity is accessed.

Closure of the Paramedian Incision

The peritoneum and posterior rectus sheath are sutured together as one layer with nonabsorbable continuous sutures. The rectus sheath is kept in its normal position. Now the anterior rectus sheath is closed with continuous nonabsorbable sutures. Skin is closed with sutures or clips.

Problems of Paramedian Incisions
- More chance for hematoma and infection
- More chance for incisional hernia because of the denervation of the rectus muscle
- Takes more time compared to the midline incision.

LATERAL PARAMEDIAN INCISION

This is a stronger paramedian incision because the rectus sheath is opened in such a way that the integrity of the rectus sheath is better maintained. The vertical incision is made over the junction of middle and outer third of the rectus muscle region over the skin and the anterior rectus sheath is also opened vertically, a bit laterally compared to the paramedian. Then, the posterior rectus sheath and peritoneum are opened in the same vertical plane after retracting the muscle laterally.

Advantages

- Integrity of the rectus sheath is better maintained
- Lower risk for wound dehiscence
- Lower chance for incisional hernia.

TRANSVERSE INCISION

Upper Abdominal Transverse Incision

The transverse incisions are used usually in children for laparotomy. The transverse upper abdominal incisions give access to pancreas, adrenal gland, gallbladder, etc. Sometimes, during upper midline or paramedian laparotomies, for wider access, a transverse cut may be employed, especially for splenectomy. The layers after skin and subcutaneous tissue are:
- Medially, anterior rectus sheath and rectus muscle
- Laterally, external oblique muscle, internal oblique muscle, and transversus abdominis muscle
- The posterior rectus sheath along with peritoneum is incised and opened laterally.

Closure

The peritoneum is closed with absorbable synthetic suture material like polyglactin (Vicryl). The posterior rectus sheath, internal and transverses muscles are sutured with continuous nonabsorbable sutures like polypropylene or delayed absorbable like polydioxanone (PDS). The cut end of the rectus muscles are sutured with polypropylene. The external oblique muscle and the anterior rectus sheath are sutured with continuous polypropylene/PDS.

Advantages

- Cosmetically a better scar
- Less chance for infection
- Less chance for incisional hernia.

Pfannenstiel Incision (Hermann Johannes Pfannenstiel)

This incision is used for most of the gynecological operations, hysterectomy, pelvic operations, and bladder and prostate operations. A 10–12 cm long transverse, curved suprapubic incision is made along the skin line. After the skin incision, the two layers of the superficial fascia are divided, namely (1) the superficial fatty layer (fascia of Camper) and (2) the deep membranous layer (fascia of Scarpa). The vessels are ligated and secured on either side. The anterior rectus sheath is incised on either side and the rectus abdominis muscles are exposed. The anterior sheaths are elevated from the underlying rectus both upward and downward by sharp dissection. The rectus are widely separated and held retracted. The transversalis fascia and peritoneum are then incised in a vertical direction.

For bladder exposure, the transversalis fascia and peritoneum are swept upward and the prevesical fascia is divided.

Closure

The peritoneum is closed. The rectus muscle may be approximated in the midline and the skin can be either sutured or clipped.

Lanz Incision

This is a transverse incision at the McBurney's point region, lateral to the rectus abdominis border. This is used for appendicectomy in young patients. It gives a cosmetic scar compared to the McBurney's gridiron incision. The rest of the steps are similar to the gridiron incision, described below.

Suprapubic Transverse Incision

The incision is made 2 cm above the pubis. The layers are similar to the Pfannenstiel, except for the fact that the peritoneum is not opened. The lateral extension of the incision is limited. It is used for bladder surgery and prostate surgery.

OBLIQUE INCISIONS

Gridiron Incision

The gridiron incision was first described by *McArthur*. It is made at right angles to the spinoumbilical line at the junction of medial two-thirds and lateral one-third in center being the *McBurney's point*. The incision will extend upward for two-thirds and downward for one-third. This is used for the conventional appendicectomy. The incision is a *muscle splitting incision*. It is called gridiron because the abdominal muscles are arranged in the form of a gridiron of the keel of a ship.

The layers are:
- Skin, subcutaneous tissue, and fat are divided.
- External oblique muscle is split along the direction of the muscle fibers, with the help of an artery forceps (as though one is putting the hand into the front pocket of a trouser).

- The internal oblique muscle is next split along the direction of the muscle fibers with the help of artery forceps (the direction of the muscle fibers is as though one is putting the hand on the back pocket of a trouser). One should be very careful at this stage of splitting this muscle because the nerves and vessels are seen between the internal and transverses muscles. If the bleeding vessels are not tackled, it will produce hematoma and infection. The nerve damage will lead onto future inguinal hernia on the same side.
- The transversus muscle is also split along the direction of the muscle fibers.
- Now the peritoneum is exposed which is held between two artery forceps and opened vertically.

(The appendix is identified by tracing the taenia coli, which will converge on the base of the appendix. The appendicular vessel is identified and clamped in the mesoappendix and ligated. The appendicectomy may be done with or without a purse string suture).

Closure

The peritoneum is closed with absorbable suture material. There is no need to close the internal and transversus muscles. The external oblique muscle aponeurosis is closed with polyglatin. Skin closure is usually with subcuticular sutures or skin clips.

Problems of gridiron incision are:
- It can be used only when the diagnosis of appendicitis is sure
- The access is minimal and limited medially by the rectus sheath
- If further access is required, it can be extended laterally and upward by dividing the muscles or make another right paramedian or midline incision, after closing the first incision
- It gives poor access for exploration of the upper abdomen in the event of a wrong diagnosis
- Cosmetically, it is a poor incision and, therefore, nowadays a Lanz or modified Lanz incision is recommended.

Kocher's Subcostal Incision

This is the standard incision for the conventional cholecystectomy. The incision is put 2.5 cm below and parallel to the right costal margin. A similar incision is put on the left side for splenectomy. The incision extends from the midline laterally. The lateral extend may be decided after opening the medial part.

The layers are:
- Skin, subcutaneous tissue, and fat
- Anterior rectus sheath and rectus muscle medially

- External oblique, internal oblique muscles laterally
- Posterior rectus sheath along with peritoneum and transversus abdominis muscle is opened.
  If more access is required, all the layers laterally may be further divided.

Closure
- The peritoneum along with the posterior rectus sheath is closed by continuous suturing.
- The divided rectus abdominis muscle is approximated.
- The anterior rectus sheath and the oblique muscles are sutured with nonabsorbable or delayed absorbable suture material.

Rooftop Incision
Bilateral subcostal incision is connected by a transverse incision below the xiphisternum. It is usually done for pancreatic surgery and liver surgery.

Rutherford–Morrison Incision
This is an oblique muscle cutting incision. The lateral extend reaches just above the anterior superior iliac spine and the medial extend is about 3 cm above the pubic tubercle. All the tissues are divided in the same line. The inferior epigastric vessels are ligated during the course of division. The incision is used for lower ureter, colon, inferior vena cava (IVC) on right side, and retroperitoneum. When it is used for ureter and retroperitoneal structures, the peritoneum is not opened, which is reflected anteriorly.

INCISION FOR KIDNEY EXPOSURE

Lumbar Subcostal Approach (Retroperitoneal Approach)
Position of the Patient
The patient is placed on his/her sound side laterally with the loin overlying the kidney bridge of the table, so that the space between the costal margin and the iliac crest is increased. The hip and knee of the limb on the side of the table are kept fully flexed and the upper leg is extended. Additionally, a sandbag is placed behind the patient so that the patient will not fall by rolling over. The arm on the upper side is supported on an armrest. The patient may require additional strapping, so that the patient would not fall down.

Incision
An oblique incision is made starting from the angle between the last rib and erector spinae muscle. The incision is carried downward and forward obliquely toward 4–5 cm above the anterior superior iliac spine. For wider exposure, incision can be extended as far as the lateral border of the rectus

muscle. After incising the skin and subcutaneous tissue, posteriorly you encounter the latissimus dorsi muscle and anteriorly the external oblique muscles. Both these muscles are divided. Then the serratus posterior inferior muscle will be visible posteriorly and the two oblique muscles anteriorly. All the three are divided. Thus, five muscles are divided namely, latissimus dorsi and serratus posterior inferior muscle posteriorly and the three flat muscles anteriorly. Posteriorly, the quadratus lumborum muscle will be seen. The lumbodorsal fascia which is seen lateral to the quadratus lumborum is seen. This fascia is incised transversely, exposing the extraperitoneal fat by gently inserting two fingers into this space and the peritoneum is separated from the deep surface of the transversus abdominis muscle. The division of the transversus and the internal oblique muscle is deferred until this stage. The subcostal nerve and vessels (passing downward and forward in the deep layers of the internal oblique) can be retracted. The kidney is exposed by incising the renal fascia. Further procedure will depend upon the nature of the renal surgery.

Closure

The muscles are repaired in two layers with interrupted synthetic absorbable suture material. The kidney bridge of the table is lowered before tightening the sutures in the muscle. A drain can be inserted in the perinephric space if required and the skin is sutured.

Kidney can also be exposed transperitoneally, especially for tumor cases where there is extension of tumor thrombus into the IVC.

BREAST INCISIONS (FIG. 2)

The recommended incisions are:
- Periareolar
- Circumareolar
- Circumferential
- Submammary incision of Gaillard-Thomas
- Radial incision (radial incisions are recommended only at 3 and 9 o'clock positions); in other areas, it would produce a cosmetically bad scar
- Transverse or oblique elliptical incision for mastectomy.

Incision for Breast Biopsy

Make an incision as recommended in the **Figure 3** in such a way that in the case of a histological surprise of a malignancy, the scar can be included in the transverse elliptical incision for a mastectomy without compromising much of skin. If the lump is clinically suspicious for malignancy, always try to do a wide excision with at least 1 cm margin around it. After the skin is incised, grasp the lump with Allis forceps. Excise the tumor using a combination of scalpel, scissors, or diathermy.

Surgical Incisions

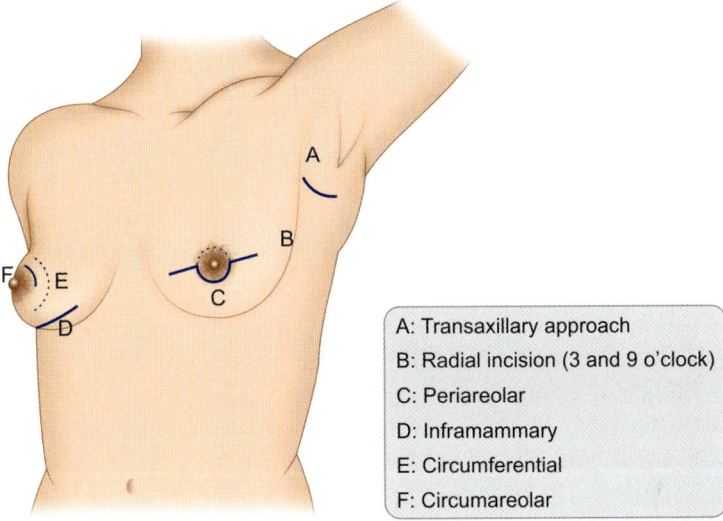

A: Transaxillary approach
B: Radial incision (3 and 9 o'clock)
C: Periareolar
D: Inframammary
E: Circumferential
F: Circumareolar

Fig. 2: Breast incisions.

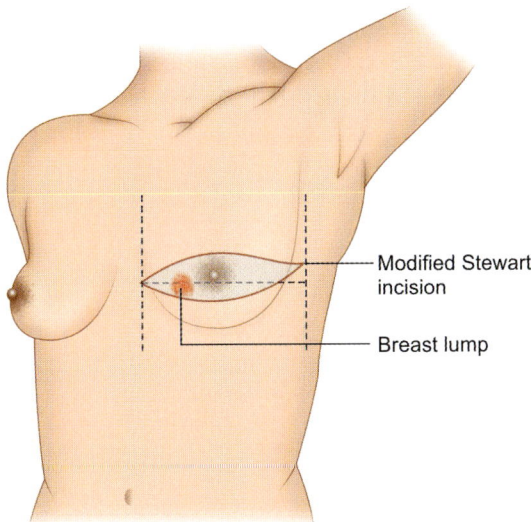

Fig. 3: Incision for mastectomy: Incision for modified radical mastectomy usually a transverse elliptical incision including the nipple areola complex and the skin over lying the tumor included in the eclipse is the incision of choice preferably the medial end at a lower level than the lateral end.

Closure

Always go for adequate hemostasis. If there is suspicion of further oozing, a suction drain may be inserted which is brought outside through a separate stab incision. While obliterating the cavity, see that it is not producing dimpling and distortion of the breast. The inside approximation is done by absorbable suture material like polyglatin and the skin is closed with subcuticular sutures.

GENERAL INSTRUCTIONS FOR SUTURE REMOVAL IN VARIOUS PLACES

Sutures can be removed earlier than what is mention below. Once it is removed, if there is a tendency for gaping, adhesive skin tapes can be used. The more the suture is in place, the more scar formation will be seen. Wherever the wound is sutured under tension, it is preferable to delay the suture removal. For inguinal region, it is preferable to avoid skin sutures because every skin suture will be a potential tract for infection. It is better to do subcutaneous sutures or skin tapes in the inguinal region:

- *Scalp*: 4–5 days
- *Face and neck*: 3–4 days
- *Abdomen*: 7–10 days
- *Limbs*: 5–7 days
- *Amputation stumps*: 10–14 days
- *Feet*: 8–10 days.

17 Sutures

John S Kurien

SUTURE MATERIALS

The earliest mention of sutures is in the Ebers Papyrus. Sushruta used both silk and cotton sutures and the Aztec Tribe in South America used large ants to hold wound edges together, by making the ants bite the two edges and then cutting off their bodies.

Sutures are divided into absorbable and nonabsorbable types. The tensile strength of a suture means the strength by which it keeps the tissues together and this lasts up to half its degradation time.

Regarding Properties of a Suture

Knot holding is best in braided sutures. Malleability is a good property. Elasticity should be minimum and memory (retaining of the coiled shape in the packet) should be minimum for a good suture. All monofilament sutures have poor knot holding property and have more memory.

ABSORBABLE SUTURES

Natural

- *Catgut*: It is made from the intestine of cattle or sheep. It was originally known as kitgut because it was used as strings for a musical instrument called "kit." And later, it became catgut. It is made of protein and so it is degraded by proteolysis. It is also from another species and so when used, for the second time in a patient, may cause rejection, stitch abscesses, and sensitivity reactions. But the cost is much lower than synthetic sutures:
  - *Plain catgut*: Tensile strength is 3 days and it gets degraded in 7 days. So, it is useful only for subcutaneous tissue **(Fig. 1)**.
  - *Chromic catgut*: When catgut is immersed in chromic acid, the tensile strength becomes 3 weeks and it gets degraded in 6 weeks. So, it can be used for subcutaneous tissue, muscle, small intestine, stomach, the biliary tract, and the urogenital tract.
- *Kangaroo tendon*: The tail of the kangaroo is also used for manufacturing sutures in Australia, and the tensile strength and degradation times are similar to the chromic catgut.

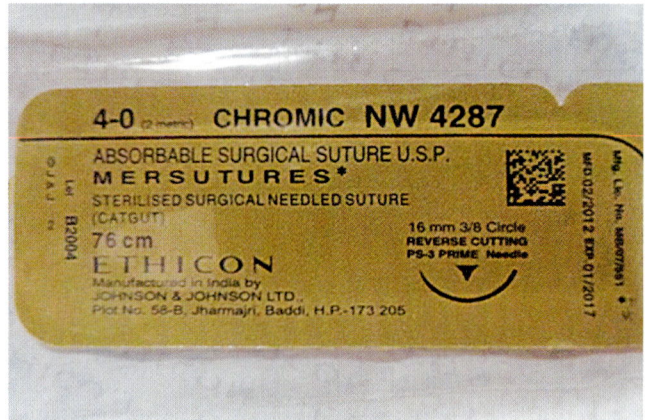

Fig. 1: Chromic catgut suture.

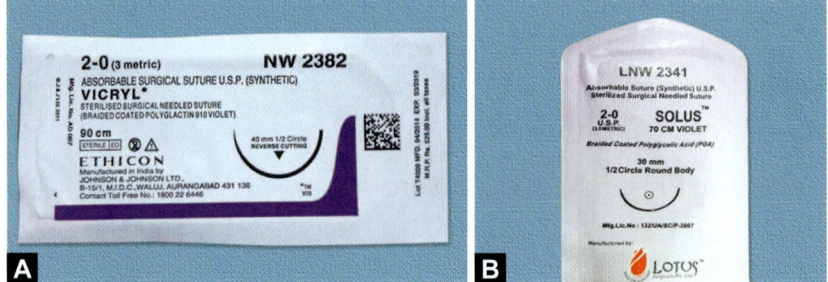

Figs. 2A and B: (A) Polyglactin sutures; (B) Polyglycolic acid sutures.

Synthetic

All synthetic absorbable sutures are degraded by hydrolysis. So they do not cause any tissue reaction and the chance of rejection is minimal. They are however costly:

- *Polyglactin*: This is a combination of glycolide and lactate in the ratio 910:90 and so the Ethicon Company who devised it named it "Vicryl 910" **(Fig. 2A)**. The tensile strength is 3 weeks and it gets degraded in 6 weeks. It is braided and hence knot holding property is very good and so surgeons love it.
- *Polyglycolic acid*: This is a braided monomer devised by the United States Surgical Corporation who named it "Dexon." Tensile strength is similar to polyglactin. Both polyglactin and polyglycolic acid are colored violet for visibility and identification **(Fig. 2B)**.
- *Poliglecaprone*: Poliglecaprone is a monofilament, launched by Ethicon, brown in color and the tensile strength and degradation are similar to polyglactin.
- *Polydioxanone*: This is a monofilament with increased memory and colored violet. Tensile strength lasts for 6 weeks and it gets degraded by

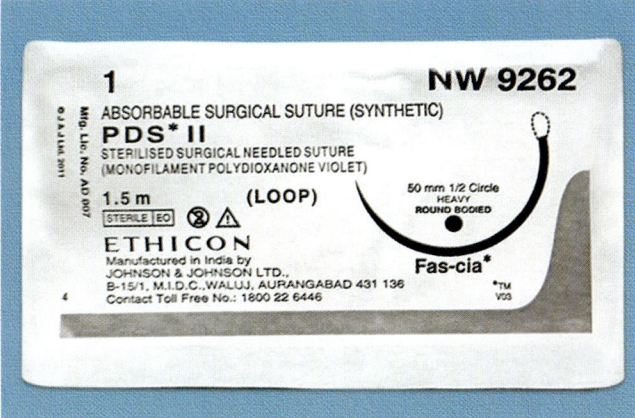

Fig. 3: Polydioxanone sutures.

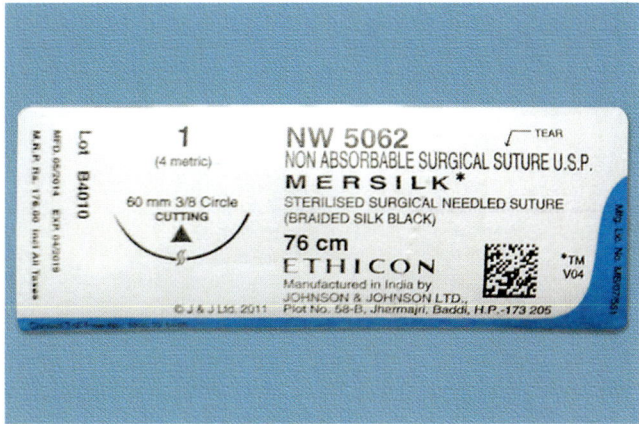

Fig. 4: Silk suture.

3–4 months. Hence, it can be used for the biliary tract and for closure of subcostal and Pfannenstiel incisions in addition to its use wherever polyglactin can be used. It was devised by the Ethicon Company **(Fig. 3)**.

NONABSORBABLE SUTURES (FIG. 4)
Natural
- *Silk*: Silk is a protein called sericin, made from the silkworm cocoon. It is braided and colored black for visibility. It gets degraded by the third year. It loses 30% strength when wet and should not be reautoclaved.
- *Cotton*: Cotton is made from the cotton seed pod and is cellulose. Cellulose gains strength when wet. It lasts indefinitely in the body.
- *Linen*: Linen is made from the flax plant and is cellulose and lasts indefinitely in the body.

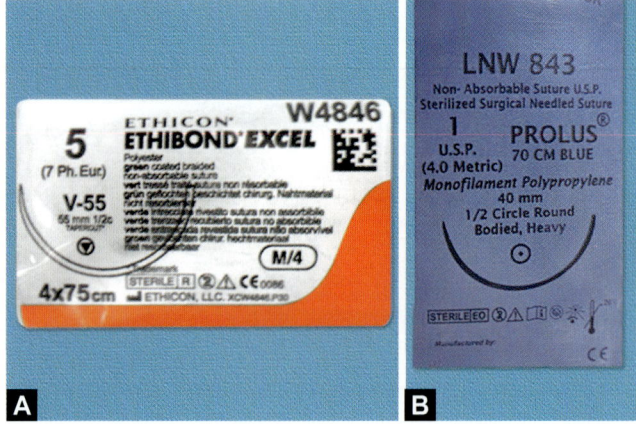

Figs. 5A and B: (A) Polyethylene sutures; (B) Polyester suture.

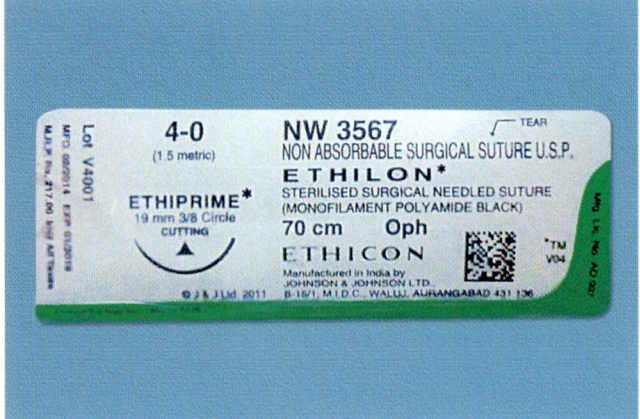

Fig. 6: Polyamide sutures.

Synthetic

- *Polypropylene*: It is a monofilament. It has increased memory but lasts indefinitely in the body and hence is the best suture for hernia repair, esophageal, colonic and rectum suturing, and closure of the anterior abdominal wall because these structures take 1 year to regain their original strength **(Fig. 5A)**.
- *Polyamide*: It is also known as nylon. It loses 10% strength per year. It is a monofilament and has memory but it is still a cheap substitute for polypropylene and is mainly used for skin suturing. Only a monofilament should be used for skin suturing as use of a braided suture will allow skin commensals such as *Staphylococci* to migrate along the suture by "wick effect" and colonize the suture tracts **(Fig. 6)**.
- *Polyester*: It is a braided suture coated with polybutylate mainly used in cardiovascular, ophthalmic, and neurosurgeries. It lasts indefinitely **(Fig. 5B)**.

- *Stainless steel*: It is available in all sizes and last indefinitely. Sizing is done by the brown and sharp gauge sizes.

NEEDLES

There are *straight needles, curved needles, compound curved needles, ski needles* (used in laparoscopy), *spatulate needles* (for corneal suturing), and *Port needles* (for closing laparoscopy port incisions).

Atraumatic needles have a hole in the base of the needle into which the suture is inserted and pressed. This process is called swaging.

Atraumatic sutures produce only minimum trauma because they do not possess an eye and so the diameter of the needle is same as the diameter of the suture.

Suturing with a curved needle involves pronation and supination and can be done by drawing a circle with the wrist.

The United States Pharmacopeia (USP) is used to denote the sizes of needles. The largest needle is number 6 which is used for the sternal closure and the size successively decreases toward zero and then 1-0 (same as 0) going up to 12-0. Beyond 5-0, a loupe is needed to suture. Since these sutures are sold in France also, the metric size is also written on the suture foil.

Circular needles form part of a circle. Three-eighth needles are used for skin and subcutaneous tissue. Half circle needle is a universal needle and five-eighth needle is used for suturing structures in the depth of the abdomen and the pelvis.

The length of the suture and the length of the needle are chosen depending on the tissue to be sutured. If sutures have needle at only one end it is called single armed and if needles are present at both ends, it is called double armed (tendon and vascular sutures).

Round bodied needles: The cross-section is circular and is used for soft tissues and intestine.

Cutting needles: The cross-section is triangular with the cutting edge on the concave side. It is used for tough tissues.

Reverse cutting needles: The cross-section is triangular with the cutting edge on the convex side. It is better than a cutting needle in all aspects but is costlier and is specifically used for tendon suturing.

STERILIZATION

Synthetic absorbable sutures are sterilized using ethylene oxide. Synthetic nonabsorbable sutures can be sterilized by either ethylene oxide or gamma irradiation. Catgut is preserved in alcohol. Sutures are checked by the manufacturer for tensile strength, color leaching, and sterility and they usually have a shelf-life of 5 years.

Surgical Knots: Different Types

Muhammed Muneer

SURGICAL KNOTS

A knot (strictly a bend or hitch, since a knot is a node or knob) is an intertwining of threads for the purpose of joining them.

The *half-hitch* or an overhand hitch forms the basis of most knots **(Fig. 1A)**. A half-hitch is formed by crossing one thread over the other to form a closed loop **(Fig. 1B)** and the two ends are to be tied and tightened on the opposite.

Granny Knot

If you tie the first half-hitch, the left thread was passed in front of the right one, then underneath, to emerge in front on the right side. For the second half-hitch, the new left thread (the former right thread) is also passed in front of the new right thread (the former left thread) and emerges in front on the right side.

In the granny knot, the threads of the two half-hitches cross and shortening the length of contact **(Figs. 2A and B)**.

A granny knot has much greater holding power.

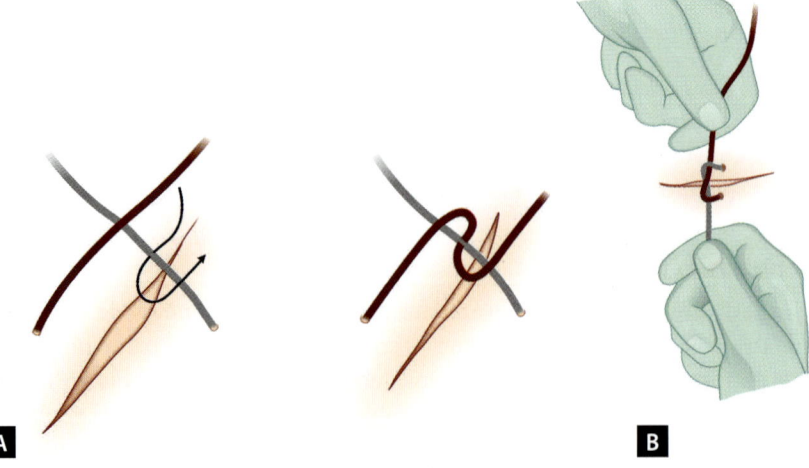

Figs. 1A and B: Half-hitch.

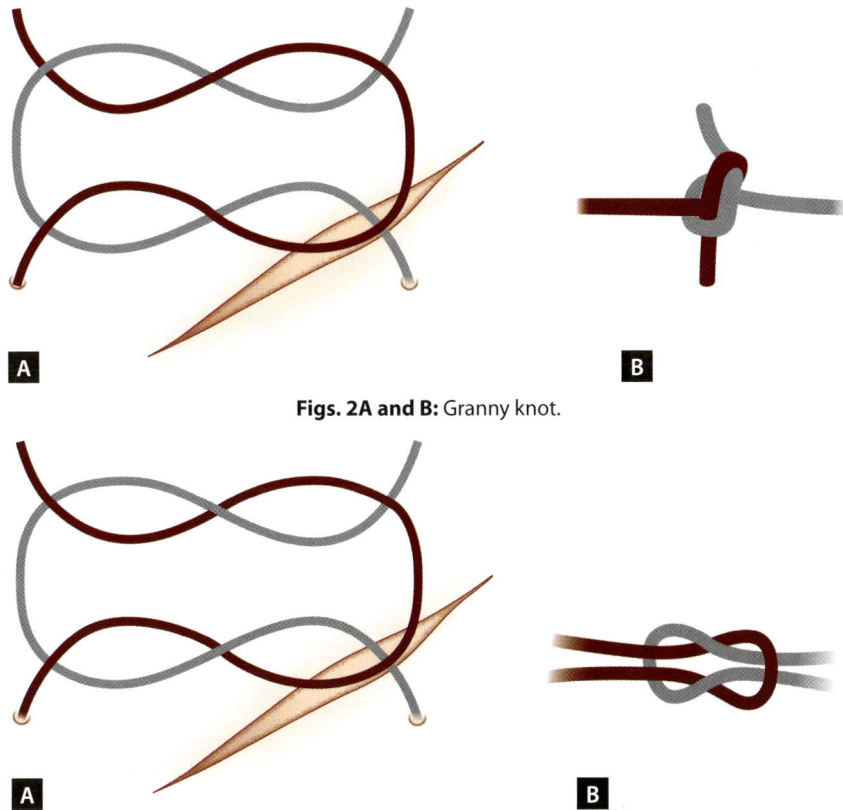

Figs. 2A and B: Granny knot.

Figs. 3A and B: Reef knot.

Reef Knot

To form a reef knot, left thread was passed behind the right thread for the first half-hitch, then under it through the loop and taken to the right. The right thread emerges on the left. For the second hitch, the new left thread passes in front of the new right and passes under it to emerge on the right **(Fig. 3A)**. In the reef knot, the threads of the two half-hitches run parallel to the standing parts; in a granny knot, the ends tend to lie at right angles to the standing part **(Fig. 3B)**.

Slip Knot

Slip knot is tied by the same half-hitches as for a granny and a reef knot but keep one thread taut. Ship sailors used these reef knot because it was not only secure but also it could be released easily and rapidly **(Fig. 4)**.

Triple Throw Knot

After tying a reef knot, form a third half-hitch, creating a reef knot with the second half-hitch, to produce a triple throw knot **(Fig. 5)**. This is more reliable and is used in surgery when security is essential.

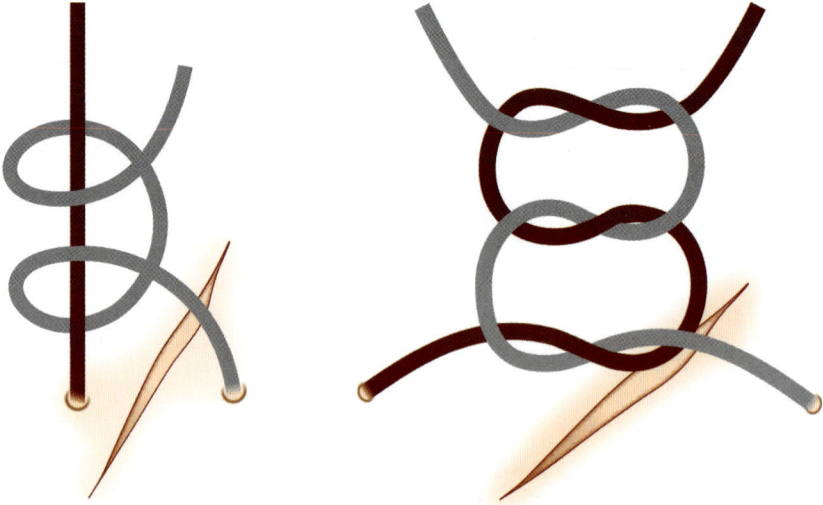

Fig. 4: Slip knot. **Fig. 5:** Triple throw knot.

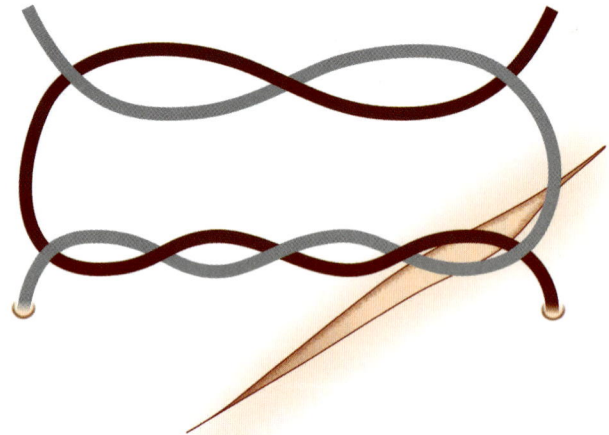

Fig. 6: Surgeon's knot.

Surgeon's Knot

In case of true surgeon's knot, the first half-hitch has two "throws" or turns. The second is a standard half-hitch. It should be finished off with a third half-hitch that forms a reef knot with the second half-hitch **(Fig. 6)**.

LEFT HANDED KNOT TIE

In this technique, knot is tied with the left hand while holding an instrument in the right hand. This is a perfectly good knot. One hand is used for forming knot but it is two-handed for tightening. Hold one hand still, form and tighten the hitches around it and create a slip knot.

- There are two types of half-hitch—(1) *index-finger hitch* and (2) *middle-finger hitch*. Both hitches must be tied alternately to produce a reef knot:
    - *Index-finger hitch*: When the short end is away from you, pick up the short end with the thumb and the middle finger of the left hand and hold it vertically. Flex the wrist so your left hand hangs from it, then supinate your hand, and extend the index finger to create a loop of the short thread over it **(Fig. 7A)**:
        - Pick up the long thread with your right hand and hold it vertically in front of the short thread so that it crosses the short thread in the section between the index finger and the grasp of the middle finger and thumb of your left hand.
        - Flex the terminal interphalangeal joint of your left index finger round the long thread to reach behind the short thread **(Fig. 7B)**. The short thread lies against your nail on the dorsum of the finger. As you pronate your left hand, extend the tip of the left index finger, carrying the loop of short thread under the loop of long thread **(Fig. 7C)**.

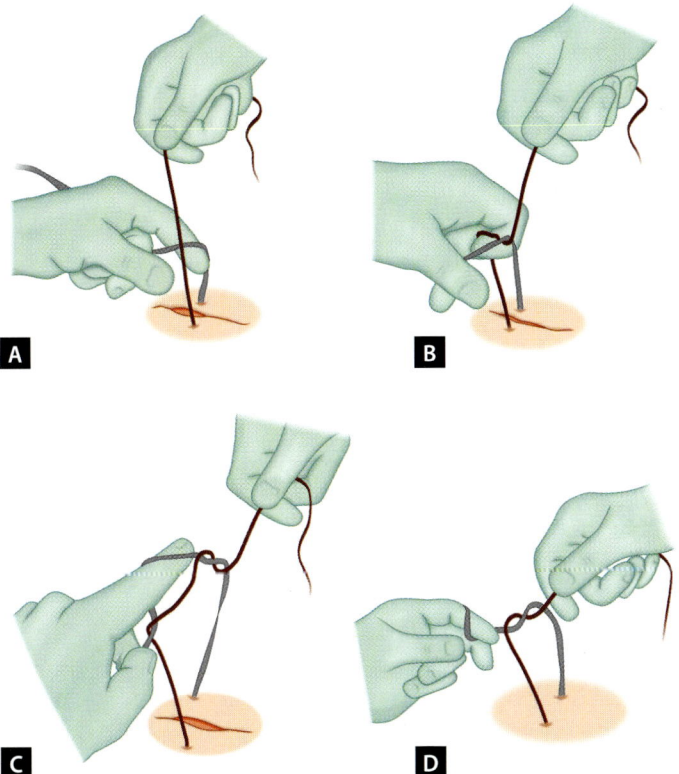

Figs. 7A to D: Steps of index-finger hitch.

- Release the middle finger contact with the thumb of the left hand to allow the end of the short thread to be carried through and use the middle finger to trap the emerging end against the index finger **(Fig. 7D)**.
- Now bring the short end toward you and take the long end away from you to tighten the hitch.

• *Middle-finger hitch* is done when the short end lies near you, pick it up between the index finger and thumb of the pronated left hand, and hold it vertically. Pick up the long thread with your right hand and hold it vertically:
  - Supinate your left hand as you extend the middle finger between the near short thread and the far long thread and pull the long thread over it toward yourself, crossing the short thread.
  - Flex the tip of your middle finger over the top of the horizontal section of the long thread and beneath the section of the short thread between the crossing of the threads and the grip of the left thumb and index finger; the nail of your middle finger lies in contact with the short thread.
  - As you pronate your left hand, extend your middle finger to carry the end of the short thread underneath the long thread, to point away from you, as you release the grip of your index finger and thumb on the tip and extend your ring finger to trap the end against the middle finger.
  - Now carry the short end away from you and bring the long end toward you to tighten the hitch **(Figs. 8A to H)**.

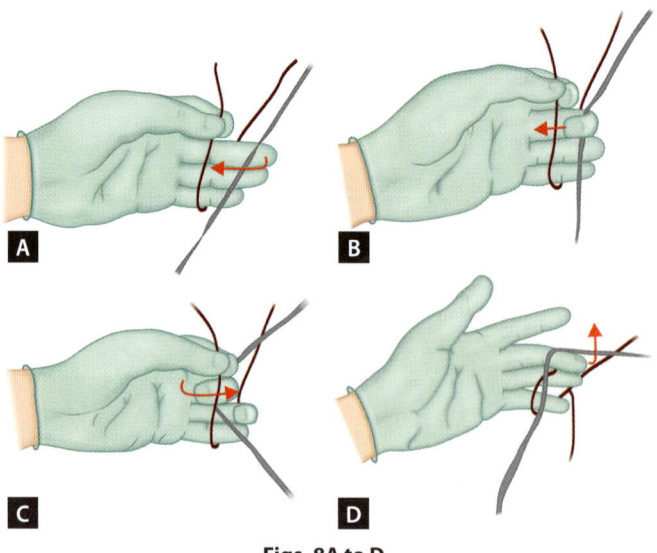

Figs. 8A to D

Surgical Knots: Different Types

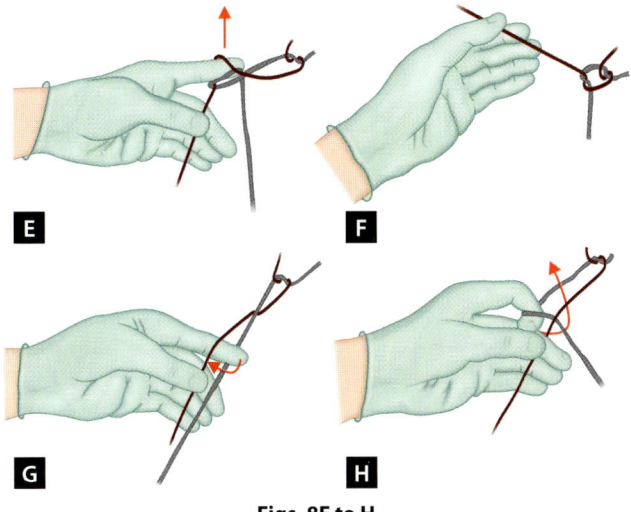

Figs. 8E to H

Figs. 8A to H: Steps of middle-finger hitch.

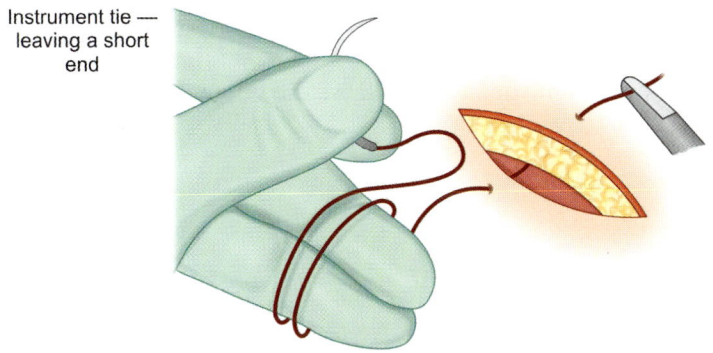

Instrument tie — leaving a short end

Fig. 9: Routine knot tying.

SURGICAL KNOTS USING INSTRUMENTS

Use instrument ties for repetitive routine knot tying.

This method is economical of suture material, since the short end need be only long enough to be grasped by the instrument **(Fig. 9)**:

- If the short end is away from you and the longer thread toward you, lay the needle holder on the long thread.
- Take the long thread closest to you and pass it over the tip of the needle holder, round it, and back toward you. While maintaining the loop, maneuver the needle holder through it so you can grasp the short end and draw it back through the loop toward you, while taking the long thread away from you to tighten it.
- Tighten the hitch by taking the short thread away from you and drawing the long thread toward you **(Figs. 10A to C)**.

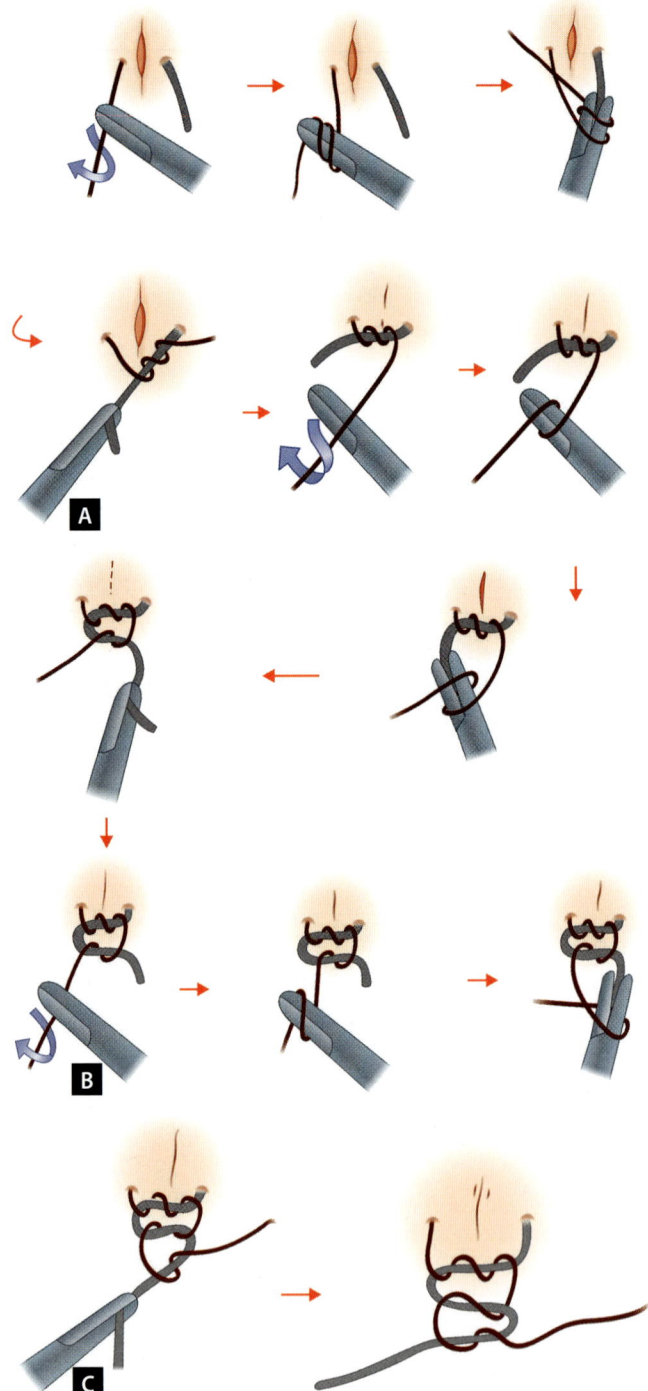

Figs. 10A to C: Steps of routine knot tying.

19. Minor Surgical Procedures of Subcutaneous Swellings

R Dayananda Babu

LYMPH NODE BIOPSY, EXCISION OF CYSTIC SWELLINGS, AND LIPOMA UNDER LOCAL ANESTHESIA

Lymph Node Biopsy

In general terms, lymph nodes in the neck, supraclavicular fossa, axilla, or groin should be biopsied under a general anesthesia. However, if they are very easily defined and the doctor is experienced, superficial lymph nodes may be excised using local anesthetic infiltration. In generalized lymphadenopathy, it is preferable to take a neck node rather than axillary or inguinal node. If inguinal and axillary nodes are enlarged, it is preferable to take axillary rather than the inguinal (inguinal lymph nodes are enlarged in bare-footed persons, and therefore, may not be significant).

Steps of Lymph Node Biopsy of Neck

- Position of the patient—small sand bag behind shoulders with a head ring for support and head tilted to the contralateral side.
- Skin antiseptic preparation and draping of the area.
- Infiltration of local anesthetic agent/general anesthesia.
- The incision should be made in the line of the skin crease over the swelling and should be at least twice the size of the node to be biopsied to ensure that the whole dissection is carried out under direct vision.
- The fat and superficial fascia should be incised in the line of the wound and the lymph node or group of nodes exposed using blunt dissection.
- If necessary, a small self-retaining retractor may be used to aid the dissection.
- The tissue that tethers the deep surface of the node will contain small blood vessels and lymphatic channels, and therefore, an artery clip is placed across this pedicle, which is then ligated and divided, leaving the clip attached to the specimen (it may be adherent to the major vein such as internal jugular vein).
- The capsule of the node should not be grasped, since this may distort the histological features. It is preferable to take a lymph node intact, rather than a part of the lymph node.

- If tuberculosis is suspected, it is better to take two nodes, one for the pathology and for microbiology department. The specimen for the microbiology is sent in saline bottle and for the pathology department, the specimen is sent in formalin.
- The wound is closed with subcutaneous absorbable sutures and 3/0 nylon to the skin.

Note:
- Remember most of the lymph nodes of the neck are deep to the deep fascia, and therefore, one has to open the deep fascia.
- Lymph nodes are distributed along the veins, and therefore, it is important to avoid injury to the internal jugular vein, if it is located near to the vein.
- While doing posterior triangular lymph node biopsy, one should take care of the spinal accessory nerve.

Excision of Sebaceous Cyst and Other Cystic Swellings

Sebaceous cysts are of two basic histological types, although the distinction has no significant practical relevance:
- Those arising from hair follicle cells are more properly called pilar cyst and occur on hair-bearing areas such as the scalp.
- Epidermoid cyst arises from nonhair-bearing areas such as the palms and soles.
- Although usually simple to diagnose, nevertheless, a sebaceous cyst can sometime be mistaken for other lesions.

Differential Diagnosis of a Cystic Swelling

- Thyroglossal cyst in the midline at the front of the neck
- Branchial cyst anterior to the sternocleidomastoid at the junction of its upper third and middle two-third
- Parotid tumor at the angle of the mandible
- Congenital dermoid cyst at lines of embryonic fusion
- Caseating lymph node
- Pulsating boney swelling of the skull—metastasis from follicular carcinoma thyroid (mistaken for sebaceous cyst at times)
- Rarely a solid subcutaneous tumor (such as secondary deposit of a malignant melanoma; thus all excised specimen should be sent for histological examination).

Site of the Cyst

Cyst in some sites of body can cause great difficulty in their removal, unless the doctor is experienced. Cyst situated in the posterior triangle of neck or behind the angle of the mandible should be done carefully because of the risk of damage to the spinal accessory and facial nerve.

Removal of cyst on the back of the neck may be more difficult and more bloodier than expected because the skin there is often thick and firm.

If possible, the cyst should be removed wholly. The cyst wall is often (but not always) attached to the deep layers of the overlying dermis. If any remnant of the cyst wall is left behind, the cyst is likely to recur. For this reason, incision and squeezing out the contents is not recommended (except when infected), although puncturing and emptying the cyst can allow the deflated cyst to be removed through a smaller incision and is an acceptable technique **(Figs. 1 to 3)**.

Swellings in the Scalp

When removing small cyst in the scalp, it is often enough to trim the hair immediately overlying the cyst itself and then to hold the rest of the hair out of the way with adhesive tapes.

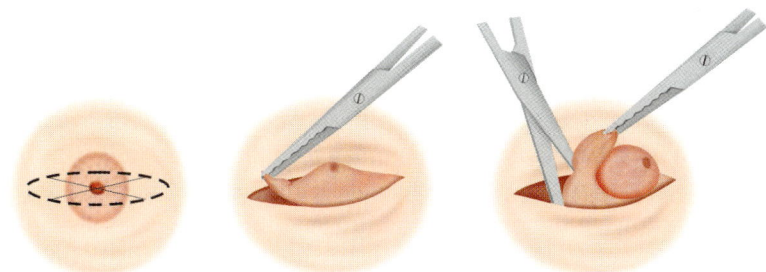

Fig. 1: Sebaceous cyst excision.

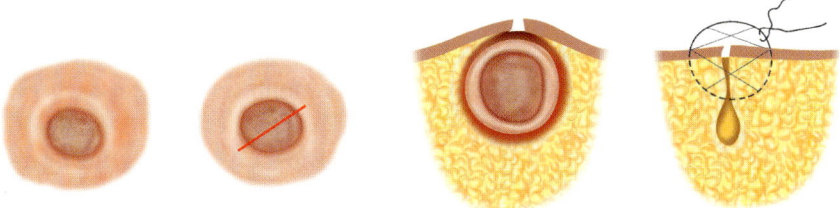

Fig. 2: Excision of a small sebaceous cyst simple incision over the dome.

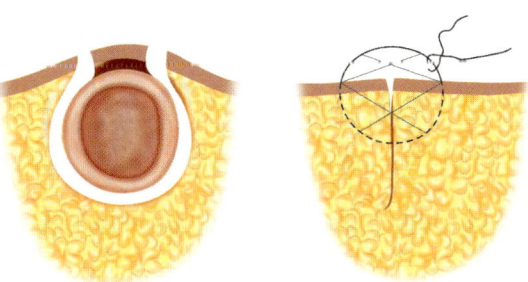

Fig. 3: Excision of a sebaceous cyst avoiding dead space.

Steps of Excision of Large Cyst under Local Anesthesia

- Position—according to the site of the swelling.
- Antiseptic skin preparation (it is preferable to clip the hair overlying the swelling and the surrounding area) and draping.
- Local infiltration.
- *Incision*: An elliptical incision is put over the swelling so that the redundant skin can be avoided during closure. This will also avoid dead space.
- The elliptical incision should be centered on the punctum with care taken not to puncture the cyst.
- The incision is carefully deepened by sharp dissection until the plane between the cyst and the subcutaneous fat is identified. Once this plane has been entered, the cyst may be easily shelled out by blunt dissection with an artery forceps or curved dissecting scissors. It may be helpful to retract one end of the skin ellipse with an artery forceps.
- Special care should be taken when dissecting the neck or face to avoid accidental damage to any underlying vessels and nerves, particularly when applying traction.
- If the cyst is accidentally incised during the initial skin incision or during the excision, subsequent dissection may be difficult and messy. In these circumstances, it may be helpful to make a fresh, slightly more lateral skin incision, allowing the dissection to proceed further away from the cyst wall and minimizing spillage of cyst content into the wound.
- Any spillage should be mopped up with a wet swab.

Inflamed Sebaceous Cyst

If the cyst is red and painful but the overlying skin is not too angry or indurated, then it is often better to excise the cyst followed by primary suture rather than subjected to incision and drainage followed by later excision. The local anesthetic takes longer time to work when there is inflammation. Excision of the inflamed cyst will always give rise to more bleeding during the procedure **(Fig. 4)**. Bleeding will be minimized when local anesthetic mixed with adrenaline is used.

Previously Infected Sebaceous Cyst

The excision of a previously infected cyst may be quite difficult and bloody because of dense fibrous tissue formed. In such circumstances, it may be impossible to shell out the cyst. Instead the cyst should be excised by sharp dissection in continuity with a block of subcutaneous tissue **(Fig. 5)**.

Lipoma

Small superficial lipoma or lipomata are easily diagnosed and shelled out under local anesthesia; however, larger lipomas may extend deep to the deep fascia and sometimes may be intermuscular. Lipomas of the back may be deeper than expected and it is safer to do it under general anesthesia **(Fig. 6)**.

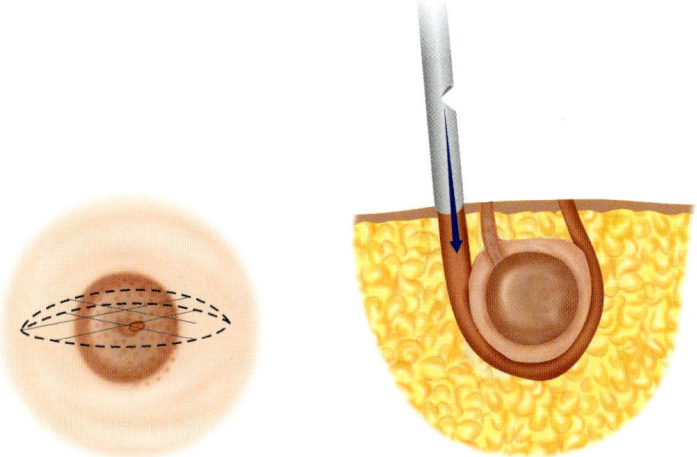

Fig. 4: Sebaceous cyst excision by secondary incision.

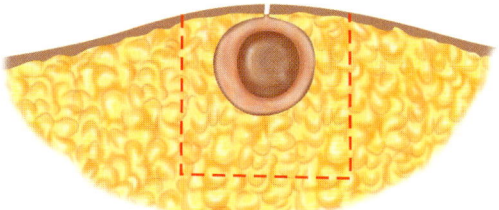

Fig. 5: Excision of previously infected sebaceous cyst.

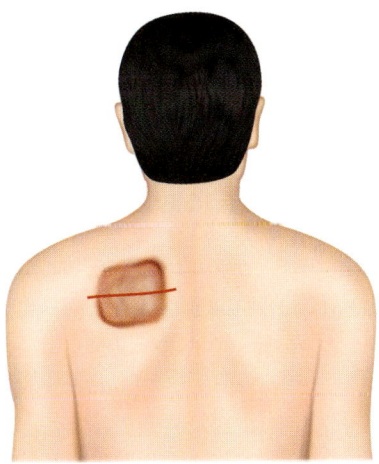

Fig. 6: Lipoma dissection.

The fat lobules of a lipoma are usually larger and are easily distinguished from those of normal subcutaneous fat **(Fig. 7)**. The tumor is usually well-defined with a very thin capsule and can be either dissected out or removed using the squeeze technique.

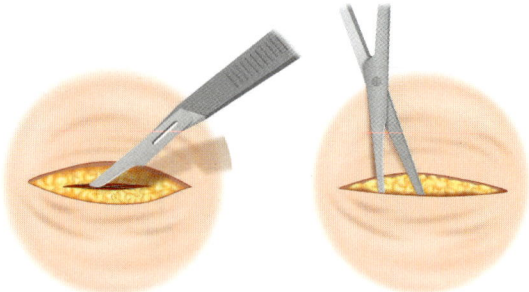

Fig. 7: Dissection of lipoma lobule.

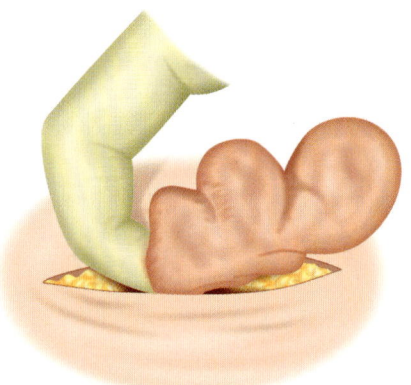

Fig. 8: Lipoma finger dissection.

Steps of Excision of Lipoma

- Position of the patient—according to the site of the swelling.
- Antiseptic skin preparation and draping.
- Local infiltration.
- Incision is made over the swelling along the skin lines of least skin tension and deepened until the lipoma is identified. The incision is needed only for two-thirds of the length of the lesion.
- Once the plane is found between the lipoma and the subcutaneous fat, then it is shelled out by blunt dissection using scissors or a finger (**Fig. 8**).
- Occasionally, there are some tethering vessels on deep surface of the lipoma and these should be ligated with absorbable sutures.
- Secure hemostasis.
- The wound should be closed taking care to avoid any dead space.
- In the squeeze method, a smaller incision is made and traction is applied to the lipoma, while digital pressure is applied around the lesion's circumference to squeeze it out of the wound. Since the wound is deliberately small, its cavity cannot be easily inspected. Therefore, particular care should be made to ligate any vessels to ensure against any bleeding inside the wound.

20. Incision and Drainage of Abscess

R Dayananda Babu

INTRODUCTION

Early acute suppurative inflammation is a prerunner of abscess and can be treated with antibiotics (even early abscesses in areas such as breast are treated nowadays by sono-guided aspiration).

Once pus is organized, needs drainage of pus to limit the extent of tissue damage.

Superficial Abscesses

Abscess may be superficial or deep, one should not wait for fluctuation in areas such as breast and parotid, because the pus will be present deep inside. Hence, sono-guided aspiration or incision and drainage should be carried out as early as possible. This is more important in immunocompromised patients such as diabetics.

Deep abscess—fluctuation will always be absent in situations such as ischiorectal fossa. Infection and abscesses in the middle of the face need prompt treatment due to risk of cavernous sinus thrombosis (dangerous area of the face).

Look for associated ascending lymphangitis and if it is present, it is suggestive of *Streptococcus pyogenes*. Rule out diabetes in all patients with abscess.

DANGEROUS AREAS FOR INCISION AND DRAINAGE

There are four areas where major vessels are present beneath the abscess. Therefore, it is important to aspirate before you put knife for drainage. Aneurysms can present exactly like abscess in the following situations:
1. Popliteal fossa
2. Inguinal region
3. Axilla
4. Neck.

Anesthesia

- Deep abscesses and perianal and ischiorectal abscesses need general anesthesia (GA). Perineum is a very sensitive and painful area.

- Superficial abscesses may be drained by dome infiltration (**Fig. 1A**).
- If doom is thin and abscess is pointing, it can be drained even without anesthesia.
- If it is thin and non-necrotic, it needs infiltration of anesthetic.
- Wide infiltration is needed if dome is thick and indurated.
- If inflammation is present, inject widely as it is painful to inject in red areas.
- Wait as it takes more time than normal for skin to get anesthetic effect, and it is also short-lived.

Steps

- Position depends on the site of abscess.
- Clean with antiseptics and drape the area.
- Local or regional anesthesia or general anesthesia.
- Abscess confirmed by needle aspiration.
- Put an incision by No. 11 blade with the tip pointing upward (No. 15 blade also may be used).
- Drain the pus in a kidney tray.
- The aspirated pus is sent for culture and sensitivity.
- Break all the loculi of the abscess cavity by a sinus forceps (in cases of big cavity, a gloved finger may be inserted for breaking the loculi).
- Abscess cavity is cleared of pus and give a thorough wash with normal saline.
- Keep the wound open with or without a gauze wick for 24 hours.
  [An alternate treatment is to give antibiotic 1 hour before incision, drainage and curettage, followed by primary suturing to obliterate the cavity. For large cavity or with skin necrosis, a *cruciate incision* (**Fig. 1B**) is made and corners are removed in areas such as sole of foot and fingers to avoid excision of the skin].

Boils are drained by a stab incision.

Carbuncle has multiple loculations of pus, pointing at number of areas. It is preferable to put a cruciate incision enclosing the entire area and lift the flaps so that all the pus loculations can be evacuated.

Pulp space abscess: Here, pus is trapped deep in the tissue and point to the surface as collar-stud abscess. Skin over the pulp is tethered to the deep bone by fibrous band. Deep pocket of pus should be drained by probing or with forceps under digital nerve block (**Fig. 1C**).

Breast abscess needs GA, if it is not responding to sono-guided aspiration. Circumareolar incisions are preferred over radial incisions. Radial incisions are recommended only in 3 and 9 o'clock positions (*see* the picture for incisions in Chapter 9, Figure 9).

Incision and Drainage of Abscess

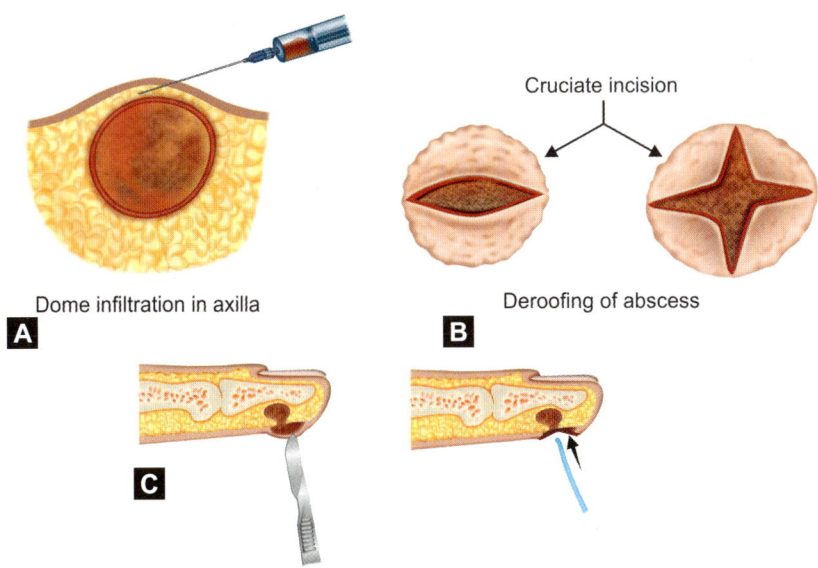

Figs. 1A to E: Incision and drainage of abscess in different parts.

Acute pilonidal abscess is drained with a special care taken to remove all the hair nests. All the sinus tracks are also excised.

Perianal abscess: Needs general or regional anesthesia. In males with anterior perianal abscess, avoid injury to the urethra by putting a Foley catheter beforehand. The patient should be warned of a future fistula formation.

Hilton's method to drain an abscess. During drainage of abscesses situated in important areas such as axilla and groin, there is a chance of injury to underlying major vessels and nerves if adequate care is not taken.

In drainage of abscesses in such location, the skin and the subcutaneous tissues are incised with a knife.

The deep fascia is not incised with a knife but pierced by thrusting a sinus forceps. The blades of the forceps are then opened up enlarging the opening in the deep fascia for easy drainage of pus.

Blair method of opening parotid abscess: A vertical incision is put just in front of the tragus. The parotid fascia is then opened horizontally. This will avoid injury to the facial nerve branches.

21 Preoperative Preparation in General for Elective Surgery

R Dayananda Babu

INTRODUCTION

A proper history and clinical examination are important for a successful outcome in any major surgery. Even though in young adults of <40 years' age group, there is not much of a role for preoperative investigations other than for the disease for which the surgery is planned. The evaluation and investigations will vary from institution to institution and the anesthesiology department.

The following points are important in history:
- History of smoking, alcoholism, and liver disease (it is preferable to stop smoking 1 month before surgery for the recovery of the collagen in cases of hernia surgery)
- Obesity (recent loss of weight)
- History of diabetes mellitus
- Hypertension
- Cardiovascular diseases (chest pain, palpitation, and dyspnea) and dyslipidemia
- Respiratory problems (dyspnea, cough, wheeze, asthma, etc.) and chronic obstructive pulmonary disease (COPD)
- History of allergy
- Neurological—history of syncope, epilepsy, cerebrovascular accident (CVA), and transient ischemic attacks (TIAs)
- Bleeding diathesis
- History of intake of antiplatelet drugs such as aspirin, clopidogrel, and warfarin [it is preferable to stop these medications for 5 days prior to surgery. When patient is on warfarin, infusion of unfractionated heparin is given when the international normalized ratio (INR) falls below 1.5. The infusion of unfractionated heparin is stopped 2 hours before the surgery. Heparin and warfarin should be started in the postoperative period]
- Urinary problems and renal dysfunction
- Risk factors for DVT [see Chapter 18 on deep vein thrombosis (DVT)]
- Tuberculosis and human immunodeficiency virus (HIV).

GENERAL EXAMINATION
- Look for pallor, icterus, cyanosis, clubbing, lymphadenopathy, and edema.
- Nutritional status [body mass index (BMI), anthropometric measurements, biochemical of which most important is albumin (<3.5 g/dL will adversely affect the outcome), hematological, and immunological tests]. A BMI of <18.5 is suggestive of nutritional impairment; <15 is associated with significant hospital mortality. Morbid obesity (BMI >35) is also associated with increased risk of postoperative complications.

Cardiovascular
- Pulse
- Blood pressure
- Heart sounds including murmurs
- Bruits
- Lower limb edema
- Raised jugular venous pressure
- Peripheral pulsations.

If the patient can climb a flight of stairs without any problem, then there is a low risk of perioperative cardiovascular morbidity and mortality. Any abnormality identified clinically or electrocardiography (ECG) wise, must be referred to a cardiologist for ECHO and further evaluation.

Hypertension
The blood pressure should be controlled to 160/90 mm Hg. If any new drug is added, 2 weeks of stabilization period should be allowed.

Coronary Artery Disease
Elective surgery should be postponed for 3–6 months after an attack of myocardial infarction. Cardiology opinion is required if the patient had coronary stents and antiplatelet therapy such as clopidogrel and aspirin.

Arrhythmias and Valvular Heart Disease
In atrial fibrillation patients on warfarin, the drug should be stopped 5 days preoperatively so that the INR will remain 1.5 or less. There is no need for anticoagulation in the perioperative period. For patients with mechanical heart valves, the warfarin should be stopped 5 days before surgery. In this situation, an infusion of unfractionated heparin is given when the INR is <1.5.

Respiratory
- Respiratory rate
- Chest expansion

- Breath sounds
- Air entry
- Tracheal shift.

The patient should be referred to a respiratory physician if a respiratory comorbidity is identified. Pulmonary function test may be required in such patients. Elective surgery should be postponed until the respiratory problems are controlled.

Neurological
- Level of consciousness, orientation, and cognitive function
- Motor and sensory system and reflexes
- Spine deformities.

Gastrointestinal
- Liver diseases
- Portal hypertension
- Ascites.

Airway Assessment
In patients requiring general anesthesia, the ease performing airway maneuvers can be assessed by modified Mallampati test by examining the findings on full mouth opening:
- Grade 1—fauces, pillars, soft palate, and uvula seen
- Grade 2—fauces, pillars, soft palate with some part of uvula seen
- Grade 3—soft palate seen
- Grade 4—hard palate only seen.

The higher the grade, the higher the risk for securing the airway. In addition, look for oral hygiene, caries teeth, loose teeth, premalignant lesions such as oral submucous fibrosis.

Diabetic Patient
As per the new World Health Organization (WHO) definition, fasting blood sugar of >126 mg/dL is diagnostic of diabetes mellitus. It is preferable to do HbA_1C level in all diabetic patients. A value of >6.5 is diagnostic of diabetes. It is ideal to control the diabetes before carrying out elective surgery. Fasting blood sugar <140 mg/dL is preferable. Patients with diabetes should be first on the operating list in the morning. They are advised to omit the morning dose of medication and breakfast. If the operation is scheduled in the afternoon, patient can be given breakfast and half the regular dose of insulin or full dose of oral hypoglycemic agents (OHAs). If the patient is taking a morning dose of insulin, the short-acting insulin is omitted on the morning of the procedure.

Oral Contraceptives

There is an increased risk of thromboembolic complications if combined pills are continued. Hormone replacement therapy should be stopped 6 weeks prior to elective surgery. Progesterone only pill can be continued. DVT prophylaxis is given separately in another chapter.

INVESTIGATIONS

Minor surgery (<30 minutes)—for minor surgery, if there are no comorbidities, not much of a role for routine investigations other than to check for serology, blood sugar, and hemoglobin estimation. If comorbidities are there, detailed evaluation is required.

Major Surgery (any Surgery Going beyond 30 minutes)

- Full blood count
- ECG for all patients above 50 years of age
- Blood glucose and HbA_1C—in patients with diabetes mellitus
- Blood urea and electrolytes for patients over 40 years with cardiovascular and renal problems
- Coagulation profile for patients with liver disease, family history of bleeding disorders, bleeding diathesis, and patients with history of eclampsia. Single test such as prothrombin time (PT) is enough rather than doing bleeding time (BT), clotting time (CT), partial thromboplastin time (PTT), and platelet count
- Chest X-ray—even though a chest X-ray is not mandatory in young individuals <40 years of age as per Western protocol, it is routinely done for all patients in our place
- Urine analysis
- Pregnancy test for premenopausal patients
- Liver function test—indicated in patients with hepatitis, cirrhosis, and poor nutritional status
- Serology—HIV, hepatitis B virus (HBV), and hepatitis C virus (HCV)
- Blood grouping and Rh typing and if required cross-matching *(preoperative transfusions are indicated for chronic anemia only if the hemoglobin level is 8 g or less)*.

Other Investigations

If any abnormality is found during the above investigations, further appropriate investigations may be carried out.

INFORMED CONSENT

A valid informed consent is necessary for all elective surgical procedures. Valid consent is one which is given by a competent person and this is possible for a normal adult. Explain the advantages, complications, prognosis, morbidity, and mortality in relation to every procedure. The language used must be simple and in patient's own language, especially in explaining the risk. The risk related to the comorbidities and anesthesia should also be explained. If high-risk consent is needed, that also should be taken after explaining the situation. Separate consent should be taken for surgery and anesthesia. The patient should be send to the preanesthetic clinic for the evaluation by anesthesiologist and taking consent from their part.

NIL PER ORAL

Even though the custom of nil per oral (NPO) midnight is practiced in most of the surgical centers, it is preferable not to allow solid food within 6 hours and clear fluid 2 hours before anesthesia. This is done to prevent the risk of acid aspiration. The infants can be given mother's milk up to 3 hours preoperatively. If the surgery is delayed, it is preferable to start intravenous fluids. H_2 receptor blockers or proton pump inhibitors are given by most of the centers in the preoperative period.

PREOPERATIVE SKIN PREPARATION/SHOWER/HANDWASHING/MASKS/DRAINS

- Open skin lesions should be allowed to heal.
- Preoperative shower with antiseptic such as povidone iodine the night before the operation.
- No shaving the night before the surgery—it is preferable to clip the hair on the day of surgery.
- Obese patients must lose as much weight as possible.

OPERATING ROOM ENVIRONMENT

- Handwash—brief rinse with soap and water followed by handrub with alcohol gel. Brush if at all used, should be only for the nail beds and not for the skin. Brushing of the skin will bring out the bacterial flora.
- Change gowns and gloves every 2 hours—20% of the surgical gloves fail during operation.
- Surgical masks should cover the nose and mouth. This is to prevent the source from chronic nasal carriers.
- Avoid hypothermia—there is increase in the risk for surgical site infection.
- Blood transfusion—increases the rate of nosocomial infection.
- Blood sugar—>200 mg at any time on the first postoperative day increases the surgical site infection. Blood glucose concentration <110 mg/dL is associated with 40% decrease in mortality, fewer nosocomial infections, and less organ dysfunction.

- Oxygenation—administration of oxygen in the postoperative period is found to be beneficial for wound healing and prevention of infection. Oxygen has been postulated to have direct antibacterial effect.
- Drains—drains should not be placed in incisions which will cause more infections. It will also prevent sealing of the wound by epithelialization and it will act as a conduit holding a portal for invasion by pathogens. They should be, therefore, used early and removed as soon as possible. There is no need for prolonged antibiotic usage to cover indwelling drains.
- Enteral feeding—every effort should be made to start enteral feeding after laparotomy and gastrointestinal surgery (within 36 hours).

22. Preoperative Preparation of Common Operations

R Dayananda Babu

ENDOCRINOLOGY

Thyroidectomy

Preoperative Evaluation

The following investigations are recommended:
- *Thyroid function tests*: Thyroid-stimulating hormone (TSH) alone is enough as a screening test. T3 and T4 are recommended in symptomatic patients.
- Ultrasound of neck and sono-guided fine needle aspiration cytology (FNAC).
- X-ray of neck anteroposterior and lateral view for assessment of the tracheal displacement and luminal narrowing.
- Laryngoscopy video/indirect for assessment of occult vocal cord palsy.
- If retrosternal extension is suspected, computed tomography (CT) of the neck.
- X-ray of chest and electrocardiography (ECG) for cardiac evaluation.
- Blood sugar estimation.
- Routine hematological and serological examination.
- *Blood grouping*: In case of large goiter, arrange one bottle of cross-match blood.

Make the Patient Euthyroid before Surgery
- In cases of hyperthyroidism, the TSH value may not come to normal levels. If the T3 and T4 are normalized, the patient can be taken up for surgery.
- Occult hypothyroidism must be corrected by thyroxine. Otherwise, it will lead on to laryngeal edema postoperatively.
- Patients treated medically with either propylthiouracil (PTU) or methimazole should take their medication on the day of surgery and should be resumed within 72 hours of surgery.
- Patients on beta-blockers must continue the drug for 1 week.
- Thyrotoxic patients requiring emergency surgery should be premedicated with beta-blockers, antithyroid drugs, and corticosteroids.
- Untreated hyperthyroid patients should have elective procedures postponed until euthyroid.

Patients with Hypothyroidism

- Clinically euthyroid patients may have their thyroid hormone withheld on the day of surgery. Postoperatively, they may resume thyroid replacement when tolerating oral intake (the half-life of T4 is 7 days).
- Profound hypothyroidism patients tolerate surgical stress poorly. These patients should receive intravenous (IV) T4 (300–500 mg) and steroids. Intraoperative hypotension should be anticipated in such patients. Other problems are fluid and electrolyte disorders, prolonged ileus, impaired febrile response to infection, and neuropsychiatric problems.

DIABETES MELLITUS

The diabetic patients experience significant stress during the perioperative period and at an increased risk of morbidity and mortality. They are immunocompromised and more prone for infectious complications and have impaired wound healing. Diabetic patients have 50% lifetime chance of a surgery. Vascular diseases are more common and a silent coronary artery disease must be ruled out.

Preoperative Evaluation

It is desirable to admit a type I diabetic patient for one or more days for stabilization of diabetes mellitus (DM) before surgery. It is preferable to bring plasma glucose level below 200 mg/dL. Type II DM patients with plasma glucose <150 mg/dL that is controlled by diet or oral agents may not require any insulin.

Investigations

- Fasting blood sugar
- HBA_{1c}
- Baseline ECG (a resting tachycardia and lack of variability of R-R interval are suggestive of autonomic neuropathy)
- Renal function test—blood urea and creatinine
- Serum electrolytes.

Type II Diabetes Patients on Oral Hypoglycemic Agents

- These patients can take the oral hypoglycemic agent (OHA) until the morning of surgery.
- On the day of surgery, skip the morning dose.
- Long-acting sulfonylureas should be discontinued for 48–72 hours. Otherwise there is an increased risk of *hypoglycemia*. Severe hypoglycemia may produce *arrhythmias and cognitive deficits*.
- They are also most prone for hyperosmolar hyperglycemic states leading on to severe volume depletion and ketoacidosis during stress.

- Metformin increases the risk of renal hypoperfusion. It is contraindicated in hepatic insufficiency. It should be cautiously used in congestive heart failure.
- They may be managed by diet alone preoperatively.
- Supplementation of short-acting insulins may be required if the glucose levels rise during surgery which is evaluated by capillary finger prick samples.
- OHA can be restarted after surgery once the patient resumes seating.
- Metformin should not be restarted in patients with renal insufficiency.

Type I Diabetes on Insulin

They are insulin deficient and insulin should not be withheld at any time. They are prone to develop ketoacidosis:
- It is preferable to schedule the surgery as first in the list.
- Patients on insulin can continue with subcutaneous insulin perioperatively.
- If the long-acting insulin is titrated properly, it can be continued.
- It is better to reduce the dose of intermediate-acting insulin on the night prior to surgery.

Minor Operations
- One-third to half of the insulin total dose is given as intermediate-acting insulin.
- Start 5% dextrose solutions at the rate of 75–125 mL/hr.
- Restart the usual short-acting insulin prior to the first meal.

Major Operations in Type I Patients
- These patients need IV insulin by the combined glucose insulin potassium solution (GKI). The rate of insulin infusion is 0.5–5 U/hr. Glucose is administered 5–10 g/hr 0.3 U of insulin is infused for each gram of glucose.
- Usually 500 mL of 10% dextrose with 10 mmol of KCl and 16 U of short-acting insulin is used in this regime which is given at the rate of 100 mL/hr (1–2 U of insulin/hr).
- Insulin infusion should be continued in those who are not able to eat postoperatively.
- Once the patient is on solid food, subsequent insulin administration is given by subcutaneous administration guided by blood glucose determination every 4–6 hours.

UPPER GASTROINTESTINAL SURGERY

Patients with evidence of gastric outlet obstruction with associated vomiting do the following:

The two most important causes for gastric outlet obstruction are gastric cancer and pyloric stenosis secondary to peptic ulcer.

Estimation of serum electrolytes blood urea and creatine. The metabolic abnormality of *hypochloremic alkalosis* is corrected by isotonic saline and the associated hypokalemia is corrected with potassium chloride in IV fluid bottle.

The patient should be *rehydrated*.

Patients with gastric cancer are usually anemic and correction may be required. *Grouping and cross-matching* of the blood and arranging blood for expected loss. Full *complete blood count* examination is required.

The stomach should be emptied using a wide bore *nasogastric tube*. Sometimes, it may be necessary to pass an *orogastric tube* for lavaging the stomach. The stomach should be completely emptied by lavage in such cases. Once it is clear, *upper gastrointestinal (GI) endoscopy* can be carried out and biopsy done, if required.

Contrast CT scan is done in cases of gastric cancer.

Nutritional assessment of the patient is important in such cases [A body mass index (BMI) *<18.5 indicates nutritional impairment and BMI below 15 is associated with very significant hospital mortality*]. *Serum albumin* of <3.5 g is also associated with wound healing problems. Vomiting may be associated with episodes of aspiration. Therefore, it is important to correct the respiratory function.

Cardiac evaluation is done for such patients to exclude any abnormality. If the patient is hypertensive, control of blood pressure is important.

Do a fasting blood sugar and HBA_{1c}, if the patient is diabetic, control diabetes.

Liver, Biliary, and Pancreatic Operations

- *Liver function tests*: Bilirubin and alkaline phosphatase—estimation of total, direct, and indirect bilirubin are important in differentiating obstructive jaundice from jaundice due to nonobstructive causes. The total and direct bilirubin will be elevated in obstructive jaundice along with a rise in the alkaline phosphatase level.
- Jaundiced patients may be deficient in the vitamin-K dependent clotting factors—II, V, VII, IX, and X resulting in bleeding tendency. *Prothrombin time (PT) and activated partial thromboplastin time (aPTT)* estimations are done. Give (vitamin K 10 mg intramuscularly or K1 10 mg intravenously) to patients with obstructive jaundice prior to surgery if the PT is abnormal.

  Fresh frozen plasma may be required for patients with significant coagulopathy requiring urgent operation.
- Preliminary investigation of choice for obstructive jaundice is ultrasound examination of the abdomen which will reveal the following:
  - Intrahepatic biliary radical dilatation

- Size of the common bile duct (CBD) and cystic duct
- Presence or absence of gallstones
- Gallbladder (GB) wall thickness
- Level of obstruction of the extrahepatic biliary system
- Any mass lesion in pancreas (difficult to detect)
- Any free fluid in the abdomen
- Liver metastasis—presence or absence.
- *Contrast CT* of the abdomen is taken to identify the mass and its operability.
- Magnetic resonance imaging (MRI) abdomen/magnetic resonance cholangiopancreatography (MRCP) may be required in some cases.
- *Upper GI endoscopy* is done in suspected periampullary carcinoma.
- *Serological tests* are done for Hepatitis B and C viral markers.
- Preoperative insertion of *biliary stents* for preoperative drainage is done in patients who are at poor risk for surgery and one can buy time. It is indicated in very elderly patients, patients with biliary sepsis and deeply jaundiced patients (bilirubin above 15 mg).
- *Adequate preoperative hydration* is very important to prevent hepatorenal syndrome.
- *Antibiotic prophylaxis*: Infective complications are common and, therefore, antibiotic prophylaxis is recommended:
  - *Acute cholangitis* demands antibiotics and urgent biliary tract drainage either endoscopically or percutaneously.
  - *Cirrhosis* is a high-risk problem. Coagulation correction with vitamin-K or fresh frozen plasma may be required. In patients with portal hypertension, operation may be technically difficult and they badly tolerate major fluid shifts. They will go in for encephalopathy and renal failure. It is better to avoid surgery in Child-Pugh patients.
  - In patients with severe pulmonary disease inducing pneumoperitoneum for *laparoscopic surgery* may render ventilation difficult.
  - Cholecystectomy.
  - No special preparations are required other than keeping the patient nil per os (NPO) midnight.
  - No need for nasogastric tube.

LARGE BOWEL OPERATIONS

The peculiarity of the colon is the precarious blood supply and the resultant anastomotic leakage and the luminal content which is fecal matter. The conventional mechanical bowel preparation is controversial and the recent studies have failed to show any benefit from it. Mechanical bowel preparations are contraindicated in patients with obstructing lesions. In such cases on table colonic lavage by infusion through the appendicostomy stump is recommended. The conventional chemical bowel preparations are replaced by prophylactic antibiotics (read the chart on antibiotics prophylaxis).

- Low residue diet is given 3 days before surgery.
- Liquid diet is given on the day before surgery.
- Sodium picosulfate 10 mg is given on the morning and night before surgery.
- Polyethylene glycol (PEG) four sachets in 4 L of water is prepared and 250 mL is given every 15 minutes.
- Mechanical washout using rectal tube is another option.
- Elderly patients may require IV hydration to compensate the fluid loss.

Consent for Colostomy
- Take consent for colostomy in all patients undergoing large bowel surgery.
- Consult the stoma care nurse to select and mark the practical site for colostomy.
- Counsel the patient undergoing rectal surgery about the risks of pelvic nerve injury, impotence, and bladder control.

APPENDICECTOMY
- No specific preparations are required for appendectomy.
- No need for nasogastric tube.

23 "Safe Surgery Saves Lives"—A WHO Initiative

R Dayananda Babu

Summary of the World Health Organization (WHO) initiative published (*World alliance for patient safety; Global patient safety challenges*).

Roughly, 1 operation is carried out per every 25 people. Every year an estimated 63 million people undergo surgery for trauma; 31 million surgeries are done to treat malignancies and 10 million operations for pregnancy-related complications. Major complications are reported to occur in 3–16% of in-patient surgical procedures. The permanent disability or death rates are approximately 0.4–0.8%. Surgical procedures are intended to save lives. Unsafe surgical care can cause substantial harm. The global patient safety challenge, "*Safe surgery saves lives,*" was launched in 2007 to improve the safety of surgical care around the world. The WHO "Surgical Safety Checklist" is an essential part of this program.

WORLD HEALTH ORGANIZATION SURGICAL SAFETY CHECKLIST

This is a simple practical tool that any surgical team in the world can use to ensure that the preoperative, intraoperative, and postoperative steps that have been shown to benefit patients, if it is done in a timely and efficient way. The checklist was developed based on a set of 10 essential objectives (or standards), for safe surgery that should be met by every surgical team. These standards were identified by the *Alliance* in consultation with surgeons, anesthesiologists, nurses, patient safety experts, and patients around the world. The implementation of the checklist was shown to lower the incidence of surgery-related deaths and complications by one-third.

It has got three steps:
1. Sign in (before induction of anesthesia)
2. Time out (before skin incision)
3. Sign out (before the patient leaves the operating room).

Sign In (Before Induction of Anesthesia)
- *Patient has confirmed*:
  - Identity
  - Site
  - Procedure
  - Consent

- Site marked/not applicable
- Anesthesia safety check completed
- Pulse oximeter on patient and functioning
- Does patient have a known allergy?
  - No
  - Yes
- Difficult airway/aspiration risk:
  - No
  - Yes, and equipment/assistants available
- Risk of >500 mL blood loss (7 mL/kg in children):
  - No
  - Yes, and adequate intravenous access and fluids planned.

Time Out (Before Skin Incision)

- Confirm all team members have introduced themselves by name and role
- Surgeon, anesthesia professional, and nurse verbally confirm:
  - Patient
  - Site
  - Procedure
- *Anticipated critical events*:
  - *Surgeon reviews*: What are the critical or unexpected steps, operative duration, anticipated blood loss?
  - *Anesthesia team reviews*: Are there any patient specific concerns?
  - *Nursing team reviews*: Has sterility (including indicator results) been confirmed? Are there equipment issues or any concerns?
- Has antibiotic prophylaxis been given within the last 60 minutes?
  - Yes
  - Not applicable.
- Is essential imaging displayed?
  - Yes
  - Not applicable

Sign Out (Before Patient Leaves Operating Room)

- *Nurses verbally confirm with the team*:
  - The name of the procedure recorded
  - That instrument, sponge, and needle counts are correct (or not applicable)
  - How the specimen is labeled (including patient name)
  - Whether there are any equipment problems to be addressed
  - Surgeon, anesthesia professional, and nurses review the key concerns for recovery and management of this patient.

This checklist is not intended to be comprehensive. Additions and modifications to fit local practice are encouraged.

In each phase, the checklist coordinator must be permitted to confirm that the team has completed its tasks before it proceeds further. While signing the checklist, coordinator will verbally review with the patient, that his or her identity has been confirmed, that the procedure and the site are correct and that the consent for surgery has been given. The coordinator will visually confirm that the operative site has been marked and that a pulse oximeter is on the patient and functioning. The coordinator will also verbally review with the anesthesia professional, the patient's risk of blood loss, airway difficulty and allergic reaction and, whether a full anesthesia safety check has been completed. Ideally the surgeon will be present for "sign in", as the surgeon may have a clearer idea of anticipated blood loss, allergies or other complicating patient factors. However, surgeon's presence is not essential for completing this part of the checklist.

For time out, each team member will introduce him/herself by name and role. If already part way through the operative day together, the team can simply confirm that everyone in the room is known to each other. The team will pause immediately prior to the skin incision to confirm out loud that they are performing the correct operation on the correct patient and site and then verbally review with one another, in turn, the critical elements of their plans for the operation using the checklist questions for guidance.

TEN ESSENTIAL OBJECTIVES FOR SAFE SURGERY

1. Team will operate on the correct patient at the correct site.
2. The team will use methods known to prevent harm from anesthetic administration, while protecting the patient from pain.
3. The team will recognize and effectively prepare, for life-threatening loss of airway or respiratory function.
4. The team will recognize and effectively prepare for risk of high blood loss.
5. The team will avoid inducing an allergic or adverse drug reaction known to be a significant risk to the patient.
6. The team will consistently use methods known to minimize risk of surgical site infection.
7. The team will prevent inadvertent retention of sponges or instruments in surgical wounds.
8. The team will secure and accurately identify all surgical specimens.
9. The team will effectively communicate and exchange critical patient information for the safe conduct of the operation.
10. Hospitals and public health systems will establish routine surveillance of surgical capacity, volume, and results.

24. Prophylactic Antibiotics in Surgery

R Dayananda Babu

INTRODUCTION

Surgical site infection is the third most common nosocomial infection and will occur in 3% of all surgical procedures and 20% of emergency intra-abdominal procedures. This causes substantial morbidity and increases the hospital stay by 7–10 days and increases the hospital cost.

The wounds are classified into four categories:
1. *Clean (Class I)*: Infection rate 1–3%.
   Definition: Atraumatic wound, no inflammation, gastrointestinal, genitourinary, respiratory, and biliary tract not entered.
   Organisms: *Staphylococcus aureus* and *Staphylococcus epidermidis*.
   For example, hernia repair and thyroidectomy.
2. *Clean—contaminated (Class II)*: Infection rate 5–10%.
   Definition: Elective operations of gastrointestinal tract (GIT), genitourinary, respiratory tract have been entered during surgery under controlled conditions.
   Organism: Endogenous microflora of the organ that has been entered.
   For example, cholecystectomy and elective bowel resection.
3. *Contaminated (Class III)*: Infection rate 15%.
   Definition: Traumatic wounds (fresh), major break in sterile techniques, gross spillage from GIT, and acute nonpurulent inflammation.
   Organism: Endogenous bacteria.
   For example, appendicectomy.
4. *Dirty (Class IV)*: Infection rate 40%.
   Definition: Old traumatic wounds, devitalized tissue, gross purulence, preexisting infection, and perforated viscera.
   Organism: Endogenous bacteria.
   For example, Hartmann's operation for perforated diverticulitis.
   Definition of prophylactic antibiotic: Prophylactic antibiotic is an antibiotic or antimicrobial administered for <24 hours postoperatively.
   Therapeutic antibiotic: When administering antibiotic for >24 hours, it is called therapeutic antibiotic.

INDICATIONS FOR PROPHYLAXIS

- All clean-contaminated and contaminated wounds (prophylaxis for clean wound is controversial).
- Insertion of prosthesis requires prophylaxis.
- In cases of craniotomy and sternotomy.

ORGANISMS FOR SURGICAL SITE INFECTION

- *S. aureus* (the most common) and *S. epidermidis*.
- *Enterococcus faecalis, Escherichia coli,* and Bacteroides.

THE CONCEPT OF ANTIBIOTIC PROPHYLAXIS

This concept was introduced by Miles and Burke in 1950. They found that the infection can be prevented only when antimicrobials are given prior to or at the time of infectious challenge. Antibiotics 3 hours after the challenge are ineffective. Concentration of organisms above 100,000/g of tissue exceeds the host defense capacity.

Single-dose prophylaxis was recommended after Strachan and colleagues' study in 1977. In their study of single dose of preoperative cefazolin versus 5-day treatment of cefazolin, it was found that the infection rate was 3% for single dose and 5% for 5-day treatment.

Six principles of antibiotic prophylaxis are as follows:
1. The antibiotic should be safe.
2. It should have a narrow spectrum.
3. It should have a short half-life—<2 hours.
4. The antibiotic should not be relied upon for clinical treatment.
5. It should be administered for a defined period.
6. It should be given within 1 hour before the time of incision.

OTHER PRINCIPLES

- Use antibiotic against the bacteria likely to contaminate.
- Use full dose of the antibiotic chosen.
- Administer the drug prophylactically.
- If the operation is prolonged >3 hours, give another dose.
- Employ antibiotic when the risk of infection is increased.
- A third-generation cephalosporin or quinolone should never be used.
- Antibiotic should not be administered to cover indwelling drains or catheters.
- Do not put antibiotic in lavage fluid.

FINAL CONSENSUS

The consensus is that a single dose immediately before operation is enough and that there are dangers not only to the hospital but also to the patient in prolonged course of prophylactic antibiotics. Resistance to antibiotics is related closely to the prolificity with which antibiotics are prescribed.

WHICH ANTIBIOTIC?

- First-generation cephalosporins—cefazolin 2 g is the ideal antibiotic for the prophylaxis.
- In case of anaphylaxis, use clindamycin.
- Vancomycin prophylaxis is advocated when the methicillin-resistant *Staphylococcus aureus* (MRSA) incidence of the hospital is >20%.
- For orthopedic and vascular surgery procedures, antibiotics can go up to 24 hours (two more doses).
- For solid organ transplantation, the antibiotic is extended for 48 hours.
- For colon, ampicillin + sulbactam or quinolone + metronidazole is recommended.

PROBLEMS OF PROLONGATION OF PROPHYLAXIS

- *Clostridium difficile*-associated disease (CDAD)—may be asymptomatic to colitis to perforation
- Later nosocomial infection unrelated to surgical site infection
- Emergence of multidrug resistant (MDR) pathogens
- Pneumonia and catheter-related infection
- Surgical site infection by MRSA.

ANTIBACTERIAL SUTURES

It is found that triclosan with polyglactin suture will give protection against wound infection. It can inhibit *S. aureus*, *S. epidermidis*, and MRSA.

REMEMBER

- "Our arsenals for fighting the bacteria are so powerful that we are in more danger from them than from the invaders."—Lewis Thomas
- Sepsis is not an antibiotic deficiency syndrome.
- The most novel antibiotics and the best supportive care are meaningless if the principles of source control are not adhered to with obsessiveness.
- Antibiotic for the fool is a tool which appears cool but somebody pays the price as a rule.

ANTIBIOTIC PROPHYLAXIS FOR COMMON OPERATIONS (TABLE 1)

Table 1: Recommendations for antibiotic prophylaxis for common operations.

Nature of operation	Likely pathogens	Recommended antibiotics	Adult dose before surgery
Gastroduodenal (high-risk patient)	Enteric Gram-negative bacilli, Gram-positive cocci	Cefazolin	1–2 g IV
Biliary	Enteric Gram-negative bacilli, Enterococci, Clostridia	Cefazolin	1–2 g IV
Colorectal	Enteric Gram-negative bacilli	Ampicillin + sulbactam and metronidazole	1.5–3 g of ampicillin + sulbactam and 500 mg metronidazole
Appendectomy (no perforation)	Anaerobes and Enterococci	IV: Cefazolin + metronidazole	Before an 8 AM operation 1–2 g IV 500 mg IV Metronidazole
Head and neck, entering oral cavity or pharynx	Oral anaerobes, enteric Gram-negative bacilli, Staphylococci	Cefazolin, ampicillin, sulbactam, clindamycin, and gentamicin	1–2 g IV (C) or 1.5–3 g IV (amp+ sulbactam) or 600–900 mg IV (clindamycin) or 60–80 mg/kg IV (gentamicin)
Cardiac: Prosthetic valve and other procedures	Staphylococci, Corynebacteria, enteric Gram-negative bacilli	Cefazolin/ vancomycin/ cefuroxime	1–2 g IV 1 g IV 1.5 g IV
Vascular: Peripheral bypass or aortic surgery with prosthetic graft	Staphylococci, Streptococci, enteric Gram-negative bacilli, Clostridia	Cefazolin/ vancomycin/ cefoxitin	1–2 g IV 1–2 g IV 1–2 g IV
Orthopedic: Total joint replacement or internal fixation of fractures	Staphylococci	Cefazolin/ vancomycin	1–2 g IV 1 g IV
Ophthalmic	Staphylococci, Streptococci, enteric Gram-negative bacilli, *Pseudomonas* species	Gentamicin, tobramycin ciprofloxacin and ofloxacin	Multiple drops topically over 2–24 hours

Contd…

Contd...

Nature of operation	Likely pathogens	Recommended antibiotics	Adult dose before surgery
Vaginal or abdominal hysterectomy	Enteric Gram-negative bacilli, *Anaerobes*, Enterococci	Cefoxitin Cefazolin	1–2 g IV 1–2 g IV
Cesarean section (high-risk patient)	Enteric Gram-negative bacilli, Anaerobes, group B Streptococci, Enterococci	Cefazolin Cefoxitin	1–2 g IV 1–2 g IV

25. Surgical Site Infection

R Dayananda Babu

INTRODUCTION

Surgical site infection (SSI) is the third most common cause for nosocomial infection. Thirty-eight percent of the surgical infections are as a result of SSI. It is the most common nosocomial infection in the surgical ward. It increases the hospital stay by 7–10 days. Wound infection is a term that has caused a lot of confusion among surgeons worldwide. As a result of this confusion, there has been a lot of disparity in the collection and comparison of data regarding wound infection in postoperative patients. To tide over this problem, the Center for Disease Control (CDC) came up with certain definition and protocols (1992) that could be used world over.

CDC DEFINITION

As per the CDC classification, there are three types of surgical site infections (SSIs) **(Fig. 1)**:
1. Superficial incisional SSI
2. Deep incisional SSI
3. Organ/space SSI.

Superficial Surgical Site Infection

The superficial incisional SSI is the most common incisional infection in modern practice and it is confined to the subcutaneous adipose layer.

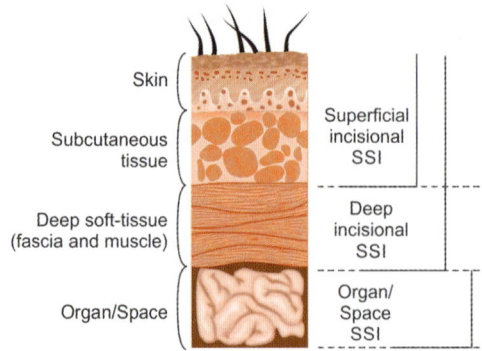

Fig. 1: Three different types of surgical site infections (SSIs).

Superficial SSI is impossible, if the subcutaneous space is left unclosed and allowed to heal by second intention.

To call an infection a superficial SSI, it should meet the following criteria:
- Infection should occur within 30 days of the surgery.
- Infection should involve the skin and subcutaneous tissue.
- Incision must meet one of the following criteria:
  - Purulent drainage from the superficial incision
  - Organism isolated from an aseptically obtained culture of fluid or tissue.
- Incision must show at least one of the following signs or symptoms:
  - Pain or tenderness
  - Localized tenderness
  - Redness or heat.
- Superficial incision is deliberately opened by a surgeon unless the incision is culture negative or diagnosis of superficial incision SSI is made by the surgeon.

The earliest sign of such an infection is induration accompanied by erythema and increasing pain.

Immediate therapy consists of opening the wound and evacuating the pus. *Antibiotics are not usually required.* Antibiotics are given only for cellulitis and systemic toxicity. Antimicrobial drugs will not accelerate the healing process and will not be sanitized (source control is mechanical, not pharmacological). Topical saline soaked wet to dry dressing is recommended. Other local applications will suppress fibroblast proliferation.

The following conditions should not be considered as SSI:
- Stitch abscess
- Infection of an episiotomy or newborn circumcision site
- Infected burn wound.

The most common organism for superficial SSI is *Staphylococcus aureus*. The patient is not seriously ill unlike deep incisional surgical site infection. Seeding of the bloodstream is rare and the complications are rarely lethal.

Deep Incisional Surgical Site Infections

Deep incisional SSIs develop less frequently, however, have more serious consequences by invading the fascia and muscles.

Infection occurring within 30 days of surgery (1-year implant in place) and infection involving deep soft-tissue and at least one of the following:
- Purulent discharge from the deep incision, but not from the organ space.
- Either fever of 38°C or greater, local pain/tenderness, and deep incision spontaneously dehisces or is opened.
- Abscess or other evidence of infection involving deep incision found on direct examination or visual/radiological/histological.
- Diagnosis by the physician/surgeon.

Note: Clinically, the plane between the deep fascia and the subcutaneous fat is lost as a result of enzymatic/ischemic destruction of the posterior adherence of fat to the fascia. The deep incisional SSI will lead onto fasciitis and myonecrosis, if untreated. The patient will be usually seriously ill unlike superficial infection and there will be seeding of bloodstream. Lethal complications are possible. Multiple organisms may be isolated with presumed synergy of action.

Treatment: Immediate reoperation for debridement of the involved tissue followed by broad-spectrum antibiotics. Specimens for gram staining and cultures of fluid and tissue should be obtained.

The superficial and deep surgical site infections are closed space infections. Mechanical conversion of closed, infected three-dimensional space to an open, contaminated two-dimensional surface.

Organ Space Surgical Site Infection

They are infections of body cavities or organs manipulated by surgeons.

Infection occurs within 30 days (1 year of implant). Infection involving any part of the anatomy other than the incision, which was opened/manipulated at the time of surgery plus one of the following:
- Purulent drainage from a drain that is placed through a stab wound in the organ/space.
- Organism isolated from aseptically obtained fluid from the organ/space.
- An abscess or other evidence of infection in the organ/space obtained during reoperation/histology/radiology.
- Diagnosis of an organ/space infection made by the surgeon.

Organ Space SSI Masquerading Incisional SSI

Imaging studies are required to rule out subfascial collection/fistula from hollow organs. Presumptive systemic antibiotics are given. If not treated promptly, it will trigger lethal multiorgan failure (MOF).

Treatment: Drainage is carried out either by reoperation or external drainage by interventional radiology.

THE RISK OF WOUND INFECTION

The rate of SSI is dependent on several variables:
- Patient (endogenous)
- Operation and perioperative environment
- Pathogen

$$\text{The risk of SSI} = \frac{(\text{Dose of contamination} \times \text{Virulence})}{\text{Host resistance}}$$

Surgical Site Infection

The Predictive Index—CDC

SENIC—Study of the Effect of Nosocomial Infection Control.

The patients are given a score of 0 or 1 for the following four factors:
1. An abdominal operation
2. An operation that lasts longer than 2 hours
3. An operation that is contaminated
4. A patient who will have three or more diagnosis at the times of discharge exclusive of wound infection.

SENIC score:
- *Score 0*: 1% infection
- *Score 1*: 3–6% infection
- *Score 2*: 9% infection
- *Score 3*: 17% infection
- *Score 4*: 27% infection.

NNIS risk index:
- *NNIS (National Nosocomial Infection Surveillance) ASA score*: 3 or more
- *Length of operation*: 75th percentile of the duration of the specific operation
- *Level of contamination*: Contaminated/dirty.

Endogenous or Patient-related Factors

- *Duration of preoperative hospitalization*: If the patient is hospitalized preoperatively for a few days, the chance for SSI is more.
- *Presence of remote infection*: More chance for SSI.
- *Diabetes mellitus*: More chance for infection.
- *Age > 50 years and <1 year*: Infection chances are more.
- Abdominal operation is associated with more SSI.
- *Malnutrition*: More chance for infection.
- *Tobacco use*: More chance for SSI.
- *Altered immune response*: More chance for infection.

Exogenous or Perioperative Factors

- *Length of operation*: If it is more than 3 hours, more chance for infection, and additional dose of prophylactic antibiotic required.
- *Operating room ventilation*: Laminar flow will prevent SSI.
- *Hair removal*: It is ideal to clip the hair on the morning of the day of the surgery. Preoperative shaving the day before surgery, there is more chance for infection.
- *Foreign materials in surgical site*: More chance for infection.
- Preoperative showering with antiseptic solution will reduce the chance for surgical site infection.

- *Surgical drains*: It is preferable to avoid surgical drains or they should be kept for minimum number of days.
- Proper skin antisepsis is important.
- *Duration of surgical scrub*: For the first time, 2–5 minutes and in-between 2 minutes is enough. It is better to avoid brushes for skin, if at all, it should be used only for the nails.
- Sterile dressings are required only for 24–48 hours.
- Use sterile techniques for dressing and also wash the hands before and after dressing change.

Hospital Surgical Surveillance Program
- Apply strict CDC definitions.
- Most patients never being admitted to the hospital in the preoperative period.
- Discharge the patient the early postoperative period.
- Inpatient and outpatient data reviewed for 30 days following surgery.
- Adequate number of infection control nurses may be employed.
- Physician specific rates of SSI should be periodically reported.

26 Intravenous Fluids and Postoperative Fluid Management

R Dayananda Babu

INTRODUCTION

Fluid balance is the relationship between fluid output and fluid intake. Under normal circumstances, fluid balance is maintained quite precisely, but in the surgical patient, it has to be monitored carefully.

Fluid loss occurs in the following ways:
- *Urinary excretion*: 1,500 mL (0.5–2 mL/kg/h)
- *Insensible loss*: 900 mL (0.35 mL/kg/h)
- *Feces*: 100 mL
- *Total*: 2,500 mL/day

Normal daily requirement for an adult is as follows:
- *Water*: 2,500 mL (30–40 mL/kg/day)
- *Sodium*: 100–180 mEq/24 hours (1–2 mEq/kg/day)
- *Potassium*: 40–60 mEq/24 hours (0.5–1 mEq/kg/day)
- *Glucose*: 100 g (minimum required to ward off ketosis).

POSTOPERATIVE FLUID MANAGEMENT

Practical Fluid Balance for the Operated Patient

The calculation is based on:
- The initial estimated loss (i.e., the perioperative fluid loss)
- The maintenance requirement
- The ongoing loss.
  Usually 50% of the calculated loss is corrected in the initial 24 hours.

Four Indications for Fluid Therapy—4 Rs + 5th R—Reassessment as per the National Institute for Health and Care Excellence Guidelines

- *Resuscitation*
- *Routine maintenance*
- *Replacement*
- *Redistribution*
- *Reassessment.*

Maintenance

This will provide daily physiological fluid and electrolyte requirements. For example, a patient who is unable to drink with no ongoing fluid and electrolyte losses needs maintenance. Such a patient will require the following prescription:
- *Water*: 25–35 mL/kg
- *Sodium*: 1 mmol/kg
- *Potassium*: 1 mmol/kg
- *Dextrose*: 100 g/day.

1. This is estimated after all the operative losses have been calculated and dealt with.
2. This is based on the estimated normal requirements of the patient. For example, a normothermic 60 kg adult with a normal metabolic rate would require about 2,000 mL of water, 100 mEq of sodium, and about 50 mEq of potassium per day. Thus, this patient requires a daily fluid maintenance, under uncomplicated circumstances, consisting of:
   - 1,500 mL of isotonic water as 5% dextrose
   - 500 mL of 0.9% normal saline (NS)—*154 mmol of sodium per liter*
   - 60 mEq of potassium (K).

The National Institute for Health and Care Excellence Recommendation for Routine Maintenance

- 25–30 mL/kg/day of water
- 1 mmol/kg/day of potassium, sodium, and chloride
- 50–100 g/day of glucose.

Less fluid should be recommended in patients who are older or frail (20–25 mL/kg/day).

Restricted intravenous (IV) fluid maintenance regimen with reduced sodium chloride compared to the standard regimen was found to reduce mortality and hospital stays in two randomized controlled trials. Similarly lower chloride fluids were associated with lower mortality and morbidity. Therefore, they recommend *daily monitoring of serum chloride*. Therefore, for normal maintenance, 0.5 L of 0.9% saline is enough. Hyperchloremia can cause hyperchloremic acidosis. High-plasma chloride also promotes ileus.

The problem with 0.9% sodium chloride is that it contains 154 mmol/L of sodium and chloride. The normal plasma level of chloride is only 95–105 mmol/L. Prolonged saline use will promote edematous states.

Intravenous Fluid for First 72 hours after Surgery

Only water is required in the first 24 hours:
- Stress-induced release of *antidiuretic hormone (ADH)*, aldosterone, and cortisol causes *retention of sodium* and water and increased renal excretion of potassium.

Intravenous Fluids and Postoperative Fluid Management

Powerful sodium retention mechanisms are regulated by *renin-angiotensin* mechanism in addition. The capacity to excrete sodium is poor in the body. There will be dilutional hyponatremia when excess glucose or glucose saline is given. Postoperative hyponatremia is prevented by decreasing the total fluid except in conditions of sodium loss (*high total body sodium* is the end result).

- Endogenous release of potassium from traumatized tissues and catabolism warrants restriction of potassium.
- Therefore, in the first 24 hours, the patient requires no salt and less of water than normal.
- 2,000 mL of 5% dextrose is sufficient (when all the operative losses have been replaced).
- By the *second 24 hours*, metabolic response diminishes: Patient requires 2,000 mL of 5% dextrose and 1,000 mL of *isotonic saline* in 24 hours.
- From the *third postoperative* day and thereafter:
  - 20 mEq of *potassium* is added to each 500 mL of IV fluid to give a total of *60 mEq* in 24 hours (activation of aldosterone enhances high urinary loss. Catabolic release of amino acids, which are negatively charged, is accompanied by positively charged potassium ions).
  - *Whole body potassium depletion* is seen when there is additional gastrointestinal tract (GIT) potassium loss.
  - *Malnutrition is common in surgical patients*: There is reduction in cell membrane pumping and consequently sodium and water will move into the cell and potassium, magnesium, calcium, and phosphate will move out and they are lost in the urine. So, the malnourished individuals will also show low phosphate and magnesium in addition to low potassium.

Ongoing Losses

Additional fluid may be required in the following circumstances:
- If blood or serum is lost through drains
- It GIT losses continue; e.g., nasogastric aspiration or fistula
- Continuing third space losses in the first 24–48 hours after major surgery
- During rewarming, if the patient has become hypothermic during surgery
- These losses are replaced as isotonic saline (0.9% NS). In lower intestinal losses, Ringer's lactate is preferred (but this is best avoided in patients with hepatic disease as lactate is not converted to bicarbonate)
- For every 1,000 mL of fluid loss, 20 mEq or potassium is added.

For example, a postoperative patient has a Ryle's tube aspirate of 1,000 mL, a biliary fistula of 1,000 mL and a urinary output of 1,000 mL. If the patient is not dehydrated, fluid calculation would be thus:

Total fluid requirement is—1,000 mL + 1,000 mL + 1,000 mL + 500 mL (insensible losses) = 3,500 mL (Of this, Ryle's tube aspirate and biliary loss is replaced as 0.9% NS: 2,000 mL).

To calculate the total fluid requirement for this patient in a day (including maintenance).

Potassium required: For each 1,000 mL of bile and gastric aspirate, 20 mEq of potassium is required—
- For ongoing losses = 40 mEq
- For maintenance = 60 mEq
  Total = 100 mEq

Potassium is usually available as potassium chloride (*KCl*). It is always administered by *slow IV infusion* diluted in 0.9% sodium chloride. And, it should not exceed 40 mEq/L of fluid and it should be administered over 4 hours. Do not exceed 10 mmol/h. Mix thoroughly the potassium and sodium chloride solution by inverting the infusion bottle or bag at least five times. Direct injection of potassium will lead on to cardiac arrest. When potassium is given through the peripheral vein, it will be very painful and may produce thrombophlebitis. Potassium also can be given through the central line with syringe pump infusion with electrocardiogram (ECG) monitoring (potassium is available in ampules of 20 mEq).

Hypokalemia (K level < 3.5 mEq/L): Common causes—
- Inadequate intake
- *Gastrointestinal loss*:
  - Diarrhea and malabsorption
  - Gastric, pancreatic, biliary, or intestinal drainage
  - Abuse of laxative
- *Urinary loss*:
  - Diuretics
  - Diabetic ketoacidosis
  - Recovery phase of acute renal failure
- *Fluid losses*:
  - Large wounds
  - Burns.

Hypokalemia is clinically manifested mainly as neuromuscular effects and cardiovascular effects such as weakness, adynamic ileus, encephalopathy, arrhythmias, etc.

Electrocardiogram changes in hypokalemia:
- Increased amplitude and width of P wave
- Prolongation of PR interval
- T-wave flattening and inversion (low T wave)
- ST depression

- Prominent U waves (best seen in precordial leads)
- Apparent long QT intervals due to fusion of T and U waves.

Treatment as mentioned above.

Hyperkalemia (serum K > 5.5 mEq/L): Common causes—
- Excess potassium intake (drugs, diet, IV fluids, and blood products)
- Translocation of potassium from intracellular space (hemolysis, insulin deficiency, acidosis, drugs such as succinylcholine)
- Decreased renal excretion of potassium as in primary renal disease and potassium-sparing diuretics.

Clinical features are mainly cardiac arrhythmias including asystole and ventricular fibrillation. Other signs and symptoms are anxiety, weakness leading to flaccid paralysis, and hypotension.

Electrocardiogram changes in hyperkalemia:
- Tall, peaked T waves with a narrow base (best seen in precordial leads)
- Loss of P wave
- Widening of QRS complex
- Ventricular tachycardia, fibrillation, or asystole.

Treatment: Three approaches—
1. Antagonize cardiac toxicity by IV calcium salt (quick effect)—10% calcium gluconate, 2 mL/min with ECG monitoring.
2. Shift K into the cell—using sodium bicarbonate (7.5% sodium bicarbonate IV 100 mL) or insulin and glucose—1 unit of regular insulin in 5 g glucose.
3. Remove excess K with exchange resins or dialysis.

Glucose required: A minimum of 100 g (500 mL of 5% dextrose contains 25 g of glucose). Hence, the patient's total requirement of 3,500 mL can be administered as:
- 1,500 mL of 0.9% NS
- 1,500 mL of DNS
- 500 mL of 5% dextrose
- 100 mEq of K (5 ampules).

ASSESSMENT OF ADEQUACY OF FLUID AND ELECTROLYTE REPLACEMENT

- *Clinical and biochemical parameters*:
  - General condition and sensorium
  - Signs of dehydration
  - Hemodynamic stability; vital signs—pulse, blood pressure, etc.
  - Hematocrit, serum electrolytes, BUN, and urine osmolality.
- *Urine output*:
  - A very sensitive index

- The ultimate goal of hydration is to obtain a minimum urine output of 0.5 mL/kg/h.
- *Central venous pressure (CVP)*:
  - Normal level is 4–8 cm of water
  - Provides realistic information about fluid volume
  - Low CVP means decreased blood volume
  - High CVP means increased blood volume
  - Should be monitored half-hourly
  - Should be evaluated in the background for other data such as pulse, blood pressure, respiration, etc. For example, an increase in CVP parallels an increase in systolic BP indicating adequate fluid volume replacement.

After major surgery, assessment of fluid and electrolytes is best achieved by the measurement of urine output, CVP, and serum electrolyte concentration.

Judicious and appropriate administration of fluids in the postoperative period will reduce morbidity and mortality. Surgical patients are prone to salt and water overload in the postoperative phase.

Replacement

This will provide maintenance requirements and replacement for ongoing fluid and electrolyte losses in situations such as vomiting, intestinal fistulae, and diarrhea.

Replacement for blood loss is usually by 0.9% sodium chloride along with packed red cells. Replacement for GI loss will depend upon the chemical composition and usually given by saline, glucose with saline or balanced crystalloid solutions with additional potassium.

Resuscitation

Administration of fluid and electrolytes to restore intravascular volume in situations such as trauma, acute postoperative hemorrhage, and sepsis. The fluids used for resuscitation are crystalloids, colloids, and human albumin solutions. 1 liter of crystalloid is given initially as a bolus.

The following points should be always borne in mind with regard to IV fluid therapy:
- IV fluids are the first-line treatment for hypovolemia. Initial treatment with these fluids may be lifesaving and provide some time to control bleeding and obtain blood for transfusion, if it becomes necessary.
- Crystalloid maintenance fluids, which contain dextrose, are not suitable for resuscitation. Only crystalloid solutions with a similar concentration of sodium to plasma (NS or balanced salt solutions) are effective as resuscitation fluids. These should be available in all hospitals where IV fluids are used.

- Crystalloid resuscitation fluids should be infused in a volume at least three times the volume lost in order to correct hypovolemia.
- All colloid solutions (albumin, dextrans, gelatins, and hydroxyethyl starch solutions) are resuscitation fluids. However, they have not been shown to be superior to crystalloids in resuscitation. They are more expensive and there are potential problems of renal dysfunction, allergic responses, and disturbed coagulation.
- Theoretically, colloids are iso-oncotic with plasma.
- Colloid solutions should be infused in a volume equal to the blood volume deficit.
- Plasma should never be used as a replacement fluid.
- Plain water should never be infused intravenously. It will cause hemolysis and will probably be fatal.
- In addition to the IV route, the intraosseous, oral, rectal, or subcutaneous routes can be used for the administration of fluids.

Intravenous Resuscitation Fluids

Crystalloids: Crystalloids are composed of crystalline substances such as dextrose or sodium chloride, which, when dissolved in water, form a clear solution of electrolytes or sugars. These are aqueous solution of small molecules, which easily pass through capillary membranes, e.g., NS and balanced salt solutions.

Crystalloid replacement fluid contains a similar concentration of sodium to that of plasma. This ensures that they are excluded from the intracellular compartment since the cell membrane is generally impermeable to sodium. However, they readily cross the capillary membrane from the vascular compartment to the interstitial compartment to become rapidly distributed throughout the whole extracellular compartment.

Normally, only a quarter of the crystalloid solution remains in the vascular compartment.

Crystalloids should be infused in a volume at least three times the blood volume deficit in order to correct hypovolemia.

When large volumes of crystalloids fluid are administered, edema develops as a result of the fluid that passes (or "leaks") from the circulation into the interstitial compartment. Careful monitoring of the patient's clinical condition is therefore essential. Crystalloid maintenance fluids, which contain mainly dextrose, are not recommended for use as replacement fluids.

The dextrose rapidly becomes metabolized leaving only water, which readily crosses the capillary and cell wall membranes to become distributed throughout the extracellular and intracellular compartments. Only a small fraction remains in the vascular compartment, as shown in **Figure 1**.

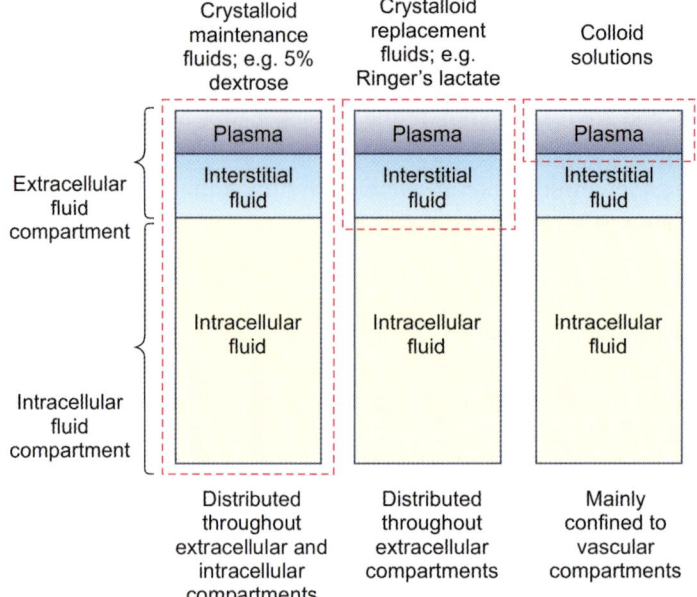

Fig. 1: Distribution spaces of various intravenous fluids.

Dextrose (glucose) solutions do not contain sodium and are poor resuscitation fluids. Do not use them to treat hypovolemia unless there is no other alternative.

Examples of crystalloid solutions are (*see* the content of each solution in the chart):
- NS (sodium chloride 0.9%)
- Ringer's lactate
- Hartmann's solution.

0.9% saline (NS or physiological saline or indifferent saline): It is not exactly known how 0.9% saline came to be used in clinical practice. It was the work of Hamburger, who showed that RBCs were least likely to lyse and compared to many other concentrations of the salt (saline). He called this solution *indifferent saline* because it had effect on RBCs. This terminology got corrupted over the years resulting in the names like *normal* and *physiological saline*. This solution is not at all physiological since it contains *154 mmol/L of sodium* and *154 mmol/L of chloride*, which is higher than the extracellular fluid. However, 0.9% saline became the most prescribed crystalloid in clinical practice. It is excreted more slowly compared to the balanced crystalloid such as Hartmann's solution and Ringer's lactate **(Fig. 1)**. However, blood volume expansions are similar. Saline will overload the interstitial space leading onto more edema.

Physiological changes of saline in the body:
- Mechanism of excretion of saline excess is not effective as a result of the suppression of the renin–angiotensin–aldosterone axis

- Toxic effect on the endothelial glycocalyx
- Hyperchloremic acidosis
- Postoperative hyperchloremia (serum chloride more than 110 mmol/L)
- Renal edema
- Decreased glomerular filtration rate (GFR).

Problems of hyperchloremia: However, recent studies show that 0.9% saline caused more side effects because of the *high-chloride* content, which will cause harm to the kidneys. The chances for hyperkalemia and metabolic acidosis are also there. Infectious complications and dialysis requirement (because of postoperative renal dysfunction) are more in saline treated patients compared to *chloride-restricted* fluid such as Hartmann's solution.

It is preferable to use balanced crystalloid solution and restrict the use of saline.

Check the daily chloride level in patients receiving NS.

Colloids: Colloid solutions are composed of a suspension of particles that have a much larger molecular weight than crystalloids. These particles are generally too big to pass through the capillary membrane and initially tend to remain within the vascular compartment. They are used as a replacement fluid, e.g., gelatins, dextrans, and hydroxyethyl starch. The effect of these particles in the circulation is to mimic plasma proteins, thereby maintaining or raising the colloid osmotic pressure of blood.

The molecular weight and number of particles in a colloid solution are important in determining its properties. The larger the particle sizes, the longer the duration of action of the solution in the vascular compartment. Also, the higher the number of particles in the solution, the greater the osmotic effect.

Solutions with an oncotic pressure greater than that of plasma have the capacity to draw water from the interstitial compartment into the blood. The increase in blood volume may thus exceed the infused volume.

Theoretically, colloids should have 100% efficiency in expanding the blood volume. But, in practice, 60–70% of the infused volume stays in the intravascular compartment. Infusion of colloids to euvolemic subjects will lead onto damage to the endothelial glycocalyx unlike in a hypovolemic subject.

Colloids can be classified as:
- *Plasma-derived (natural)*: Prepared from donated human blood or plasma (e.g., albumin 4%). These should not be used simply as replacement fluids.
- *Synthetic*: Prepared from another source (e.g., bovine cartilage)—
  - Gelatins (Haemaccel and Gelofusine)
  - Dextran 60 and Dextran 70
  - Hydroxyethyl starch (Hetastarch or *HES*)
  - Pentastarch.

6% HES: Recent meta-analysis has led to *ban on the use of HES in the UK* because of the increased mortality in patients treated with HES in the ICU. In the UK only, *gelatin and albumin* (4%) are the colloids licensed for use.

Colloids require smaller infusion volumes than crystalloids. They are usually given in a volume equal to the blood volume deficit.

However, in many conditions where the capillary permeability is increased, they may leak out of the circulation and produce only a short-lived volume expansion. Supplementary infusions will be necessary to maintain blood volume in conditions such as:
- Trauma
- Acute and chronic sepsis
- Burns
- Snake bite (hemotoxic and cytotoxic).

Properties of an Ideal Intravenous Replacement Fluid

The most important property of an IV replacement fluid is simply to occupy volume in the vascular compartment. An ideal replacement fluid should do this for a sufficient length of time and without interfering with the normal functions of the blood. Furthermore, it should be:
- Easily available and inexpensive
- Nontoxic
- Free of allergic reactions and risk of infection
- Totally metabolized or eliminated from the body.

Unfortunately, no fluid yet satisfies all these requirements. It is important, therefore, to be familiar with the properties and characteristics of the replacement fluids used in the hospital and to be able to use them safely.

The Crystalloids or Colloids Controversy

Much has been written about the crystalloids or colloids controversy, but it can be summarized as follows. Most clinicians agree that in hypovolemic patients, it is essential to restore blood volume with replacement fluids. However, they disagree on the type of fluid that should be used. Both crystalloids and colloids have advantages and disadvantages, as shown in **Table 1**.

However, ensuring that an adequate volume of replacement fluid (of whatever type) is administered to a hypovolemic patient is more important than the choice of fluid.

There is no evidence that colloids solutions are superior to NS or balanced salt solutions in resuscitation.

If the supply of infusion fluids is limited, it is recommended that wherever possible, the crystalloid NS (sodium chloride 0.9%) or a balanced salt solution such as Ringer's lactate or Hartmann's solution should be available in all hospitals where IV replacement fluids are used.

Intravenous Fluids and Postoperative Fluid Management

Table 1: Advantages and disadvantages of crystalloids and colloids.

	Advantages	Disadvantages
Crystalloids	• Few side effects • Low cost • Wide availability	• Short duration of action • May cause edema
Colloids	• Longer duration of action • Less fluid required to correct hypovolemia	• No evidence that they are more clinically effective • Renal dysfunction • Disturbed coagulation • Allergic response • Higher cost • May cause volume overload • May interfere with clotting • Risk of anaphylactic reactions

Before giving any IV infusion:
- Check that the seal of the infusion fluid bottle or bag is not broken.
- Check the expiry date.
- Check that the solution is clear and free from visible particles.

Plasma-derived Colloids

These are prepared from donated blood or plasma. They include:
- Plasma
- Fresh frozen plasma
- Liquid plasma
- Freeze-dried plasma
- Albumin (4%).

These products should not be used simply as replacement fluids. They can carry a similar risk of transmitting infection such as HIV and hepatitis, as whole blood. They are also generally more expensive than crystalloid or synthetic colloid fluids.

Table 2 shows the composition of fluids and plasma.

The National Institute for Health and Care Excellence Guidelines for Resuscitation

- Crystalloids containing sodium in the range of 130–154 mmol/L should be used for resuscitation rather than colloids.
- Initial bolus of 500 mL should be given over < 15 minutes.
- Tetra starches should no longer be used.
- Albumin could be considered in severe sepsis.

Redistribution

Many surgical patients have marked internal fluid and electrolyte distribution changes after major surgical interventions. Many patients develop high

Table 2: Composition of replacement fluids and plasma.

Fluid	Na^+ Nmol/L	K^+ Nmol/L	Ca^{2+} Nmol/L	Cl^- Nmol/L	Base mEq/L	Colloid osmotic pressure (mm Hg)
Crystalloids:						
• Normal saline sodium chloride (0.9%)	154	0	0	154	0	0
• Balanced salt solutions (Ringer's lactate/Hartmann's solution)	130–140	4–5	2–3	109–110	28–30	0
Colloids: Gelatine (urea linked), e.g., Haemaccel	145	5.1	6.25	145	Trace amounts	27
Gelatine (succinylated), e.g., Gelofusine	154	<0.4	<0.4	125	Trace amounts	34
Dextran 70 (6%)	154	0	0	154	0	58
Dextran 60 (3%)	130	4	2	110	30	22
Hydroxyethyl starch 450/0.7 (6%)	154	0	0	154	0	28
Albumin (5%)	130–160	<1	V	V	V	27
Ionic composition of normal plasma	135–145	3.5–5.5	2.2–2.6	97–110	38–44	27

(V: varies between different brands)

transcapillary escape resulting in whole body sodium and water excess. This will result in pulmonary and peripheral edema. It can lead onto weight gain and compartment syndrome. It can also lead onto poor wound healing, edema of the intestine, and leakage of anastomosis. The low intravascular volume will result in renal dysfunction. IV fluid prescriptions are extremely difficult in such situations.

Reassessment (5th R)
- Daily reassessment of fluid intake and output should be checked
- Daily clinical assessment
- Weight measurement twice weekly
- Laboratory monitoring of urea, creatinine, and electrolytes daily
- Measurement of chloride in patients getting saline
- Intermittent monitoring of urinary sodium.

Intraoperative Flow-directed Fluid Therapy

Intraoperative hypotension or occult hypovolemia will lead onto reduced splanchnic perfusion and oxygenation. The healthy patients can tolerate 25–30% reduction in blood volume without changes in BP and heart rate. However, splanchnic hypoperfusion can occur after 10–15% reduction in blood volume. Intraoperative flow-directed fluid therapy was developed to improve the stroke volume, cardiac index, and splanchnic perfusion. Transesophageal Doppler (TOD) is one such device used for intraoperative measurement of stroke volume corrected flow time in the descending aorta. Bolus of 200–250 mL of colloid solution is given over 5–10 minutes when the flow time (FTc) is < 0.35. A stroke volume increase of more than 10% or FTc <0.35 is indicative of intravascular hypovolemia and further bolus is given. Significant reduction in overall complications, GI complications, and reduction in hospital stay was observed in patients receiving flow-directed fluid therapy. The need for ICU stay was also reduced in such patients. It is useful in high-risk patients with expected blood loss more than 500 mL. Therefore, it is preferable to practice *restrictive fluid therapy* in the postoperative period.

FACTORS AFFECTED BY ACID-BASE IMBALANCE

As a result of acid-base imbalance, the following four clinical entities can occur.

Respiratory acidosis may be produced by any condition or combination of conditions that result in inadequate ventilation (atelectasis, pneumonia, and airway obstruction). The clinical signs or restlessness, hypertension, and tachycardia in the postoperative patient may indicate the presence of hypercapnia. Treatment consists of providing adequate ventilation and correcting the pulmonary problem when possible.

Respiratory alkalosis in the surgical patient is caused, usually by hyperventilation secondary to apprehension, pain, brain injury, or overventilation by mechanical respirators. If the condition is mild, no therapy is required. When the cause of hyperventilation can be determined and corrected, the problem is eliminated.

Metabolic acidosis may occur as a result of acute circulatory failure or renal damage, chloride excess, loss of lower gastrointestinal fluids, administration of unbalanced salt solutions, and uncontrolled diabetes mellitus. Correction of protracted metabolic acidosis may require the use of sodium bicarbonate. When cardiopulmonary arrest occurs, restoration of blood flow, pulmonary ventilation, and administration of sodium bicarbonate is required.

Metabolic alkalosis usually occurs when some degree of hypokalemia exists. It occurs when there is an uncomplicated loss of acids (H^+ ion) or retention of bases. Because of the associated hypokalemia, cardiac arrhythmias, paralytic ileus, digitalis intoxication, and tetany may develop.

Dangerous hyperkalemia (>6 mEq/L) is unusual, if kidney function is normal. Generally, it is unwise to administer potassium during the first 24 hours postoperatively unless there is a definite hypokalemia. These deficits should be replaced after an adequate urine output is obtained. The daily replacement of potassium for renal excretion is 40 mEq plus 20 mEq for gastrointestinal loss, if indicated; it should not be administered parenterally in concentrations of >40 mEq per liter as potassium chloride.

27 Intestinal Anastomosis

Madhu Muralee

INTRODUCTION

The success and failure of any gastrointestinal surgery depends on the sound techniques and methods adopted to do resection and anastomosis of intestinal segments. The understanding of principles of bowel healing and evolution of techniques and technology has helped us to improve the outcomes of intestinal anastomosis. Still, it remains one of the cornerstones in gastrointestinal surgery, which all surgical residents have to master.

SURGICAL ANATOMY

Understanding the anatomy and vascularity of bowel wall is of paramount importance as far as safe intestinal anastomosis is concerned. The four layers of the bowel wall are:
1. Mucosa
2. Submucosa
3. Muscularis propria
4. Serosa.

The submucosa is the "STRONG MAN" of the anastomosis and the outcomes of all anastomosis depend on how this layer is handled with the exception of esophagus where the mucosa is considered to be the strong man. The age-old dictum goes that the submucosa must be included in every suture pass while doing an anastomosis **(Fig. 1)**.

Anatomic Peculiarity of Esophagus

Contrary to most other hollow viscus, the esophagus is devoid of serosa. The mucosa is considered to be the strongest layer of the esophagus. The most common anastomosis done in esophagus is the esophagogastric tube anastomosis done either in the thorax as in the case of Ivor Lewis operation or in the neck as in case of McKeown operation.

Anatomical Peculiarity of Stomach

The vascular supply of the stomach is much more robust than that of the small intestine **(Fig. 2)**. The left and right gastric arteries along with the

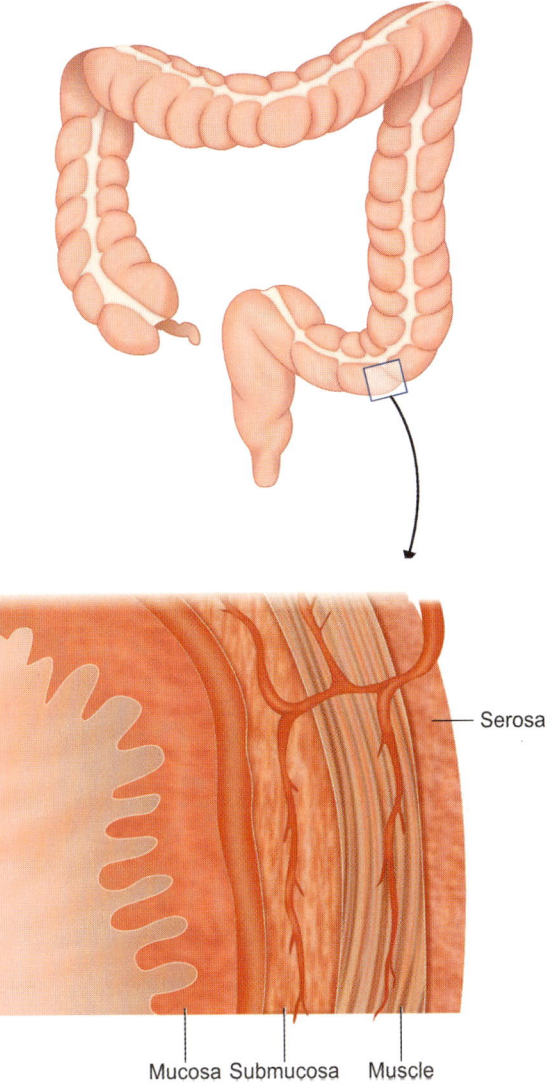

Fig. 1: Anatomy of the bowel wall.

gastroepiploic arcades form a rich plexus of vessels within the various layers of the stomach wall. Ischemia of the cut ends or the anastomosing ends is almost never a reason for failure of a gastric anastomosis.

Anatomical Peculiarity of Small Intestine

The vascular supply to the small intestine is as shown in **Figure 3**. The mesenteric artery gives rise to the arcuate system and from the arcuate system arises vessels known as vasa recta, which supply the small intestine. The vasa recta are considered to be end arteries. It is obvious that the antimesenteric

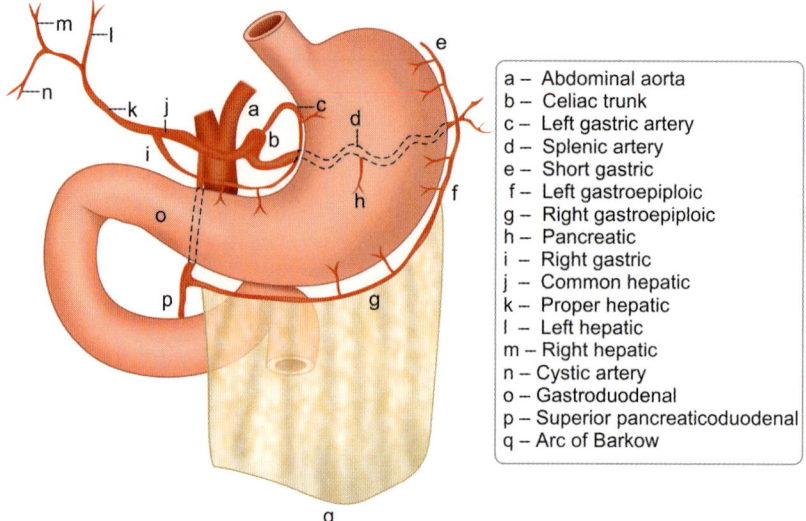

Fig. 2: Vascular anatomy of the stomach.

a – Abdominal aorta
b – Celiac trunk
c – Left gastric artery
d – Splenic artery
e – Short gastric
f – Left gastroepiploic
g – Right gastroepiploic
h – Pancreatic
i – Right gastric
j – Common hepatic
k – Proper hepatic
l – Left hepatic
m – Right hepatic
n – Cystic artery
o – Gastroduodenal
p – Superior pancreaticoduodenal
q – Arc of Barkow

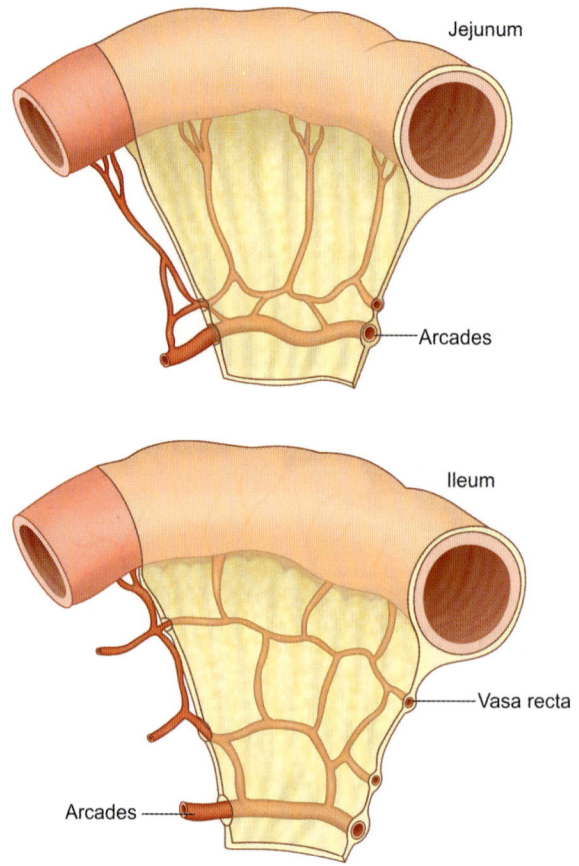

Fig. 3: Vascularity of the small bowel.

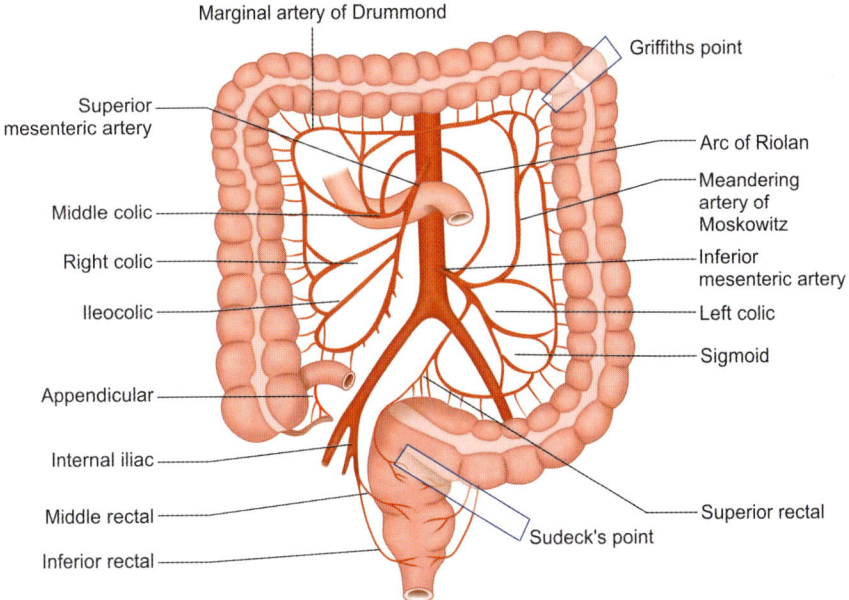

Fig. 4: Mesenteric vascular arcades and critical points of ischemia.

borders of the bowel are at the highest risk for ischemia. This fact should be borne in mind whenever an anastomosis is being planned.

Anatomical Peculiarity of Large Intestine

The vascular anatomy of the large intestine is special in that it draws its blood supply from the superior mesenteric arterial system and inferior mesenteric arterial system, which are vessels of the midgut and hindgut, respectively. Interconnecting these arterial systems is what are known as mesenteric arcades as shown in **Figure 4**. However, there are areas prone for ischemia in the large bowel known as the Griffiths point and the Sudeck's point **(Fig. 4)**.

SUTURE TYPES

A thorough knowledge of the suture materials being used can go a long way in choosing the ideal suture material for a particular anastomosis **(Box 1)**. There is no evidence to suggest that one suture type is better than the other in terms of creating a successful anastomosis.

There are certain basic medical terminologies associated with the nature of a suture material that all surgeons need to understand for the proper selection of suture material. The properties associated are given in **Table 1**.

The natural sutures are silk, cotton, linen, and the catgut. But, most of these suture materials are not commonly used these days and are being

Box 1: Features of an ideal suture material.
- Easy to handle
- Minimal tissue injury or tissue reaction
- Secure knotting (no fraying or cutting)
- High tensile strength
- Favorable absorption profile
- Resistant to infection
- Can be used in any tissue

Table 1: Properties of a suture material.

• Absorbable	Progressive loss of mass and/or volume of suture material; does not correlate with initial tensile strength
• Capillarity	Extent to which absorbed fluid is transferred along the suture
• Knot pull tensile strength	Breaking strength of knotted suture material (10–40% weaker after deformation by knot placement)
• Memory	Inherent capability of suture to return to or maintain its original gross shape
• Plasticity	Measure of the ability to deform without breaking and to maintain a new form after relief of the deforming force
• Pliability	Ease of handling of suture material; ability to adjust knot tension and to secure knots

Table 2: Classification of suture materials.

Natural	Synthetic
Absorbable	Nonabsorbable
Monofilament	Multifilament

replaced by synthetic sutures **(Table 2)**. This is because of the fact that the properties can be modified according to the need. The tensile strength, elasticity, plasticity, and absorption properties can be altered based on the necessity in case of a synthetic suture. Moreover, it has the added advantage that it can be coated/impregnated with antibiotics, which can lead to a reduction in the incidence of surgical site infections.

Synthetic sutures can be monofilament sutures or multifilament sutures with each having its own advantages and disadvantages as given in **Box 2**.

How to choose a right suture material?

When you choose a suture material, it should satisfy the following conditions:
- Choose the smallest suture that holds the tissue edges
- Tensile strength of the suture should never exceed the tensile strength of the tissue
- The relative loss of suture strength over time should be slower than the gain of tissue tensile strength.

Box 2: Advantages and disadvantages of monofilament and multifilament sutures.

Monofilament sutures:
Advantages:
- Have less tissue drag
- Do not have interstices that may harbor bacteria

Disadvantages:
- Impairs handling and knot tying more difficult
- Nicking or damaging them with forceps or needle holder weakens them and predisposes them to breakage

Multifilament sutures:
Advantages:
- More pliable and flexible than monofilament sutures
- Results in considerably better knot-holding security

Disadvantages:
- High capillarity
- Have a rough surface

Table 3: Nature of tissue and choice of suture material.

Nature of healing	Nature of tissue	Choice of suture
Slowly healing tissues	Skin, fascia, and tendon	Nonabsorbable
Rapidly healing tissues	Mucosa	Absorbable sutures

Table 4: List of sutures—absorbable.

Generic name	Characteristic	Profile
Chromic surgical gut	Multifilament and organic	14–21 days
Polyglactin	Multifilament and synthetic	60–70 days
Polyglycolic acid	Absorbable, multifilament, and synthetic	60–90 days
Poliglecaprone 25	Monofilament and synthetic	100–120 days
Polydioxanone	Monofilament and synthetic	200–230 days

Table 5: List of sutures—nonabsorbable.

Generic name	Characteristic
Silk	Multifilament and organic
Polyester	Multifilament and synthetic
Polyamide (nylon)	Monofilament and synthetic Multifilament and synthetic
Polypropylene	Monofilament and synthetic
Stainless steel wire	Monofilament or multifilament, metallic

The nature of the tissue that we intend to suture also has to be taken into consideration when choosing the suture material. The general principles are outlined in **Tables 3 to 5**.

GENERAL PRINCIPLES OF GASTROINTESTINAL SUTURING

The success of a bowel anastomosis depends on:
- *Good blood supply*: Bright red and pulsatile bleeding from the cut edges is a prerequisite for a safe anastomosis. If the vascularity of the cut edges is in doubt then the edges have to be cut back.
- *Tension free anastomosis*: Tension at the anastomotic site should be avoided at all cost. The proximal and distal ends should be adequately mobilized so that they come together without any tension.
- *Meticulous technique*: Careful tissue handling during the suturing process is of utmost importance. Holding the mucosa with instruments should be avoided as far as possible.

SINGLE-LAYER VERSUS DOUBLE-LAYER ANASTOMOSIS

A hand-sewn anastomosis can be done in single layer or two layers. If a single layer anastomosis is done as in a colocolic anastomosis, then a nonabsorbable suture material is preferred. But, if a two-layer anastomosis is being done, then the inner layer is usually an absorbable suture material and the outer layer a nonabsorbable material.

As far as the evidence is concerned, there is nothing to choose between a hand-sewn single-layer and double-layer anastomoses. Both have been compared in a 2012 Cochrane review. There was no difference between the two in terms of anastomotic failure, morbidity, and mortality rates. The only difference was that single-layer anastomosis was faster than double-layer anastomosis.

Types of Anastomosis

- *End-to-end*: An end-to-end anastomosis is considered to be the most "physiologic" one because the normal i.e. of the gut and motility is regained here.
- *End-to-side*: End of one loop is anastomosed to the side of the other loop. The end of one loop of bowel is anastomosed to the antimesenteric border in case of small bowel loop and to the taeniae in case of large bowel. This technique is used to overcome the size mismatch between bowel loops.
- *Side-to-side*: This again is a technique to overcome the size mismatch between the loops. Moreover, the advantage is that you avoid the end, which is at the highest risk of ischemia in such an anastomosis.

Overcoming Size Disparities between Bowel Ends

There are situations where there is a significant size mismatch between the bowel loops that needs to be anastomosed. Options of anastomosis in such a situation are:
- *Side-to-side or end-to-side reconstructions*: In a side-to-side anastomosis, the ends of the bowel are closed and a side-to-side anastomosis is created

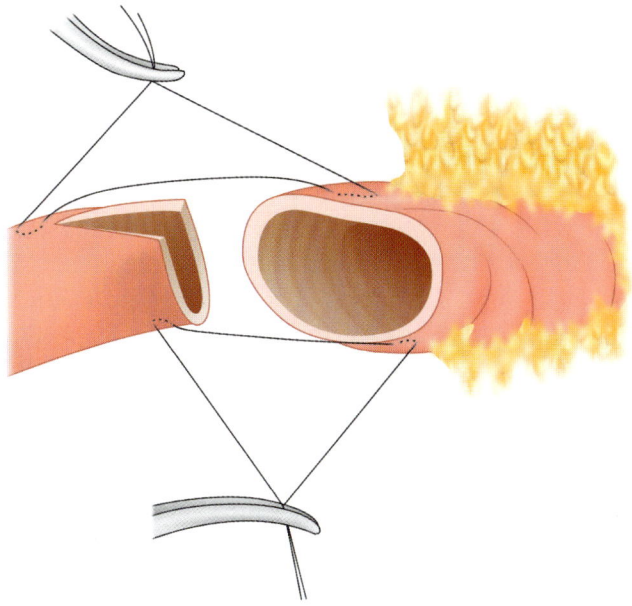

Fig. 5: Cheatle cut on the antimesenteric border.

so that the size mismatch is overcome. In an end-to-side anastomosis, end of one loop is anastomosed to the side of the other loop.
- *Stealing*: Small size mismatches can be overcome by what is known as the technique of "stealing". This is achieved by differential suture travel on each side of the bowel.
- *Cheatle cut*: Larger mismatches can overcome by making a small incision, a longitudinal slit on the antimesenteric border of bowel of the smaller caliber **(Fig. 5)**. This will effectively augment the circumference of the smaller caliber bowel so that it matches the caliber of the bowel with larger lumen to permit an end-to-end anastomosis.
- *Emergency bowel surgery*: In an emergency situation such as trauma or obstruction, the bowel anastomosis is fraught with increased chance of complications. This is because of the fact that the bowel is edematous and friable. There may be a mismatch between the luminal diameter of the segment proximal to the obstruction and distal to the obstruction. Even though there are no randomized control trials to guide the choice of suture and technique of suturing in such a situation, it is generally believed that hand-sewn anastomosis is better than a stapled anastomosis.

TECHNIQUES OF HAND-SEWN ANASTOMOSIS

End-to-End Hand-sewn Anastomosis

The first step in any anastomosis is to approximate the ends together. This can be achieved by stay sutures placed at the mesenteric and

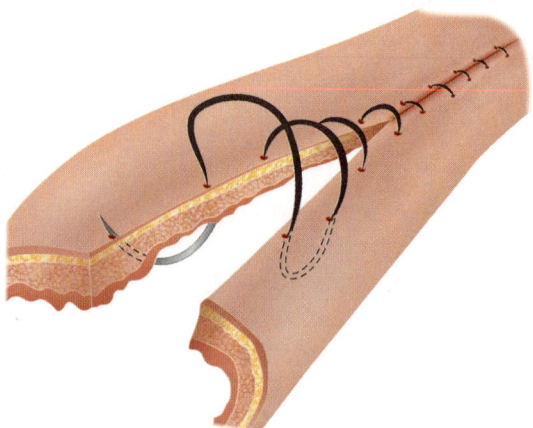

Fig. 6: Connell sutures.

antimesenteric borders. Once they are aligned together, the anastomosis can be done in single layer or double layer. If a double layer is being done, the inner layer can be continuous or interrupted.

No studies have shown the superiority of one technique over the other. But, it is a universally accepted fact that mucosal inversion has to be made sure while carrying out the anastomosis. The age-old dictum of "More of Serosa and less of Mucosa" should be the guiding principle of any anastomosis.

Lembert Sutures

If a second layer is being done, it is by means of the seromuscular Lembert sutures. The anastomosis integrity can be checked by gently squeezing both ends of the anastomosis to ensure no enteric spillage. The patency of the lumen also should be checked. At the end, the mesenteric defect is closed to prevent internal herniation.

Too tight a suturing and too many sutures also can be dangerous, as they can produce ischemia. The bite on each side of the bowel is roughly equal to the thickness of the tissue (i.e., 3-6 mm) and the sutures are spaced approximately twice this distance apart (i.e., 6-10 mm). The general rule is to take sutures 0.5 cm from the edges and 0.5 cm away from the previous suture to ensure that they are neither too close not too far.

The Connell Suture

The Connell technique of suturing was devised to invert the mucosa and get a watertight closure. The basic principle is as shown in **Figure 6**. The suturing goes by *"outside in-inside out on one side followed by outside in-inside out on the other side"* thereby ensuring complete mucosal inversion. This is usually done when a single layer anastomosis is being planned. This can be reinforced by a second layer as well.

Esophagogastric Anastomosis

As mentioned earlier, this can be done in the thorax as part of Ivor Lewis surgery or in the neck as part of McKeown surgery. It can either be a stapled anastomosis or hand-sewn anastomosis or a hybrid anastomosis:

- *Hand-sewn anastomosis*: When a hand-sewn anastomosis is planned between the esophagus and the stomach tube, it is usually an end-to-side anastomosis (end of esophagus to side of stomach tube). It can be a single-layer or double-layer anastomosis.
  If it is single layer, the choice of suture material can be a 3/0 polypropylene suture or polydioxanone. In case a double-layer anastomosis is planned, the inner layer is a continuous absorbable suture material and outer layer is an interrupted nonabsorbable suture material.
- *Stapled anastomosis*: If an intrathoracic end-to-side anastomosis is being done as in case of Ivor Lewis surgery, the stapler of choice is a circular stapler of size 25 **(Fig. 7)**.
- *Hybrid anastomosis*: In case of a neck anastomosis as in case of McKeown surgery, it can be a hybrid anastomosis called modified Collard anastomosis **(Fig. 8)**. Here, the posterior walls are anastomosed side-to-side using linear cutter and the anterior wall is stapled by a double-layer suturing technique.

Esophagojejunal Anastomosis

This is usually done after a total gastrectomy. This again can be a hand-sewn anastomosis or a stapled anastomosis. In case of a hand-sewn anastomosis, a double-layer anastomosis with an inner 3/0 interrupted polydioxanone and outer 3/0 continuous polypropylene is preferred by many surgeons. But, the most commonly performed anastomosis in esophagojejunostomy at the authors' center is a stapled end-to-side anastomosis suing a circular stapler of size 25.

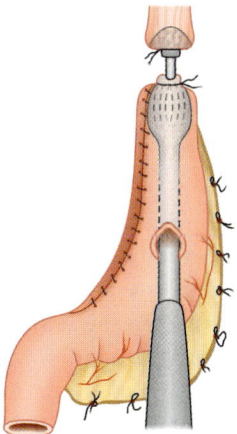

Fig. 7: Intrathoracic esophagogastric anastomosis using circular staplers as in Ivor Lewis operation.

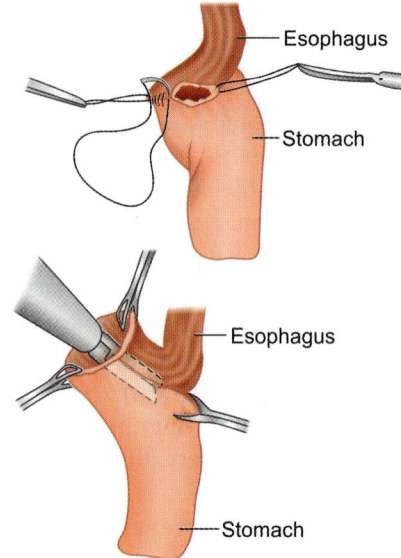

Fig. 8: Modified Collard anastomosis as in McKeown operation.

Gastric Anastomosis

A gastrojejunostomy is the most common anastomosis done after a resectional surgery of the stomach. Here again, it can be hand sewn or stapled. A hand-sewn anastomosis is always a two-layer anastomosis with inner 3-0 absorbable continuous and outer nonabsorbable interrupted sutures. This is classically called the four-layer anastomosis:
1. The first layer being the posterior interrupted seromuscular layer.
2. The second being the inner continuous full-thickness layer.
3. The third being the outer continuous full-thickness layer, which actually is a continuation of the second layer.
4. The fourth layer being the anterior interrupted seromuscular layer.

In case of stapled anastomosis, it is a side-to-side anastomosis with a liner cutter. The point to be noted is that stomach being a thick-walled structure, a stapler with thicker pins is preferred (green staplers).

Ileocolic Anastomosis

An ileocolic anastomosis is usually done after a right or extender right hemicolectomy or as a bypass procedure. As there is a size disparity between the ileum and colon, the anastomosis usually is made in a side-to-side manner. This can be a hand-sewn anastomosis or a stapled anastomosis.

But, an end-to-side (end of ileum to side of colon) or end-to-end anastomosis using a Cheatle cut made on the antimesenteric border of ileum is possible.

The side-to-side ileocolic anastomosis is one where the evidence is in favor of a stapled anastomosis. The 2011 Cochrane review showed that the stapled anastomoses were associated with lesser leak rate compared with hand-sewn anastomoses. The side-to-side hand-sewn anastomosis is usually done in a double layer.

Colocolic Anastomosis

Colocolic anastomosis is usually an end-to-end anastomosis and a hand-sewn anastomosis is preferred by most surgeons. It can be a single-layer anastomosis using a nonabsorbable 3/0 suture material and in such a case, it is interrupted sutures that are placed. In case of a double-layered anastomosis, the inner layer is a continuous absorbable suture material and outer layer is an interrupted nonabsorbable suture material.

Colorectal Anastomosis

This is usually done after an anterior resection or sigmoid resection. Colorectal anastomosis can be end-to-end as well as side-to-end (side of colon to end of rectum). This can be done using a circular stapler. Hand-sewn and stapled colorectal anastomoses for a colorectal anastomosis have been compared in a 2012 Cochrane review. There was no significant difference in the anastomotic failure rate regardless of the level of anastomosis. But, as we go lower down in the pelvis as in the case of low anterior resection or ultralow anterior resection, a circular stapler is preferred over hand-sewn anastomosis. The size of the circular stapler is decided based on the size of the lumen. Usually, a 28/29 size stapler is used in females and a 31/33 is preferred in males.

Large Bowel Anastomosis and Bowel Preparation

Unprepared or loaded large bowel as experienced during emergency surgery can be a major problem while doing a large bowel resection and anastomosis. Most surgeons prefer a prepared bowel while carrying out a large bowel anastomosis. There are evidences for and against bowel preparation before a colonic surgery. But it remains a fact that while resecting and carrying out the anastomosis, there should not be any spillage of bowel content because it can lead on to an increased incidence of surgical site infection.

STAPLERS IN SURGERY

Surgical staplers used for bowel resection and reconstruction can be broadly classified as follows:
- *Transverse anastomosis (TA) staplers*: Even though they are called transverse anastomosing staplers, they are not actually anastomosing staplers. They are basically linear staplers without cutting properties. After stapling with a TA stapler, the specimen needs to be divided manually. They can also be used for closing ostomies.

- *Linear cutting staplers*: These are anastomosing staplers, which have cutting properties. Two to three rows of staplers are fired on both sides and the cutting mechanism cuts in-between these rows to complete the transection.
- *Circular staplers*: These are anastomosing staplers with cutting properties. They can be used as end-to-end as well as side-to-end anastomosing staplers. The stapling and cutting take place intraluminally.

The staplers are made of titanium. The size, stapler thickness, and length of staple lines vary from manufacturer to manufacturer. The stapler thickness and length/circumference is color coded but unfortunately they differ from manufacturer to manufacturer.

Some general principles followed while choosing the stapler:
- *Thick-walled bowel*: Green staplers
- *Thin-walled structure*: Blue staplers
- *Vascular staplers*: White staplers.

COMMON ANASTOMOSIS IN A NUTSHELL

Common anastomoses are described in **Table 6.**

Table 6: Common anastomoses.

Cervical esophagogastric anastomosis (McKeown)	Side-to-side	*Modified Collard anastomosis*: Posterior wall stapled with linear cutter and anterior wall with two-layer hand-sewn anastomosis	
Intrathoracic esophagogastric anastomosis (Ivor Lewis)	End-to-side	Circular stapler—size 25	
Esophagogastric anastomosis	End-to-side	Circular stapler—size 25	
		Hand-sewn end-to-side two layer	Inner 3/0 absorbable interrupted Outer 3/0 nonabsorbable interrupted
Gastrojejunostomy	Side-to-side	Hand sewn	Inner 3/0 absorbable interrupted Outer 3/0 nonabsorbable interrupted
		Stapled	Linear cutter green
Ileocolic anastomosis	Side-to-side	Hand sewn	Inner 3/0 absorbable interrupted Outer 3/0 nonabsorbable interrupted
		Stapled	Linear cutter blue
Colocolic	End-to-end	Single layer	Nonabsorbable 3/0
Colorectal	End-to-end	Circular stapler	28/29 or 31/33

Note: Two other areas where staplers are used in surgery are stapled hemorrhoidectomy and skin staplers.

28

Vascular Anastomosis

RC Sreekumar

INTRODUCTION

Earliest name in the history of vascular anastomosis and organ transplantation is Alexis Carrel, who is also known as the father of vascular anastomosis. He was way ahead of his time when he developed the fine suturing methods that he learned from textile embroiders at his native of France, after being moved by the death of the French president, Sadi Carnot. Carnot had a stab injury to the portal vein which could not be repaired by the physicians.

As early as 1896, Jaboulay had published an article on end-to-end anastomosis of the carotid artery which abolished the earlier idea that sutures placed on blood vessels could lead to their early thrombosis, hence furthering the damage.

From 1904 to 1906, Alexis Carrel worked at the University of Chicago along with Charles Guthrie perfecting the technique of vascular anastomoses and the use of vein graft for damaged arteries. Alexis Carrel's work is remarkable in that he had ventured into the field of vascular surgery even before the era of anticoagulants. His concepts of gentle tissue handling and the technique of triangulation for vascular anastomosis were critical to the development of vascular surgery. It was for these contributions that he received Nobel Prize for Medicine in the year 1912.

Kunlin had introduced a revolutionary technique to join a vein graft to artery by end-to-side interposition.

BASICS OF VASCULAR RECONSTRUCTION

The essential components of vascular anastomosis include:
- Blood vessel exposure
- Blood vessel dissection
- Anticoagulation
- Blood vessel control
- Creation of a blood vessel incision (arteriotomy)
- Preparation of a patch or a bypass
- Construction of the suture line
- Securing hemostasis
- Evaluating the vascular reconstruction

- Postoperative surveillance and care
- *Blood vessel exposure*: In general, the skin incisions placed along the longitudinal axis of the vessel to be exposed to facilitate proximal and distal extension of the same. Anatomic landmark and pulse are the usual guides.
- *Blood vessel dissection*: Vessels are dissected sharply using blunt-tipped scissors or a 15 blade is used in case of scarred tissue as in redo surgeries. Inadvertent injury caused by blade is easier to repair than that caused by scissors. Once vessel is seen, adequate exposure is made sure by using self-retaining retractors, applied carefully. Debakey vascular forceps are used to hold the adventitia and gentle traction and countertraction given so that avascular plane between the vessel and surrounding structures appears and dissection is continued parallel to the vessel wall. Although dissection is done circumferentially, it is not always needed as in case of infrarenal aorta. The vessels should be handled gently, only adventitia should be grasped. A "no-touch" technique by using silastic loops to handle the vessels can be practiced. Thorough knowledge of the course of an artery and the position of its branches should be known and hence the vessel should be traced. Branches should be preserved as many as possible as they may represent major collateral channels.
- *Anticoagulation*: Systemic anticoagulation is necessary before clamping the vessels for reconstruction to prevent distal thrombosis during cross-clamping. A loading dose of 75–100 U/kg of heparin is used often for vascular procedures. Cross-clamping is done after waiting for 3–5 minutes and a supplemental dose is administered if clamp time exceeds 2 hours. Activated clotting time is used to guide heparin dosing intraoperatively. Antiplatelet agents are usually started preoperatively and continued in the postoperative period. Warfarin may be added with caution in certain patients with prothrombotic state, graft occlusion, etc.
- *Blood vessel control*: The artery should be gently palpated for presence and location of atherosclerotic plaque using index finger or pinching between index and thumb or against a right-angled clamp. Manipulation should be gentle as it can cause embolization. Several methods are available for controlling blood vessels like use of atraumatic vascular clamps, tapes with Rumel tourniquet silastic vessel loops, internal occluders, or external pneumatic tourniquet. The vascular clamp should be applied in a manner that would oppose the soft wall of the artery against the hard plaque without breaking the plaque or tearing the artery. In the presence of posterior plaque, the vascular clamp is applied to oppose the anterior and posterior walls together. In the presence of a plaque on the sidewall, the vascular clamp is applied to oppose the lateral and medial walls against each other. A Rumel tourniquet can be used to achieve vascular control in medium-sized arteries such as the common femoral or common carotid arteries. Thick silk or umbilical tape is looped around the vessel, brought

out through a short rubber catheter using a snare, and tightened against vessel using artery clamp. Single or double loop of silastic loop can be used to control small vessels as "no-touch" technique. Undue tension with silastic loop will not open up the arteriotomy and problem could be avoided by replacing the distal vessel loop with an aneurysm clip. It may not adequately occlude diseased/calcified vessels/large vessels. Internal occluders are used for small caliber vessels and maintain flow distally.

- *Creation of blood vessel incision*: An 11 blade is usually used to start the longitudinal incision in the blood vessel. The blade is introduced at a 45º angle and then advanced in a forward movement carefully, not touching the posterior wall creating sufficient space for Potts scissors to enlarge the incision. Heavily diseased vessels may be opened with teasing incision over the anterior wall using 15 blades. For common procedures like embolectomy, transverse arteriotomy is made, usually with 15 blade. Care should be taken to keep the arteriotomy size to nearly half the diameter of the vessel, more than which makes primary closure difficult and almost always causes stenosis.

- *Preparation of bypass graft*: Before starting the suture line, the size of the opening in the bypass should be checked to match appropriately the length of incision in the blood vessel. Always splice the graft after creating arteriotomy. If the arteriotomy is found to be more than the graft incision, meeting the size discrepancy is more demanding.

- *Suture line construction*: Magnifying loupe of 2.5–3.5 power is recommended for vascular reconstruction. We should introduce the needle from intimal side toward adventitia (in-out) and the reverse will cause creation of flap or dissection due to separation of intima. In soft nondiseased arteries, the needle can be safely placed from the adventitial side of the wall. The needle should enter the wall at right angle and followed along its curvature. The needle tip should never be held as it destroys the needle and hence further bites also.

  The full thickness of wall should never be held even with most atraumatic forceps and only adventitia should be grasped to open up the wall or fine suture stays can be placed. In general, bites on aorta are 3-4 mm deep and 2-3 mm apart whereas in medium and small vessels, 1-2 mm deep and 1 mm apart. Bites far apart can cause bleeding, crumpling of suture line, and later pseudoaneurysm. Adventitia should be cleared off the suture line as it is thrombogenic. Assistant should always maintain adequate tension on the suture and nerve hook can be used to adjust the final tension in the suture line before tying.

- *Securing homeostasis*: Before tying the suture line, the vessel lumen is irrigated with heparinized saline to flush out any debris. Forward and backward bleeding should also be rechecked before completing the suture line. The distal clamps are released first. The proximal clamps are then partially released to identify obvious leaks when extra sutures can be

taken or loose sutures tightened. Weeping suture line usually settles with heparin reversal and pressure. Flow is opened to least critical outflow vessel to let air/debris to pass into that instead of vital circulation (e.g., external carotid artery before internal carotid artery).
- *Evaluating the vascular reconstruction*: Although presence of distal pulse is the most satisfying sign for operating surgeon, other noninvasive modalities like handheld Doppler and duplex ultrasound are employed to confirm the technical adequacy of bypass. In case of hybrid operating rooms, an angiogram can be done to visualize the distal outflow and flow in bypass graft.
- *Postoperative surveillance and care*: The leg should be kept warm. Wound care is needed in some patients. Ankle brachial index should be monitored serially in the postoperative period starting from day 1. Antiplatelets should be continued along with anticoagulation as the case may be. Development of hematoma should be watched out for and evacuated promptly if causing compression on the bypass graft. Infection and lymphorrhea are major problems in groin wounds, especially in uncontrolled diabetics and should be treated aggressively more so if there is prosthetic graft.

CLOSURE OF ARTERIOTOMY

An arteriotomy can be closed primarily where the walls are sutured directly to each other or by using a vein/prosthetic patch to bridge the defect between the walls termed as patch closure/patch angioplasty. The method depends on the size of the artery, the direction and the shape of the arteriotomy, and the presence of atherosclerotic plaque. The basic principle of arteriotomy closure is to avoid luminal compromise or to create a lumen slightly larger than the native diameter.
- *Primary closure of transverse arteriotomy*: Undiseased arteries can be closed primarily even with 1.5–2.0 mm diameter such as the radial or the posterior tibial artery. Similarly, most longitudinal incisions in undiseased arteries with a diameter >5 mm such as the common carotid artery or the common femoral artery can also be closed primarily. Some degree of narrowing of the lumen is likely to occur with primary closure and could threaten the patency of the reconstruction, especially in longitudinal incisions. Patch closure should be considered in such cases.

It is usually performed with continuous running suture introduced first from the adventitial surface of one wall usually along the direction of flow and then from the intimal surface of the opposite wall avoiding any dissecting flap by pushing the plaque away from the wall. The depth and advancement of the bites should be even throughout the length of the suture line. Bites too thin will cut through the arterial wall while too deep a bite causes focal narrowing of lumen. In small vessels and heavily diseased arteries, interrupted sutures can be taken for closure.

- *Patch closure of longitudinal arteriotomy*: It is warranted by technical factors like a jagged incision, a very tortuous artery, a longitudinal incision in an artery <5 mm in diameter and the presence of calcified plaque at the arteriotomy site, nonapproximation of walls due to scarring, obstructive pathology like neointimal hyperplasia that cannot be excised, etc. Nontechnical factors include recurrent thrombosis/stenosis. In patch closure, the needle can be introduced constantly from the adventitial aspect of the patch and then from the intimal aspect of the arterial wall. Good-size bites can be taken in patch and artery without causing luminal compromise. Aneurysmal dilatation could occur when the width of the patch significantly exceeds the diameter of the vessel to be repaired. Patch can be anchored or parachuted down and sutures continued or two anchoring sutures can be placed at each end of the patch tied down and sutured to either side.

TECHNIQUES OF ANASTOMOSIS

- *End-to-side anastomosis*: The proximal and distal anastomoses are constructed in an end-to-side fashion for most bypasses performed for peripheral occlusive diseases. It allows inflow to be taken from least diseased area of the vessel while maintaining the native flow. The distal anastomosis helps to create antegrade and retrograde flow.

  The geometry of an end-to-side anastomosis depends on the diameters of the bypass and the artery and the length of the anastomosis, which will influence the angle of transection of the bypass. As the diameter of the distal vessel does not change, the hemodynamics greatly depends on the size of arteriotomy. The length of arteriotomy in common femoral artery is about 1–2 cm usually. Some say, the length should be twice the diameter of the artery.

  It may be anchor technique or parachute technique:
    - *Anchor technique* (**Fig. 1**): It is ideal for large vessels that are not placed deep. It starts by placing a suture at the heel which is tied down and each arm of the suture is run in continuous manner on either side of the heel and tied to complete the anastomosis. Most common, second suture is used and tied down at the apex and each limb run toward the suture from the heel end and tied on each side. There are many variations to this. Most common is horizontal mattress suture at the heel instead of simple suture or the apical sutures can be interrupted, especially in small vessels. Another variation is regarding the location of the first suture. It can be placed anywhere along the arteriotomy and not always the heel or toe end.
    - *Parachute technique* (**Fig. 2**): It is ideal for small vessels placed at a depth. Main difference is that multiple (usually five) sutures are taken around the heel and are not placed down initially, but kept at a distance till the sutures are taken and finally brought down by

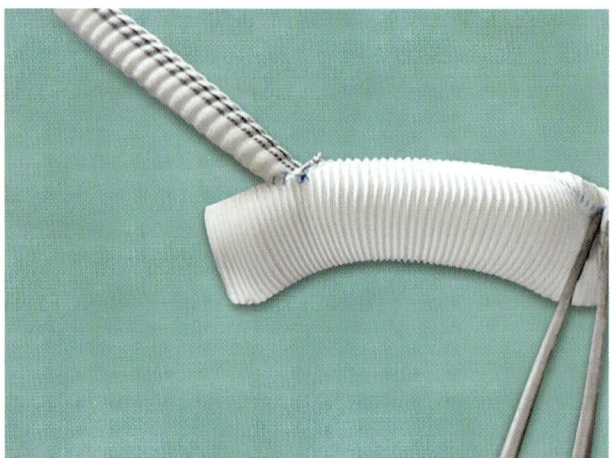

Fig. 1: Anchor technique.

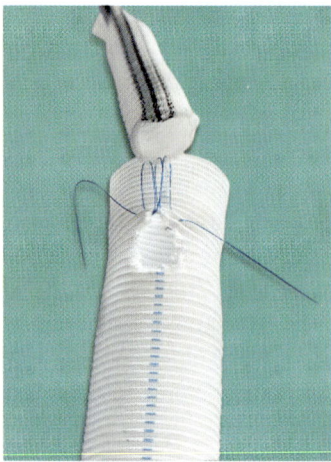

Fig. 2: Parachute technique.

giving gentle traction on either end of suture in "seesaw" fashion. The central loop can be pulled using nerve hook for keeping the sutures taut. Better visualization and placement of the sutures at the heel and the apex can be facilitated by the use of this technique. The main variation relates to the site where the suture is started. The suture may be started exactly at the center of the heel or a few bites off the center of the heel. Other variation is using an anchor technique for the heel portion and a parachute technique for the apical portion or vice versa.

- *End-to-end anastomosis (Fig. 3)*: It is usually performed in trauma when the injured vessel is trimmed and anastomosed primarily if not under tension or using an interposition graft (vein/prosthetic conduit), aneurysmal disease, composite bypass, replacing a diseased portion of

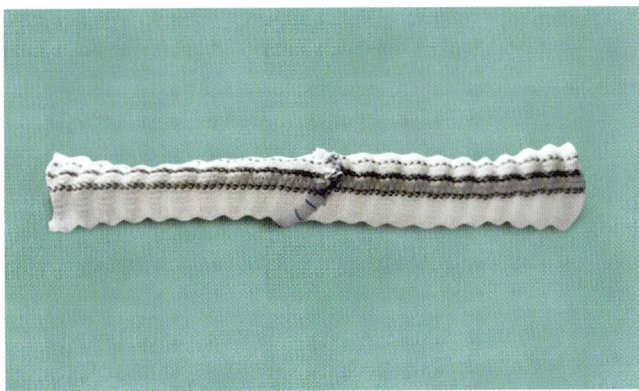

Fig. 3: End-to-end anastomosis.

graft, and situation where preservation of retrograde flow is not essential, e.g., renal or mesenteric bypass:
- *Large vessels of comparable diameter (>8 mm)*: The vessel transection and suture line are created perpendicular to long axis of vessels.
  If both segments are freely movable, the anastomosis can be done in two parts—anterior and posterior walls by tying diametrically opposite sutures and doing anterior part first, flipping the vessel by 180° and completing the posterior part. If the segments are not freely movable, posterior wall can be sutured first (parachute or anchor technique), followed by anterior. A modification of this is the "triangulation" technique propounded by Alexis Carrel in which anastomosis is divided into three parts by tying sutures at one-third of circumference (classically 12, 4, and 8 o'clock position). This method prevents uneven advancements between the sutures on either side of the vessels, especially when dealing with large vessels of comparable but unequal diameters.
- *Small vessels of comparable diameter (<6 mm)*: Usually, an anchoring suture is taken at the heel and sutured on either side of heel, second suture started at apex and continued on either side toward heel. When constructing an end-to-end anastomosis between two small vessels, a beveled or spatulated anastomosis is necessary to avoid compromising the lumen. If the vessel is thin, first suture can be done by parachute technique to spread the tension evenly. An additional technique employed is anterior patch angioplasty. It is done when the cut ends of the vessels cannot be joined but be only approximated and doing so anterior walls are divided and aligned creating an arteriotomy which can be closed with vein patch. This method avoids the use of interposition graft.
- *Vessels of unequal caliber*: The smaller caliber is trimmed to minimum, long spatulated and anastomosed to provide smooth transition.

If the diameter mismatch is very large, an option is to oversew and close the end of the larger artery followed by anastomosing the small vessel onto the side of the larger vessel (end-to-side). This is termed as "functional" end-to-end anastomosis.
- *Side-to-side anastomosis*: This is usually performed in the creation of portacaval shunt in portal hypertension, radiocephalic arteriovenous fistula for chronic hemodialysis, and the creation of a side-to-side arteriovenous fistula distal to an infrainguinal prosthetic bypass as an adjunctive procedure to decrease the outflow resistance (rarely) and creation of the second anastomosis of a sequential bypass when multiple segments of a limb require revascularization. The vessels are dissected and mobilized adequately to lie adjacent to each other. The walls in direct contact are sutured first and continued to the opposite side.

VASCULAR SUTURES

Vascular reconstructions are usually done with nonabsorbable sutures to provide the tensile strength essential to secure the walls of the vessels together until healing is completed. This is very important in case of prosthetic grafts because anastomosis never heals completely and the tensile strength provided by the sutures is needed for the duration of the patient's life.

The suture materials commonly used for vascular reconstructions include monofilament sutures such as polypropylene and polytetrafluoroethylene (PTFE).

Polypropylene Sutures (Prolene, Surgipro, and Surgilene)

Prolene sutures have gained a wider popularity and are probably the most commonly used suture material in vascular reconstructions. Made of a monofilament strand of a synthetic linear polyolefin, these polypropylene sutures tend to maintain their tensile strength over time. Polypropylene sutures are very smooth. Seven throws are usually placed to secure the knot and avoid unraveling.

Polytetrafluoroethylene Sutures

Polytetrafluoroethylene sutures also have excellent handling characteristics. They have been developed with the intention of minimizing needle-hole bleeding, which is often seen when polypropylene sutures are used with PTFE grafts or patches.

Use sutures appropriately sized for your reconstruction. The following guidelines are suggested for the choice of suture size:
- *2-0, 3-0*: Aorta
- *4-0*: Iliac arteries
- *5-0*: Axillary, common carotid, common femoral, and superficial femoral arteries

- *5-0, 6-0*: Internal carotid, popliteal and brachial arteries
- *7-0, 8-0*: Tibial or inframalleolar arteries.

VASCULAR INSTRUMENTS

Scissors
- Potts scissors **(Fig. 4)**—extension of incisions in medium vessels
- Castroviejo scissors **(Fig. 5)**—extension of incisions in small vessels.

Tissue Forceps
DeBakey tissue forceps **(Fig. 6)**—medium and large blood vessels (tip 1, 1.5, and 2 mm).

Needle Holders
- Mayo-Hegar needle holder **(Fig. 7)**—<4-0 sutures

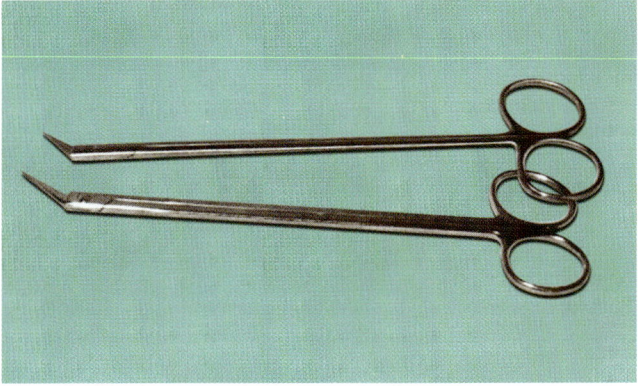

Fig. 4: Potts scissors.

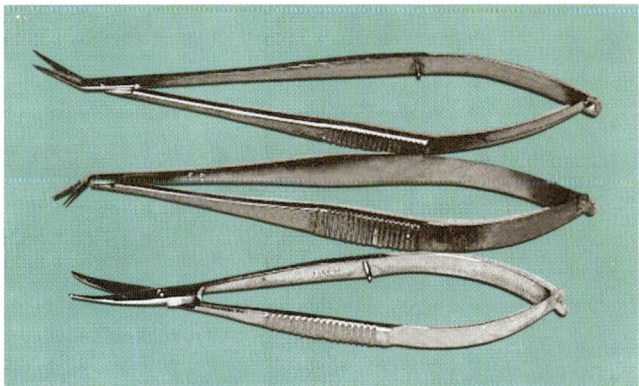

Fig. 5: Castroviejo scissors.

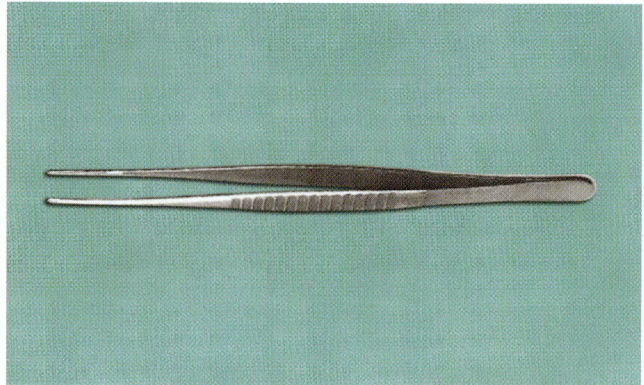

Fig. 6: DeBakey tissue forceps.

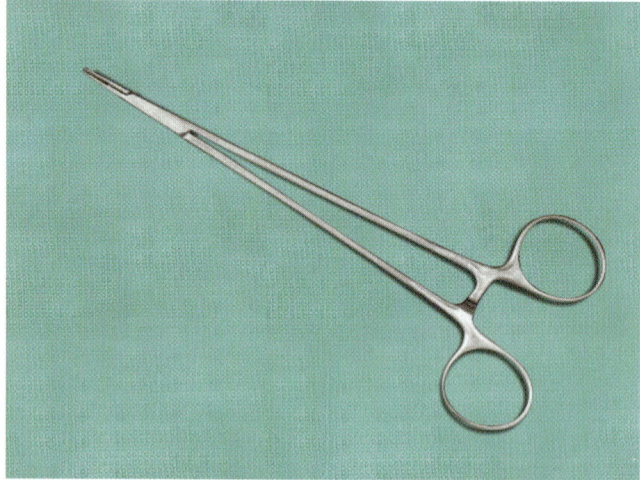

Fig. 7: Mayo-Hegar needle holder.

- Castroviejo needle holder **(Fig. 8)**—5-0, 6-0, and 7-0 sutures (with or without locking handle).

Totally Occluding Vascular Clamps
- DeBakey aortic aneurysm clamp for supraceliac and infrarenal aorta (side-to-side apposition of aortic wall) **(Fig. 9)**
- DeBakey-Bahnson aortic aneurysm clamp for infrarenal aorta **(Fig. 10)**.

Partially Occluding (Side-biting) Vascular Clamps
- Satinsky clamp for clamping aorta, vena cava **(Fig. 11)**
- Cooley pediatric clamp for clamping common femoral artery, saphenofemoral junction **(Fig. 12)**.

Vascular Anastomosis

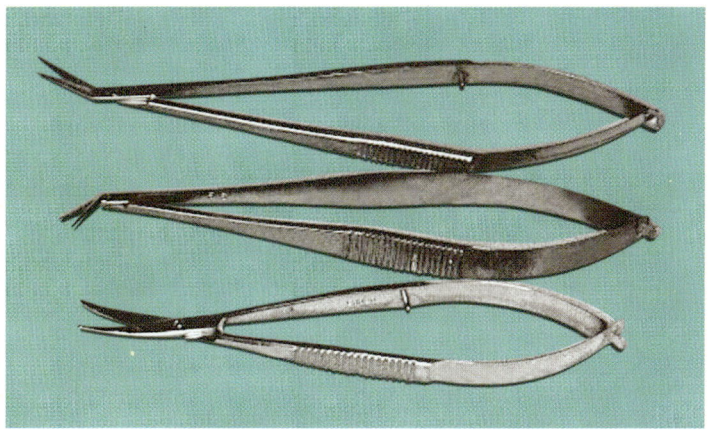

Fig. 8: Castroviejo needle holder.

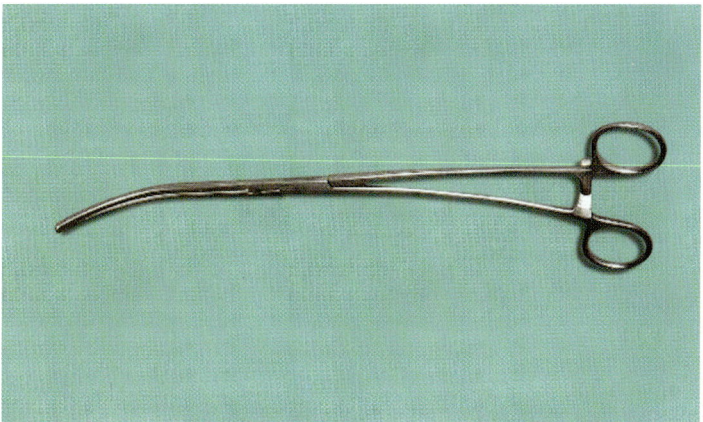

Fig. 9: DeBakey aortic aneurysm clamp.

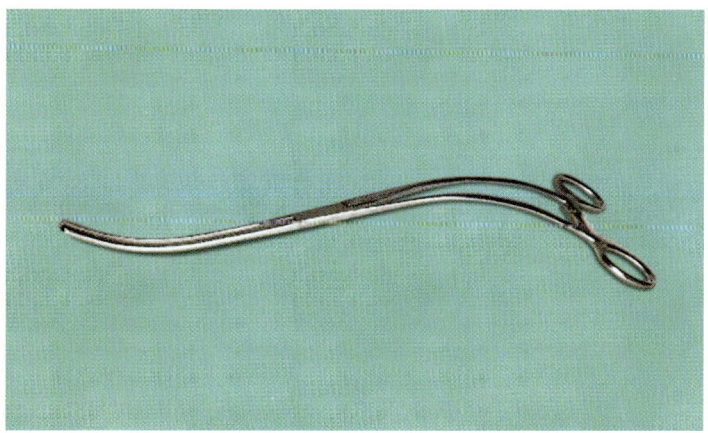

Fig. 10: DeBakey-Bahnson aortic aneurysm clamp.

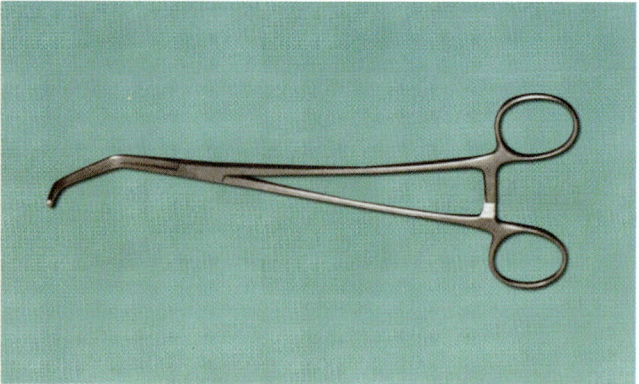

Fig. 11: Satinsky clamp.

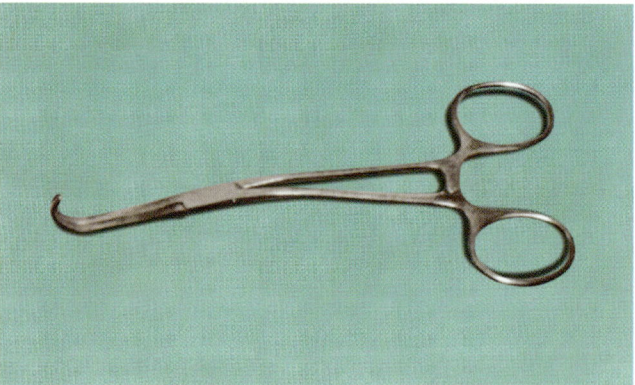

Fig. 12: Cooley pediatric clamp.

COMPLICATIONS OF VASCULAR ANASTOMOSIS

- *Embolization of atheroma, thrombus, or both*:
  - *Preventive methods*:
    - Distal and proximal vessels should be dissected and clamped before manipulating the diseased segment of the vessel.
    - When placing a vascular clamp, palpate the vessel first to be sure it is soft and collapsible.
    - When operating on an abdominal aorta with intraluminal thrombus near the renal arteries, first clamp above the renal, open the infrarenal aorta to remove thrombus, and then move the clamp to the infrarenal position.
- *End-organ ischemia*:
  - Brain—4 minutes
  - Kidney—warm ischemia—30–60 minutes
  - Muscles of the leg—up to 6 hours.
  - *Preventive methods*:
    - Revascularization within golden hour

- ◆ Prophylactic fasciotomy in case of revascularization in class 2b acute limb ischemia.
- *Arterial thrombosis after a vascular reconstruction*:
  - Most common cause—inadequate outflow may be the cause
  - Most common cause of inadequate outflow—technical failure
  - Most common technical problems that lead to thrombosis—injury to the artery from a vascular clamp resulting in an intimal flap
  - Other causes—residual stenosis, retained plaque, kinking of a vessel or graft, and inadequate inflow.
  - *Preventive methods*:
    - ◆ Avoid any configuration that leads to turbulent blood flow which indirectly cause deposition of platelets, embolization, and thrombosis
    - ◆ Meticulous reconstruction of the vessel
    - ◆ Careful assessment after restoring flow with handheld Doppler, ultrasonography, or angiography
    - ◆ Postoperative anticoagulation in selected cases of severe outflow disease.
- Bleeding, hematomas.

29. Nutrition in Surgical Practice

Murali Appukuttan, Vinitha V Nair

INTRODUCTION

Surgical residents should have the preliminary understanding about nutrition in surgical patients. The importance of nutritional assessment, care, and supplementation in surgical patients cannot be overemphasized. It should be a part of surgical training to ensure knowledge on adequate nutritional care to improve the perioperative course of events and outcome.

A thorough understanding of the basic metabolism of nutrients in the body coupled with metabolism in starvation and stress forms the fundamentals before venturing to understand the nutritional assessment and supplementation in postsurgical patients.

COMPOSITION OF HUMAN BODY

Body composition in a 70 kg adult is summarized in **Table 1**.

METABOLISM IN A WELL-FED STATE

A 70 kg adult normally needs about an average of 2,000–2,800 kcal/day depending on his activities which is met by carbohydrates (40–60%), lipids (30–40%), and proteins (10–15%). In a hospitalized patient, basic energy requirement may be ~ 1,300–1,800 kcal/day. Average physical activity raises

Table 1: Composition of human body.

	Male	Female
Weight (kg)	70	60
Total water (L): • Intracellular • Extracellular	42 28 14	31 19 12
Total solids (kg): • Fat • Protein • Minerals	28 12.5 12.5 3	28.8 17 9 3

the metabolism by 40-50% above the basal metabolic rate (BMR). BMR falls about 10% during sleep and 40% during prolonged starvation. 1 g of carbohydrate yields 3.4 kcal energy, protein yields 4 kcal energy, and fat yields 9 kcal energy after metabolism. In the fed state, glucose absorbed from carbohydrates in the diet forms major source of energy for tissues. Different tissues preferentially use different sources of energy, although the major source is glucose. Erythrocytes completely and neurons predominantly depend on glucose whereas heart and skeletal muscle can strive with fat as energy source as required and enterocytes and lymphocytes can metabolize the amino acid glutamine (overview of catabolism is shown in **Flowchart 1**).

Carbohydrates are the primary source of calories and are divided into simple carbohydrates (monosaccharides—one sugar unit, disaccharides—two sugar units) or complex carbohydrates (oligosaccharides—3-10 units of sugar, polysaccharides—>10 units of sugar). Carbohydrate digestion starts in the oral cavity with the action of salivary amylase hydrolyzing polysaccharide bonds to amylose and amylopectin that constitute starch. Further breakdown

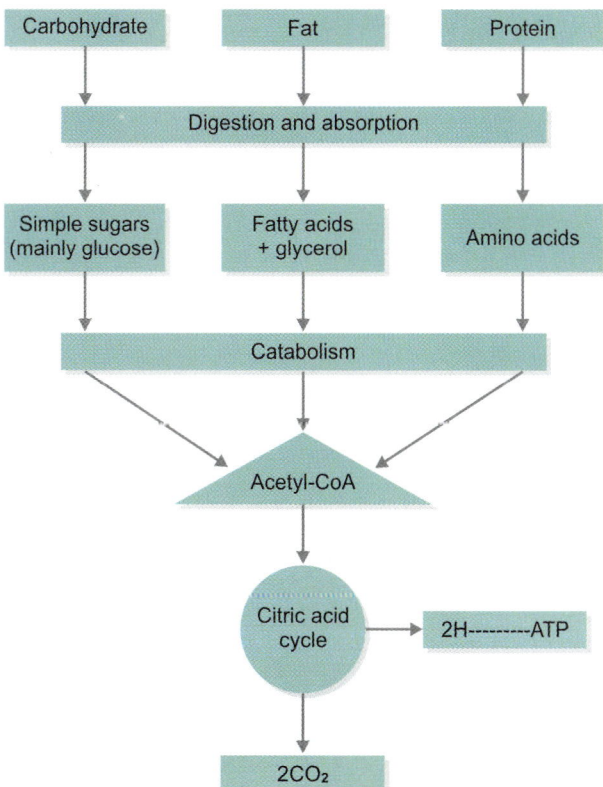

Flowchart 1: Overview of catabolism.

(ATP: adenosine triphosphate; CO_2: carbon dioxide)

occurs in gut through the actions of pancreatic amylase and the brush border enzymes sucrase, lactase, maltase, and isomaltase to yield monosaccharides (glucose, fructose, and galactose—mainly D isomers) which are absorbed and transported to liver. In the colon-resistant starch and nonstarch, polysaccharides are fermented by colonic bacteria producing short-chain fatty acids (mainly butyrate which is the preferential fuel for colonocytes). Normal fasting level of plasma glucose in peripheral venous blood is 70–110 mg/dL (3.9–6.1 mmol/L) and in arterial blood plasma glucose level is 15–30 mg/dL higher. Obligatory glucose requirement is around 2 g/kg/day even under conditions of prolonged fasting (up to 200 g/day).

In normal carbohydrate metabolism, absorbed glucose is channeled to one of the following pathways **(Flowchart 2)**:

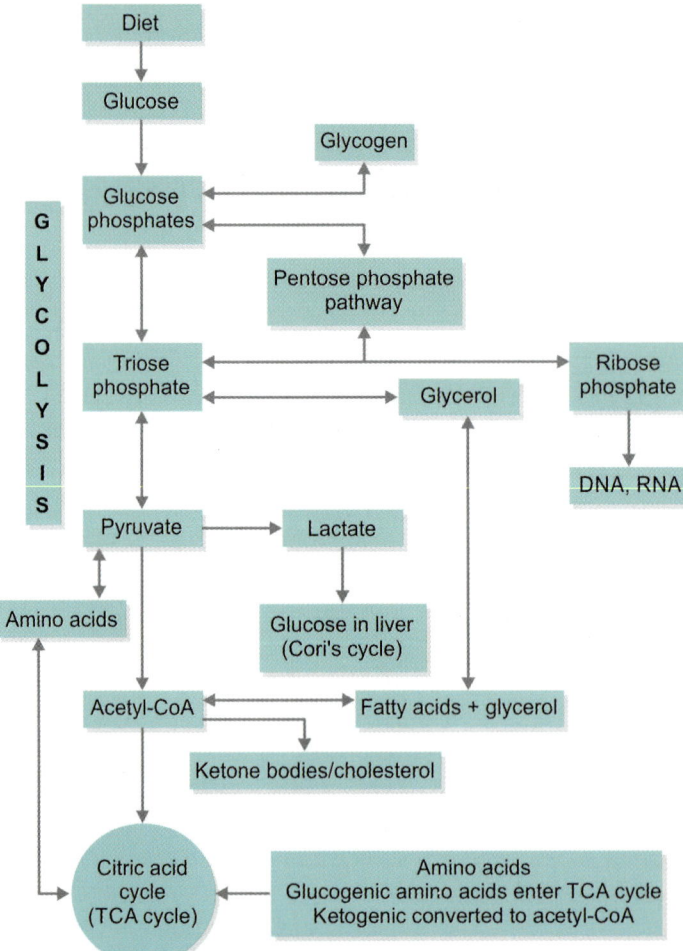

Flowchart 2: Overview of carbohydrate metabolism.

(DNA: deoxyribonucleic acid; RNA: ribonucleic acid; TCA: tricarboxylic acid)

- *Glycolysis—conversion to pyruvate*: The aerobic tissues convert this to acetyl-CoA which forms the precursor for many other synthetic pathways. Under lack of oxygen, pyruvate is converted to lactate. This lactate is converted back to pyruvate in the liver by Cori cycle.
- *Glycogenesis*: Synthesis of the storage polymer in liver and skeletal muscle.
- *Lipogenesis*: Fatty acid synthesis from excess glucose, stimulated by insulin (physiologic maximum that glucose can be oxidized is 4 mg/kg/min which is equivalent to 1,500 kcal/day in a 70 kg man. Rest nonoxidized glucose will be converted to fat).

Insulin secreted by the pancreas controls the glucose uptake by muscle and adipose tissues by modifying the glucose transporter type 4 (GLUT4) transporters. Around 90% of portal venous glucose is removed from the blood by hepatocytes through carrier facilitated diffusion (GLUT2). Stored form of glucose in the liver and skeletal muscle is glycogen. Liver is the predominant site for glucose homeostasis (lesser extent renal cortex) including glycogenesis, glycogenolysis, and gluconeogenesis (glycogen synthesis, glycogen degradation, and glucose synthesis, respectively) from noncarbohydrate sources. In a 70 kg man, carbohydrate reserves total about 2,500 kcal, stored in 400–500 g of muscle glycogen, 100 g of liver glycogen (65 g/kg liver tissue), and 20 g glucose in extracellular fluid. Hepatic synthesis of glycogen begins with a core composed of a high-density protein primer glycogenin (with 1:4α and 1:6α glycosidic linkages) with glycogen synthase which catalyzes the final synthetic step as the rate-limiting enzyme. This enzyme is activated by insulin/glucose inhibited by glucagon/epinephrine. During fasting, glycogenolysis leads to release of glucose with the rate-limiting enzyme glycogen phosphorylase being activated by glucagon and epinephrine (inhibited by insulin). Glucagon can act only in hepatic glycogenolysis (elevate blood glucose without raising lactate levels) while epinephrine can act on both skeletal and liver causing elevation of blood sugar levels along with hyperlactatemia. Glycogen stores get exhausted in 12–24 hours of fasting and lean body stores are mobilized to maintain adequate glucose levels by gluconeogenesis to maintain supply to brain. Substrates for this pathway include all gluconeogenic amino acids (except leucine and lysine which are ketogenic only, i.e., produce acetyl-CoA as end product and cannot produce glucose), glycerol derived from degradation of triacylglycerol (TAG) in adipose tissue, and lactate produced from anaerobic glycolysis (Cori cycle).

Lipids are hydrophobic molecules that include fatty acids, phospholipids, glycerolipids, sphingolipids, eicosanoids, and vitamins. They have a key role in cell structure and function, formation of biologic membranes, energy storage and expenditure, and cell signaling. Triglycerides (TGs) which are the stored form of lipids are the greatest and most potent source of energy in the body ~ 1.12 lac kcal (12–13 kg fat in the body of a 70 kg individual). Dietary

TG get emulsified and hydrolyzed to monoacylglycerol (MAG) and free fatty acids (FFAs) by a mixture of lipases found primarily in biliary, pancreatic, and intestinal secretions from glands along the gastrointestinal tract (GIT). 20% of digestion and absorption along with emulsification starts at stomach by gastric lipases and emulsified TGs entering duodenum stimulate contraction of gallbladder releasing bile and pancreatic fluids containing lipase, colipase, phospholipase A2, and cholesterol esterase. Bile acids and colipase enable pancreatic lipase to act on TGs to produce diacylglycerol (DAG) and MAG along with FFA.

Lipids, absorbed as FFAs and glycerol, are secreted into the lymphatic system as chylomicrons (largest plasma lipoproteins) along with fat-soluble vitamins (A, D, E, and K). After hydrolysis (by lipoprotein lipase), it can either be oxidized to fuel or esterified to TAG for storage. Chylomicron remnants are cleared by the liver. The main sources of long-chain fatty acids are either dietary lipid or de novo synthesis from acetyl-CoA from carbohydrates or proteins in adipose tissue and liver. Fatty acids may get oxidized to acetyl-CoA (beta-oxidation) or esterified with glycerol, forming TAG as body's main fuel reserve. Adipose tissue TAG is the main fuel reserve of the body. Adipose triglyceride lipase (ATGL—first step) and hormone-sensitive lipase (HSL) along with a series of lipases cause hydrolysis of TAG into FFA and glycerol in the adipocyte cytosol. Glycerol is a substrate for gluconeogenesis. FFA bound to albumin is being taken up by all tissues [except red blood cell (RBC) and brain] where it is esterified into TAG for storage or oxidized as a fuel. The newly synthesized TAG and TAG from chylomicron remnants are secreted into circulation as very-low-density lipoprotein (VLDL) which undergoes a same similar to that of chylomicrons. Partial oxidation of fatty acids in liver leads to ketone body formation and exported to extrahepatic tissues in starvation and prolonged fasting to provide as a fuel. During fasting, glucocorticoids increases lipolysis.

Acetyl-CoA formed by beta-oxidation has got three fates **(Flowchart 3)**:
1. As with acetyl-CoA arising from glycolysis, it is oxidized to carbon dioxide (CO_2) and water by citric acid cycle.
2. It can be precursor for synthesis of cholesterol and other steroids.
3. In liver, it is used to synthesize ketone bodies, acetoacetate, and 3-hydroxybutyrate which are important fuels in prolonged fasting and starvation.

Fatty acids and ketone bodies formed from them cannot be used for the synthesis of glucose. The reaction catalyzed by pyruvate dehydrogenase forming acetyl-CoA is irreversible and for every two carbon units from acetyl-CoA that enters the Krebs cycle, there is loss of two carbon atoms as CO_2 before oxaloacetate is reformed (i.e., acetyl-CoA and any substrates that yield acetyl-CoA can never be used for gluconeogenesis). The relatively rare fatty acids with an odd number of carbon atoms yield propionyl-CoA

Flowchart 3: Overview of fat metabolism.

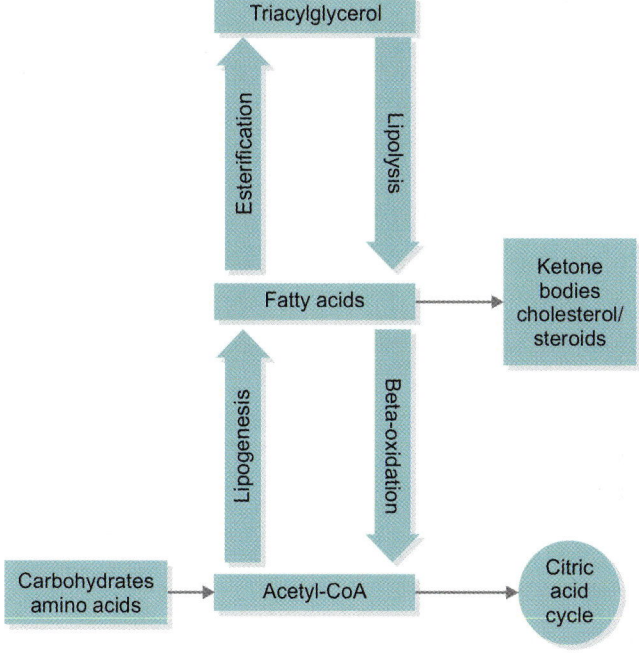

as the product of final cycle of beta-oxidation (which can be converted to succinyl-CoA which is a Krebs cycle intermediate) and this can be a substrate for gluconeogenesis, as glycerol released by lipolysis of adipose tissue TAG reserves. From the viewpoint of energetics, formation of any one mole of any acyl-CoA compound is equivalent to the formation of one mole of adenosine triphosphate (ATP). Around 129 molecules of ATP are being produced from one molecule of fatty acid palmitate.

Proteins are essential to the function and structure of every cell and participate in cell signaling, adhesion, and immunogenicity. The breakdown of proteins to peptides starts at stomach through acid denaturation and action of pepsin. Further digestion to tripeptides, bipeptides, and amino acids occurs at duodenum through proteases secreted from the pancreas and peptidases from brush border of intestines and absorbed at small intestine. There are 20 amino acids of which eight are essential (not produced de novo from amino acids—must be obtained from diet), six are conditionally essential (may not be synthesized at rates not meeting requirement, especially in illness or childhood requiring supplementation), and remaining six are nonessential (synthesized internally) **(Box 1)**.

Amino acids are required for protein synthesis. Fates of amino acids through diet are as follows **(Flowchart 4)**:
- Apart from supply of essential and nonessential amino acids through diet, dispensable amino acids can be formed from metabolic intermediates by

> **Box 1:** Different types of amino acids.
>
> *Essential amino acids/Indispensable amino acids:*
> - Valine
> - Leucine
> - Isoleucine
> - Lysine
> - Methionine
> - Threonine
> - Phenylalanine
> - Tryptophan
>
> [Valine, leucine, and isoleucine are the branched-chain amino acids (BCAAs) constituting 40% essential amino acids and their metabolism happens predominantly in muscle, breakdown of BCAA in muscle produces alanine and glutamine, leucine and lysine are the only ketogenic amino acids, and histidine and arginine can be essential in infants]
>
> *Conditionally essential amino acids:*
> - Arginine
> - Histidine
> - Tyrosine
> - Cysteine
> - Glutamine
> - Proline
>
> *Nonessential amino acids/Dispensable amino acids:*
> - Alanine
> - Asparagine
> - Aspartate
> - Glutamate
> - Glycine
> - Serine
> - Ketogenic amino acids—leucine, lysine
> - Ketogenic and glucogenic amino acids—isoleucine, tryptophan, tyrosine, and phenylalanine
> - Aromatic amino acids (AAAs)—phenylalanine, tryptophan, and tyrosine
> - Fischer ratio—BCAA/AAA—normally 3–4.2, decreased in liver diseases

  transamination using amino groups from other amino acids (all amino acids, except lysine and threonine participate in transamination at some point in their catabolism and these two amino acids lose their amino groups by deamination).
- After *deamination*, amino nitrogen is excreted as urea and the carbon skeletons that remain after transamination may:
  - Get oxidized to CO_2 via Krebs cycle
  - Used to synthesize glucose (gluconeogenesis), glycogen
  - Form ketone bodies or acetyl-CoA, which may be oxidized or used for fatty acids synthesis
  - Amino acids not used in biosynthetic reactions are burned as fuels.
- Several amino acids are precursors of other compounds like purines, pyrimidines, porphyrins, creatinine, hormones like epinephrine, thyroxine, and various neurotransmitters.

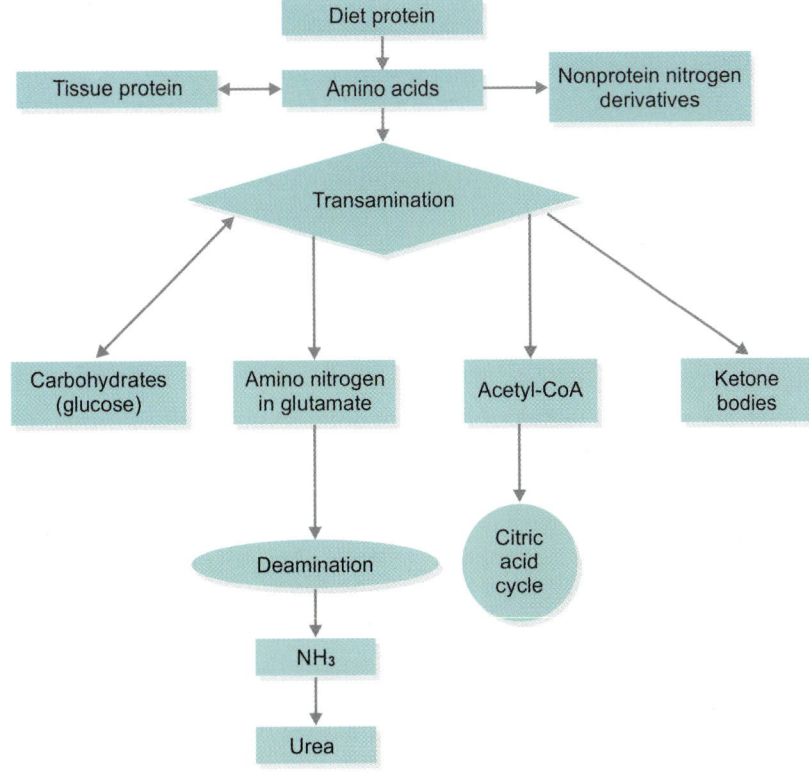

Flowchart 4: Overview of protein metabolism.

(NH$_3$: ammonia)

Alanine and glutamine are generated during branched-chain amino acid (BCAA) breakdown in skeletal muscles. Alanine is released from skeletal muscle that can be used by the liver and is a preferred precursor for gluconeogenesis as part of glucose-alanine cycle. Alanine is provided by either amino acids in the diet or provided by muscle during protein turnover. Lactate produced in the muscle during anaerobic glycolysis is converted to lactate in liver by Cori cycle.

Proteins, absorbed as amino acids from diet, are taken up through the portal vein into the circulation and are handled by the liver for the following pathways—25% of the amino acids maintain the plasma pool, 55% are converted to urea to be excreted, 6% is utilized to synthesis the plasma proteins, and the rest 14% become integrated as liver protein. Protein turnover is the simultaneous synthesis and degradation of protein molecules. In healthy, fed adults, total amount of protein remains constant (~400 g/day, synthesis = degradation). So, in a 70 kg man with 100 g/day protein intake, amino acid pool is around 90–100 g. This amino acid pool is supplied by three sources—(1) amino acids from degradation of body proteins, (2) amino acids from dietary proteins, and (3) nonessential amino acids synthesized from simple intermediates of metabolism. Liver and skeletal muscles together account for ~ 50% of daily protein turnover. Though the skeletal muscle on contrary to liver has got large mass, but it has low turnover rate (1–2% only). Liver has a relatively low mass (~1.5 kg), but high protein turnover (10–20% per day). Protein synthesis is 50:50, i.e., 50% renewal of structural proteins and 50% synthesis of export proteins of which albumin is the major export protein (albumin renewal 10% per day). Transcapillary escape rate (TER) of albumin is 10 times the rate of synthesis (5% per hour) and short-term changes in albumin concentration are mostly due to increased capillary permeability. For these reasons, serum albumin concentration is fastly affected to a greater degree by physical effects of redistribution and dilution than by nutritional or metabolic effects on synthesis or breakdown. Albumin TER may be increased threefold following major injury/sepsis.

Urea accounts for 90% nitrogen-containing components of urine (one nitrogen of urea produced in liver is supplied by free ammonia and other by aspartate).

Two mechanisms are available in humans for transport of ammonia from peripheral tissues to the liver for conversion of urea (not exclusive to skeletal muscle):

1. First uses glutamine synthase to combine ammonia with glutamate to form glutamine (largest pool of amino acids in the body), a nontoxic form of ammonia. In liver, glutamine is cleaved by glutaminase to glutamate and ammonia. The glutamate is oxidatively deaminated to alpha-ketoglutarate and ammonia by glutamate dehydrogenase. The ammonia is converted to urea.
2. Second transport mechanism involves formation of alanine by transamination of pyruvate produced from both aerobic glycolysis and metabolism of succinyl-CoA generated by catabolism of BCAA isoleucine and valine. Alanine in liver is transaminated to pyruvate by alanine transaminase (ALT) [serum glutamate pyruvate transaminase (SGPT)] and it can get converted to glucose which again can be transported to muscle for further usage through glucose-alanine cycle.

METABOLISM AT ORGANISM LEVEL (FED STAGE AND STARVATION)

Human body exists in different states of metabolism during healthy state—the *fed* stage, the *fasting* stage which can be *early* fasting or starvation stage (postabsorptive stage)/*late* fasting or starvation stage (preabsorptive stage), and the *refeeding* stage:

- *Fed stage*—it represents the time when the body is digesting and absorbing nutrients. Here anabolism exceeds catabolism. Body is preparing to store for lean body mass (LBM). The main regulator of this phase is insulin. Glucose and parasympathetic system stimulate insulin release from beta-cells of pancreas. It stimulates glycogenesis, glycolysis, fatty acid synthesis, and muscle building. It inhibits gluconeogenesis, glycogenolysis, and fatty acid and muscle breakdown. It also increases the absorption of BCAA.

- *Fasting stage*—this state occurs after nutrition has been digested, absorbed, and stored (3–5 hours after fed phase). Glucagon is the signal for starvation state. Fasting state is broken into an early fasting/early starvation phase and late fasting/late starvation phase. Since glucose level decreases causing for decrease in insulin release, counterregulatory hormone glucagon increases and sympathetic activation increases other counter hormones—epinephrine and cortisol. Early fasting state is when blood glucose levels begin to decrease. Initially, body relies on body glycogen stores once glucose is not present and glucagon triggers glycogen breakdown mainly in liver (glucagon cannot act on skeletal muscle). Glucagon receptors are expressed not only in liver, but also in kidney, intestinal smooth muscle, brain, adipose tissue, heart, pancreatic beta-cells, and placenta. Other counterregulatory hormones like epinephrine (activation of beta-adrenergic system) and cortisol promote glycogenolysis and gluconeogenesis inhibiting glycolysis and glycogenesis. Epinephrine and cortisol help in mobilizing the muscle glycogen (~400–500 g) which cannot be directly consumed. By glycolysis in skeletal muscle, lactate formed get converted to glucose in liver by Cori cycle and get utilized. The liver becomes an organ of glucose production in fasting since many organs including red and white blood cells and renal medulla can initially utilize only glucose for their metabolic needs. So, secondary to the demands of the peripheral tissues, blood glucose is maintained between 70 and 120 mg/dL.

When body is deprived of nutrition for an extended period (>12–24 hours of fasting), it goes into survival mode—called late fasting stage or preabsorptive changes. Glycogen stores get depleted and de novo glucose synthesis happens from noncarbohydrate stores in the liver. Initially, this glucose is derived from skeletal muscle amino acid breakdown, especially alanine and glutamine (up to 75 g/day). This proteolysis in simple starvation is readily reversed by providing exogenous glucose. During this phase, certain organs take priority like brain.

With prolonged fasting, increased beta-oxidation of fat releases glycerol (which can be converted to glucose) and FFA which can be utilized by most tissues as fuels. Low levels of insulin favors ketone body formation and after 48–72 hours of fasting, central nervous tissues adapt to utilize ketone bodies as their primary fuel. This conversion to a fat fuel economy reduces the need for muscle breakdown by up to 55 g/day. Another adaptation to starvation is reduction in resting energy expenditure (REE) by declining the conversion of inactive thyroid hormone [thyroxine (T4)] to active thyroid hormone [triiodothyronine (T3)]. Despite these adaptive changes, there remains an

> **Box 2:** Metabolic responses to simple starvation.
> - Low levels of insulin, increased glucagon, epinephrine, and cortisol
> - Hepatic glycogenolysis (early fasting)
> - Protein catabolism (after 12–24 hours of fasting)
> - Hepatic gluconeogenesis (after 12–24 hours of fasting)
> - *Lipolysis (prolonged fasting):*
>   – Mobilization of fat stores (beta-oxidation is increased)
>   – Overall decrease in protein and carbohydrate oxidation
> - Ketogenesis (adaptive)
> - Reduction in resting energy expenditure (REE) from 20–30 kcal/day to 15–20 kcal/day
> - Decreased T4 to T3 conversion
>
> (T3: triiodothyronine; T4: thyroxine)

obligatory glucose requirement of about 200 g/day (roughly ~ 2 g/kg/day) even under conditions of prolonged fasting **(Box 2)**:

- *Refeeding stage*—during transition from preabsorptive (late starvation) to absorptive state, fat is processed the same as in normal metabolic state. When refed, liver does not initially take up glucose and the glucose is left for the peripheral tissues. The liver remains in the gluconeogenic mode. Newly created glucose is used to reform glycogen storage. As blood glucose levels rise, liver replaces its glycogen storage and then processes excess glucose for fatty acid synthesis.

METABOLISM IN STRESS/STRESS STARVATION

Body's innate mechanism to aid in survival for moderate injury includes immobility, anorexia, and catabolism for attaining energy in the absence of medical intervention. Metabolic response to injury has been aptly described by Sir David Cuthbertson as "Ebb and Flow model" **(Table 2)**. The ebb phase starts immediately after injury (e.g., surgery) and can last for 24–48 hours. This phase injury response can be attenuated by proper resuscitation, but not completely abolished. It is characterized by decreased BMR, hypovolemia, decreased cardiac output, hypothermia, lactatemia, and acidosis. The hormones responsible for this phase are catecholamines, cortisol, and aldosterone secondary to renin-angiotensin system activation. The depth of this neuroendocrine-endocrine reflex depends on the degree of blood loss and stimulation of somatic afferent nerves at the site of injury, i.e., depth of injury. The physiologic role of this phase is to conserve both circulating volume and energy stores for recovery and repair and is aided by resuscitation.

Following resuscitation, ebb phase evolves into a hypermetabolic flow phase which corresponds to systemic inflammatory response syndrome. This involves mobilization of body stores for recovery, repair, and subsequent replacement of lost or damaged tissue. This phase is subdivided to early catabolic phase lasting for 3–10 days and late anabolic/recovery phase which

Table 2: Different phases of stress metabolism.

Ebb phase	Flow phase	Recovery phase
Resuscitation phase	Hypercatabolic phase	Anabolic phase
• Physiological role to conserve both circulating volume and energy stores for recovery and repair • Lasts for hours (up to 24–48 hours)	• Mobilization of body energy stores for recovery and repair and subsequent replacement of lost or damaged tissues • Lasts for days, usually 3–10 days	• Recovery and repair • Can last for weeks
• Hypovolemia • Decreased basal metabolic rate (BMR), decreased T3, decreased insulin, decreased IGF-1, and decreased testosterone • Decreased cardiac output • Hypothermia • Lactic acidosis • Predominant hormones—catecholamines, cortisol, and aldosterone (renin-angiotensin system)	• Early SIRS—immune activation (Th1 response)—early deterioration or recovery can happen • Tissue edema • Increased BMR • Increased cardiac output • Increased body temperature • Leukocytosis • Increased oxygen consumption • Increased counterregulatory hormones—catecholamines, cortisol, glucagon, growth hormone, ACTH, aldosterone (renin-angiotensin system), and ADH • Insulin resistance • Increased proteolysis • Increased hepatic gluconeogenesis • Adipocyte lipolysis • Hepatic acute phase protein synthesis • Pyrexia—by IL-1, TNF-alpha, IL-6, and IL-8 • Anti-inflammatory (Th2) response—(IL-1 receptor antagonists, TNF-soluble receptor, TGF-alpha, IL-4, and IL-10) producing specialized proresolving mediators (SPMs) like essential fatty acid-derived lipoxins, resolvins, protectins, and maresins which limit inflammation—CARS if prolonged response • PICS—if prolonged CARS with critical illness syndrome	• Refeeding syndrome • Altered neurohormonal response if recovering from critical illness syndrome • Nutrition and rehabilitative measures are the crux of treatment

(ACTH: adrenocorticotropic hormone; ADH: antidiuretic hormone; CARS: compensatory anti-inflammatory response syndrome; IGF-1: insulin-like growth factor-1; IL-1: interleukin-1; PICS: persistent inflammation, immunosuppression, and catabolism syndrome; SIRS: systemic inflammatory response syndrome; T3: triiodothyronine; TNF-alpha: tumor necrosis factor-alpha)

can last for weeks, if extensive repair and recovery are required following very serious injury. In the catabolic phase, there is increased tissue edema due to increased capillary permeability, hypermetabolism causing increased BMR, increased cardiac output, raised body temperature, leukocytosis, increased oxygen consumption, and increased gluconeogenesis. During catabolic phase, there is increased production of counterregulatory hormones and inflammatory cytokines like interleukin-1 (IL-1), IL-6, tumor necrosis factor-alpha (TNF-alpha), etc., resulting in significant fat and protein mobilization causing significant weight loss and urinary nitrogen loss. Though there is increased insulin production, there is characteristic insulin resistance during this phase causing for the reason for increased complications and aggravation of further neurohormonal and inflammatory stress responses causing a vicious catabolic cycle. The main purpose of these neurohormonal changes is to provide essential substrates for survival, postpone anabolism, and optimize host defense. This will help only for a short-term period, but harmful in long term especially to severely injured patient who would otherwise not have survived without medical intervention. During the metabolic response to injury, our body reprioritizes protein metabolism away from peripheral tissues (muscle, adipose tissue, and skin) toward key central tissues like liver, immune system, and wound. Hepatic acute phase response represents a reprioritization of body protein metabolism toward liver and is characterized by increasing plasma levels of acute phase reactants (like C-reactive proteins, fibrinogen, ferritin, etc.) and decreasing of negative acute phase reactants like production of export proteins like albumin. The body reacts with the initial inflammatory states with a compensatory anti-inflammatory response syndrome (CARS). Though the IL-6-induced protein catabolism continues, myeloid-derived suppressor cells (MDSCs) will get expanded and anti-inflammatory cytokines like IL-10 and transforming growth factor-alpha (TGF-alpha) result in immunosuppression, persistence of all these can cause long-term complications like chronic kidney disease. When these processes continue over weeks, a multifactorial syndrome of persistent inflammation, immunosuppression, and catabolism syndrome (PICS) occurs. This shows the need for introducing proper nutrition at the earliest even during acute inflammatory state depending on the individualized clinical scenario.

Insulin resistance, cortisol, glucagon, and catecholamines cause glycogenolysis and gluconeogenesis in acute stress. The inflammatory stress inhibits ketogenesis and metabolism turns toward aggressive protein catabolism to release amino acids as substrate for gluconeogenesis. The entry of pyruvate into the mitochondria is specifically inhibited by TNF-alpha and interleukins released during stress which favors the Cori cycle pathway converting pyruvate to lactate and finally glucose. The suppression of ketogenesis is in proportionate to the degree of inflammatory stress and this coupled with high metabolic rate (50% above the BMR) causes extreme degrees of muscle protein catabolism and loss of LBM which cannot be reversed by provision of calories **(Fig. 1)**. High levels of protein catabolism lead to nitrogen excretion in urine and net negative nitrogen balance. This leads to severe decline in LBM leading to stress-related malnutrition and

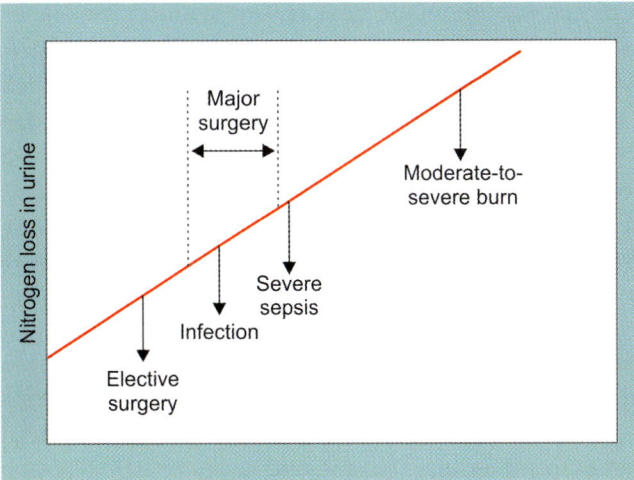

Fig. 1: Basal metabolic rate.

once the LBM loss has reached 30–40% of the total, survival is unlikely. So, unlike in simple starvation where fat/ketone bodies form the major substrate for energy production after stored glycogen stores, in stress starvation, it is the protein through hypercatabolism following a major stress in late fasting stage.

During hypermetabolism, muscle wasting occurs due to increased degradation along with decreased synthesis especially in skeletal muscles, though respiratory muscles and gut are also affected severely causing for hypoventilation, chest infections, and decreased gut motility. Cardiac muscles are usually spared. Critically ill patients resuscitated after major injury in intensive care unit (ICU) undergo massive changes in body composition by decrease in fat mass and skeletal muscle mass, with paradoxical expansion of extracellular fluid (ECF) water by 6–10 L within 24 hours contributing to increase in body weight. Aldosterone (volume loss stimulates aldosterone that reabsorbs sodium, conserve water) along with antidiuretic hormone (ADH) (volume loss increases aldosterone and ADH secretion) and adrenocorticotropic hormone (ACTH) (which augments aldosterone response) cause for salt and water retention resulting in the natural oliguria following surgery which will be further augmented by saline infusions. Ideally body weight is to be measured daily and cumulative weight gain is to be kept <2.5 kg in order to decrease mortality or morbidity in the postoperative period following the stress of surgery. Even with optimal metabolic care with nutritional support, there will be ~ 15% decrease in protein mass by next 10 days. Daily urinary nitrogen loss is around 14 g/day and it can reach up to 20 g/day or more in severe sepsis or after major injury causing for ~ 500 g loss of skeletal muscle per day (1 g nitrogen corresponds to 6.25 g protein and 36 g of wet lean tissue). As previously shown, life is not compatible once LBM loss is over 40%. So, while giving nutritional support, even hyperalimentation (increased feeding) itself is a stress and multiple studies have shown that hypocaloric feeds are well-tolerated and equivalent to normocaloric feeds (60–70% calorie vs. 100% calorie), provided proteins are supplemented with extra stress factor associated with injury grade. Enhanced recovery after surgery (ERAS) protocols advice epidural anesthesia, early enteral feed, and preoperative late carbohydrate loading to decrease the insulin resistance and increasing glycogen storages are mainly to reduce these neurohormonal responses. With a restrictive fluid strategy (with balanced solutions) as per ERAS, we can decrease excessive saline or other intravenous (IV) infusions in the intraoperative period to attain adequate fluid balances, thereby decreasing complications and length of hospital stay. Physicians should avoid factors that contribute to increased stress response like—excessive or continuous bleeding, hypothermia (avoid deadly triad of hypothermia, acidosis, and coagulopathy, also hypothermia increases cortisol and catecholamine response with two- to threefold increased arrhythmia incidence), tissue edema by restrictive fluid strategy, hypoperfusion of tissues and correction at the earliest, avoid immobility (early ambulation and mobilization), and avoid starvation and other metabolic complications and minimal access techniques in surgery, if feasible (all these are parts of ERAS protocols following surgery). Maintaining normal glycemia (~150–180 mg/dL) with insulin infusion accordingly is necessary to decrease complications, tissue edema, and unnecessary activation of endothelium-derived inducible nitric oxide synthase (iNOS)-induced nitric oxide release which augment tissue hypoperfusion and cellular hypoxia secondary to compromised microcirculation by acting along with other mediators/cytokines due to stress/sepsis.

The basic differences in simple starvation and stress starvation are depicted in **Table 3**.

Table 3: Basic differences between starvation and hypermetabolic stress.

Starvation	Hypermetabolic stress
• Glycogen store depleted early	• Same
• Protein and fat breakdown starts	• Same
• Switch to *fatty acids as sole calorie source*	• Fatty acids partial calorie source. *Protein catabolism—main source of energy*
• Resting energy expenditure (REE)↓	• REE↑↑
• Proteolysis is decreased	• Proteolysis continues unabated
• Body protein is conserved	• Body protein lost
• Protein breakdown prevented by glucose infusion	• Not prevented by glucose
• Low metabolic demand	• High metabolic demand
• No release of cytokines	• Release of cytokines
• Decreased insulin secretion	• Insulin resistance, increased cortisol, catecholamine
• Nitrogen excretion↓	• Nitrogen excretion↑↑
• Weight loss slow	• Weight loss rapid

METABOLISM AT THE SUBCELLULAR LEVEL

Mitochondria contain the enzymes for citric acid cycle, beta-oxidation of fatty acids, ketogenesis as well as respiratory chain, and ATP synthase. Glycolysis, glycogenesis, glycogenolysis, fatty acid synthesis, and pentose phosphate pathway occur in cytosol. In gluconeogenesis, substrates like lactate and pyruvate, which are formed in the cytosol, enter mitochondria to yield oxaloacetate, a precursor for the synthesis of glucose in cytosol.

The membranes of endoplasmic reticulum contain enzyme system for TAG synthesis. Ribosomes are responsible for protein synthesis. 90% of oxygen consumption in the basal state is mitochondrial and 80% of it is coupled to ATP synthesis. Around 27% of ATP is used for protein synthesis, 24% used by Na^+/K^+-ATPase, 9% by gluconeogenesis, 6% by Ca^{2+}-ATPase, 5% by myosin ATPase, and 3% by ureagenesis.

Why knowledge on nutrition is important?
- Preoperative undernutrition has higher risk of postoperative complications.
- These patients have impaired immunity and muscle strength adding to higher ventilator dependence and infections.
- Delayed wound healing and delayed mobilization prolong surgical recovery.
- Undernutrition contributes to longer ICU stay, longer hospital stay, higher readmission rates, and markedly increased healthcare costs.

Such patients require increased nutritional requirements to support wound healing and hypermetabolism associated with surgical recovery.

PREHABILITATION

Prehabilitation is the process of enhancing an individual's functional capacity to enable him or her to withstand a forthcoming stressor, e.g., major surgery.

This is an emerging concept in nutritional care of surgical patients. This includes preoperative nutritional screening for all surgical patients, identifying the high-risk group, initiation of nutritional supplementation in the preoperative period, and preparing the patient to handle the perioperative stress efficiently. Along with perioperative nutritional support, supplementation needs to be continued through the postoperative period for 2–6 months depending upon the extent of surgical stress and postoperative complications. Studies have shown that 1 $ spend on nutrition/prehabilitation preoperatively saves 52 $ postoperatively. Even in well-developed nations, though 75% surgeons understand the importance of prehabilitation, only 20% of the time prehabilitation protocols are carried out.

Assessment of Nutrition and Nutritional Screening in a Surgical Patient

Underfeeding can cause for decline in nutritional status in hypermetabolism and overfeeding can cause complications like hypercapnia, metabolic acidosis, hyperglycemia, hypertriglyceridemia, hepatic dysfunction, and azotemia. So, nutritional assessment is the starting point of any nutritional therapy **(Box 3)**. There are several conventional methods for assessment existing in the literature. Also, we need to identify the high-risk population for prehabilitation **(Box 4)**.

In the absence of pathologic fluid retention, sustained weight gain is the hallmark of recovery of anabolism following stress/surgery. The reference point of ideal body weight (IBW) is getting fade and LBM seems to be more appropriate. LBM refers to the nonadipose tissue mass, exclusive of any added mass from acute shifts in water content. Malnutrition is characterized by decreased LBM and obese malnourished patients with decreased LBM are meant to have sarcopenic obesity (decreased handgrip and slow gait are

---

Box 3: Methods of nutritional assessment.

- Clinical history
- Body weight
- *Anthropometry*—ideal body weight (IBW), lean body mass (LBM), body mass index (BMI), and adjusted body weight (AjBW):
  - Ideal body weight—men—48 kg for first 152 cm height, then 2.7 kg for each additional 2.54 cm height, women—45 kg for first 152 cm height, then 2.3 kg for each additional 1.52 cm height—<20% loss—significant
  - AjBW – IBW – 0.4 (AjBW–IBW)
  - *Body mass index (kg/m^2)*:
    - Normal—18.5–24.9
    - Underweight—16.5–18.4 (severely underweight—<16.5)
    - Overweight—25–29.9
    - Obesity—grades I/II/III—30–34.9/35–39.9/>40
- Indirect calorimetry
- Bioelectrical impedance analysis (BIA)
- Oxygen consumption, respiratory coefficient estimation
- Body composition analysis—dual-energy X-ray absorptiometry
- Biochemical measurements—albumin (t½: 21 days), transferrin (t½: 8–10 days), prealbumin (t½: 2–4 days), total iron-binding capacity, and cholesterol
- Measurements of nitrogen balance
- Measurement of immunologic function—hypersensitivity reactions, lymphocyte counts
- Sarcopenia assessment—L3 level psoas muscle area, gait assessment, and handgrip

Screening tools:
- Subjective Global Assessment (SGA) score
- Mini Nutritional Assessment (MNA)
- Malnutrition Screening Tool (MST)
- Nutritional Risk Index
- Malnutrition Universal Screening Tool (MUST)
- Nutritional Risk Screening (NRS) 2002
- Nutrition Risk in Critically Ill (NUTRIC) score

> **Box 4:** High risk for prehabilitation.
> - Chronic disease, severe undernutrition
> - Significant weight loss—>10% in 6 months or 5% in 1 month
> - Expected blood loss >500 mL during surgery
> - <20% below IBW, BMI < 18.5 kg/m²
> - Failure to thrive on pediatric growth and development curves—<5th percentile or a trend line crossing two major percentile lines
> - Serum albumin < 3 g/dL or transferrin < 200 mg/dL in the absence of an inflammatory status/hepatic or renal dysfunction
> - Those patients in whom caloric requirement for the first 7–10 days cannot be met in the early perioperative period
> - Catabolic states—sepsis, burns, trauma, pancreatitis, and postoperative complications
>
> (BMI: body mass index; IBW: ideal body weight)

> **Box 5:** Urine urea nitrogen (UUN) balance.
> - Nitrogen balance (g/day) = Total nitrogen intake (g/day) – Total nitrogen loss
> - Total nitrogen loss = Urine urea nitrogen loss (g/day) + 4 (g/day) (when low UUN, i.e., <10 g/day)
> - Total urine nitrogen loss (g/day) = UUN (g/day) + [0.2 × UUN – nonurea nitrogen (g/day)] + 2 g/day (stool/insensible loss of nitrogen) (when UUN > 10 g/day)
> - UUN (g/day) = UUN (mg/dL) × Urine output (mL/day) × 1/1,000 (g/mg) × 1/100 (dL/mL)

its characteristics) and their morbidity and mortality are associated with LBM than IBW or gross body weight. Dual-energy X-ray absorptiometry (DEXA) is used for measuring changes in body tissue composition including LBM, fat mass, and bone density. High-resolution CT scan can reliably predict DEXA assessments accurately nowadays and even bedside ultrasound can sometimes help in nutritional assessment of the patient. In patients undergoing elective surgery, preoperative albumin < 3 g/dL is highly predictive of significant morbidity (sepsis, azotemia, encephalopathy, difficulty in weaning from ventilator, cardiac arrest, pneumonia, and delayed wound healing) and mortality.

Despite the limitations, most common clinical tool to assess the adequacy of a nutritional regimen in terms of net protein anabolism is nitrogen balance. It is simply the difference between the nitrogen given to the patient and the amount lost. If positive—anabolic state and if negative—catabolic state. The nitrogen equilibrium exists between –4 and +4 (**Box 5**).

Nitrogen balance (g/day) = Total nitrogen intake (g/day) - Total nitrogen loss
Total nitrogen loss = Urine urea nitrogen loss [UUN (in g/day)] + 4 (g/day) (when low UUN, i.e., <10 g/day)

Fudge factor 4 g assumes 2 g for nonurea nitrogen in urine and 2 g for stool and insensible losses of nonurinary nitrogen (especially in low UUN loss patients <10 g/day). But in severely ill critical care or trauma patients, along with increased UUN loss (>10 g/day) in hypercatabolic states, nonurea nitrogen loss can increase up to 4–5 g/day, which can be around 15–20% of UUN. So, the above formula needs to be modified.

Total urine nitrogen loss (g/day) = UUN (g/day) + [0.2 × UUN – nonurea nitrogen (g/day)] + 2 g/day (stool/insensible loss of nitrogen) (when UUN > 10 g/day)

A 24-hour UUN is calculated as below:

UUN (g/day) = UUN (mg/dL) × Urine output (mL/day) × 1/1,000 (g/mg) × 1/100 (dL/mL)

CALORIE REQUIREMENT

Though several formulas exist in literature for calculating REE, most simplistic formula seems to be 25–30 kcal/kg/day. The major calculations are shown in **Box 6**.

In consensus with the ERAS guidelines, the American Society for Enhanced Recovery and the Perioperative Quality Initiative Joint Consensus recommend a simple too in three steps to assess the nutritional risk and initiate preoperative nutritional supplementation *[Preoperative Oral Nutritional Supplementation (PONS) score]*.

Step 1: Is the patient's BMI < 18.5 kg/m^2 (<20 kg/m^2 if age > 65 years)?

Step 2: Weight loss score—is there unplanned weight loss > 10% in last 6 months?

Box 6: Major calculations for calorie requirement.

Calculations
Simplistic formula:
Calorie requirement: 25–30 kcal/kg/day

Protein requirement:
- Normal healthy individuals—0.8–1 g/kg/day
- Hypermetabolism—1.5–2 g/kg/day depending on the extent of stress

Critically ill obese:
- 65–70% of target:
  - Body mass index (BMI) (30–40 kg/m^2): 11–14 kcal/kg *actual body weight/day*
  - Body mass index (>40 kg/m^2): 22–25 kcal/kg *ideal body weight (IBW)/day*
- Protein intake:
  - *2.0 g/kg IBW/day*: BMI 30–40 kg/m^2
  - *2.5 g/kg IBW/day*: BMI ≥ 40 kg/m^2

Calculation of estimated IBW (18 years and above) (in kg):
- **Males**: IBW = 50 kg + 2.3 kg for each inch over 5 feet or 48 kg for first 152 cm height, then 2.7 kg for each 2.54 cm
- **Females**: IBW = 45.5 kg + 2.3 kg for each inch over 5 feet or 45 kg for first 152 cm height and then 2.3 kg for each additional 2.54 cm

Chronic kidney disease:
- Without dialysis—protein—0.55–0.6 g/kg/day
- With dialysis—protein—1.2–1.5 g/kg/day

Step 3: Intake score—have you been eating <50% of your normal diet in the preceding week?

If the answer to any of these is "Yes" and/or serum albumin level <3 mg/dL, the patient needs dietary intervention in the form of oral nutritional supplementation and frequent follow-up before the surgical procedure.

Surgical ICUs should make it a policy to implement the nutritional risk assessment for all admissions and actively involved in nutritional rehabilitation. The Society of Critical Care Medicine (SCCM) and the American Society for Parenteral and Enteral Nutrition (ASPEN) recommend *Nutrition Risk in Critically Ill (NUTRIC) score* **(Tables 4 and 5)** and *Nutritional*

Table 4: NUTRIC score variables.

Variables	Range	Points
Age	<50	0
	50–75	1
	>75	2
APACHE II	<15	0
	15–20	1
	20–28	2
	>28	3
SOFA	<6	0
	6–10	1
	>10	2
Number of comorbidities	0–1	0
	≥2	1
Days from hospital to ICU admission	0–<1	0
	≥1	1
IL-6	0–<400	–
	≥400	–

(APACHE II: Acute Physiology and Chronic Health Evaluation II; ICU: intensive care unit; IL-6: interleukin-6; NUTRIC: Nutrition Risk in Critically Ill; SOFA: Sequential Organ Failure Assessment)

Table 5: NUTRIC scoring system (NRS).

Sum of points	Category	Implementation
5–9 (if no IL-6 available)	High score	Associated with worst clinical outcome (mortality/ventilation)
6–10 (if IL-6 available)		Most likely to benefit from aggressive nutritional therapy
0–4 (–IL-6)	Low score	Low malnutrition risk
0–5 (+IL-6)		

(IL-6: interleukin-6; NRS: Nutritional Risk Screening; NUTRIC: Nutrition Risk in Critically Ill)

Table 6: NRS 2002.

Impaired nutritional status		Severity of disease	
Absent: 0	Normal nutritional status	Absent: 0	Normal nutritional requirements
Mild: 1	Weight loss >5% in 3 months or food intake <50–75% of required in the preceding week	Mild: 1	Hip fracture, chronic patients with acute complications, cirrhosis, COPD, c/c hemodialysis, diabetes, and oncology
Moderate: 2	Weight loss >5% in 2 months or BMI 18.5–20.5 kg/m^2 + impaired general condition or food intake 25–60% of required in preceding week	Moderate: 2	Major abdominal surgery, stroke, severe pneumonia, and hematologic malignancy
Severe: 3	Weight loss >5% in 1 month (>15% in 3 months) or BMI < 18.5 kg/m^2 + impaired general condition or food intake 0–25% of required in preceding week	Severe: 3	Head injury, bone marrow transplantation, and intensive care unit patients (APACHE II > 10)
Score (nutritional status) + Score (disease severity) = Total score			
Adjustment for age: If age > 70 years, add 1 to total score			
Score ≥ 3: Patient nutritionally at risk, a nutrition care plan is initiated			
Score < 3: Weekly rescreening of the patient. If the patient is scheduled for a major procedure, a preventive nutritional care plan is considered to avoid the associated risk status			

(APACHE II: Acute Physiology and Chronic Health Evaluation II; BMI: body mass index; COPD: chronic obstructive pulmonary disease; NRS: Nutritional Risk Screening)

Risk Screening (NRS) **(Table 6)** *2002* (ESPEN recommends NRS 2002) to be calculated in all patients admitted to surgical ICU whose oral intake is poor. NRS seems to be the widely used screening tool based on grade 1 evidence and the only tool shown to predict morbidity and mortality reliably in acute care and GI surgery patients. High-risk patients benefit from early nutritional initiation and have better outcomes.

DECISION-MAKING FOR NUTRITIONAL THERAPY

Step 1: Does the nutritional score analysis show need for nutritional supplementation?

If yes, step 2: Is his GI tract functional?

If yes, step 3: Is there any contraindications for enteral nutrition (EN)?

If yes, start parenteral nutrition (PN), if no, start EN.

Nutritional support can be enteral or parenteral.

> **Box 7:** Indications of early enteral nutritional support.
> - Malnourished patient expected to be unable to eat >5–7 days
> - Normally nourished patient expected to be unable to eat >7–9 days
> - Adaptive phase of short bowel syndrome
> - Increased needs that cannot be met through oral intake (burns, trauma)
> - Inadequate oral intake resulting in deterioration of nutritional status or delayed recovery from illness

> **Box 8:** Contraindications to enteral nutrition.
> - Intestinal obstruction
> - Intestinal ischemia/perforation
> - Inability to access the gut
> - Severe acute pancreatitis
> - High output proximal fistula
> - Shock
> - Severe gastrointestinal (GI) bleed

Enteral Nutrition

Feeding the gut with EN is essential and the most recommended approach for almost all disease states which a surgeon can encounter. EN is more physiological, cheaper, easy available, easily implementable, and with less complications. Every effort should be made to initiate EN at the earliest in the ICU as early energy deficit is directly related to the incidence of increased infections in ICU.

Rationale for Enteral Nutrition (Boxes 7 and 8)

The basic dictum is "when gut works, use it".

Enteral nutrition maintains the intestinal villous trophicity and improves gut motility. This maintains the epithelial integrity and prevents translocation of gut bacteria to the bloodstream. The initial source of gram-negative septicemia in a critically ill patient is gut bacterial translocation due to epithelial breakdown from a nonfed patient.

How early?

All current guidelines recommend to start EN as early as 24–48 hours within admission to ICU or within a major surgical intervention, if not contraindicated otherwise. All patients after assessment of preoperative oral nutritional supplementation score in outpatient department (OPD) itself during the first visit, nutritional advice needs to be given. Supplementation needs to be started at the earliest, if oral intake is not adequate. The route of nutritional supplementation depends on the functional status of patient, type/site of surgery anticipated, how earliest surgery needs to be scheduled, and nutritional assessment scores.

Types of Enteral Feeding Formulas

- Polymeric—blenderized (kitchen feed) and commercially prepared formula feeds
- Monomeric/oligomeric
- Modular
- Disease specific
- Fiber containing
- Rehydration.

Polymeric formula: It provides intact nutrients and the energy distribution is similar to normal diet—carbohydrate 40–60%, fat 25–40%, and protein 15–25%. This is the most common formula used for tube feeding and can be either commercially prepared or kitchen feed (blenderized) **(Table 7)**.

Oligomeric formulas: These are used in critically ill patients and those with GI dysfunction who cannot digest complete nutrients. They can be supplemented with elemental or semi-elemental formulas where the nutrient is in partly digested form and can easily be absorbed. Peptide-based formulas are also included in this category.

Elemental (monomeric) formulas: Elemental formulas contain individual amino acids, are low in fat, especially long-chain triglycerides (LCTs), and as such, are thought to require minimal digestive function and cause less stimulation of exocrine pancreatic secretion. In many products, medium-chain triglycerides (MCTs) are the predominant fat source and can be absorbed directly across the small intestinal mucosa into the portal vein in the absence of lipase or bile salts; they are believed to be beneficial in malabsorptive states. They are also considered to be advantageous in patients with acute pancreatitis and in those with other malabsorptive states like critically ill patients with feeding intolerance, short bowel syndrome, chronic pancreatitis, and Crohn's disease with feeding intolerance.

Rehydration formula: This is for patients requiring optimal ratio of carbohydrate to electrolytes to facilitate fluid and electrolyte absorption, rehydration.

Modular formula: A modular formula is an incomplete liquid supplement that contains specific nutrients, usually a single macronutrient (carbohydrate,

Table 7: Common differences between blenderized food and commercial formulas.

Blenderized food	Commercial formulas
• Unknown nutritional content • Unknown osmolality • May contain lactose • Amenable to contamination • High viscosity, tube clogging common	• Complete, balanced nutrition • Low-to-moderate osmolality • Lactose and gluten free • Sterile • Excellent tube flow

protein, or fat) added to food and enteral formulas. It may also contribute to renal solute load, osmolality.

Fiber-containing formula: Formulas containing a source of fiber, reportedly beneficial for prevention/treatment of altered bowel function in enterally fed patients. Soy polysaccharide is the most common fiber additive in enteral feedings; effectiveness in treating diarrhea in tube-fed patients is unproven. Soluble fiber (guar gum, oat fiber, and pectin) may exert trophic effect on colonic mucosa and be useful in normalizing bowel function. Most enteral feedings in amounts typically used contain less than recommended fiber intake for adults (20–35 g). Patients with impaired gastric emptying should not be fed fiber-containing formula into the stomach.

Disease-specific formulas: Formulas specially made for specific conditions like kidney disease, liver disease, cancer patients, etc., are available nowadays. In renal failure patients without dialysis, standard formulas can be given if planning for oral supplementation or <5 days of nutritional plan. If >5 days, dense calorie renal formulas need to be given (2 kcal/mL). In dialysis patients, standard formulas are given for feed, but calorie dense formulas are used when tube feeding is initiated. In patients with liver disease, BCAA preparations are more in proportion to aromatic amino acid (AAA) (maintaining Fischer ratio). In patients with chronic obstructive pulmonary disease (COPD), we may have to give low carbohydrate diet in order to decrease CO_2 production. Diabetic-specific formulas are also available. Whey protein-containing formulas along with MCT preparations are preferred in those with delayed gastric emptying problems. Immunomodulatory preparations with omega-3 fatty acids and other immune nutrients are available for cancer patients to decrease the inflammatory cascade and cancer cachexia.

Enteral Formula Nutrient Sources (Box 9)

Knowledge of various nutrient sources in formulas are essential since it helps to select appropriate formulas based on the absorption and digestion criteria of each sources. The various sources of enteral formulas are depicted in **Table 8**. Protein sources are mainly soy protein and milk proteins

---

Box 9: Formula selection.

- Suitability of each formula is based on:
  - Functional status of gastrointestinal (GI) tract
  - Physical characteristics of formula (osmolality, fiber content, caloric density, and viscosity)
  - Macronutrient ratios
  - Digestion and absorption capability of patient
  - Specific metabolic needs
  - Contribution of the feeding to fluid and electrolyte needs or restriction
  - Cost-effectiveness

Table 8: Various nutrient sources of enteral formulas.

Carbohydrate (CHO)	Fat	Protein
• CHO content ranges from 40 to 90% of total calories • Typically some combination of hydrolyzed cornstarch, maltodextrins, corn syrup solids, and sucrose • *Fructooligosaccharides (FOSs):* Poorly absorbed in the small intestine, fermented in the large intestine; may promote growth of healthy bacteria in diabetic preparations • *Fiber:* Soy polysaccharide (most common) guar gum, oat fiber, and pectin	• Fat provides isotonic, concentrated energy source • Corn and soybean oil are common. Also, includes safflower, canola, and fish oil • May include medium-chain triglycerides (MCTs); more easily digested and absorbed (directly to portal vein, easy form of energy) • Fat content ranges from <10 to >50% of calories	• Whole protein, hydrolyzed protein, and free amino acids • Casein, soy protein, lactalbumin, whey, and egg white albumin • Small peptides absorbed as efficiently as free amino acids • Free amino acids are more hyperosmolar • *Arginine:* Conditionally essential amino acid with immune-enhancing properties, may be harmful in septic patients • *Glutamine:* May enhance small intestine growth and repair

(80% casein—slow absorption and digestion, 20% whey protein—fast absorption and digestion). Whey protein is the collection of protein that can be isolated from whey, a byproduct of cheese made from cow's milk.

Enteral Routes for Feeding (Fig. 2)
- Ryle's tube soft—if enteral feed expected >1 week.
- Percutaneous endoscopic gastrostomy (PEG)/Jejunostomy—if enteral feed expected >1 month.

Types of Feeding
The types of feeding are described in **Table 9**.

Open versus Closed System of Feeding
The open versus closed system of feeding is given in **Table 10**.

The various locally available products, dilutions of each products with calorie/protein content is available in a software which is available in Google Play Stores developed by a Keralite doctor/neurologist that is helpful in prescribing each product formulations easily (courtesy to the brilliant neurologist)—App name is *Feed Calc*.

Complications of Enteral Feeding
The complications of enteral feeding are given in **Box 10**.

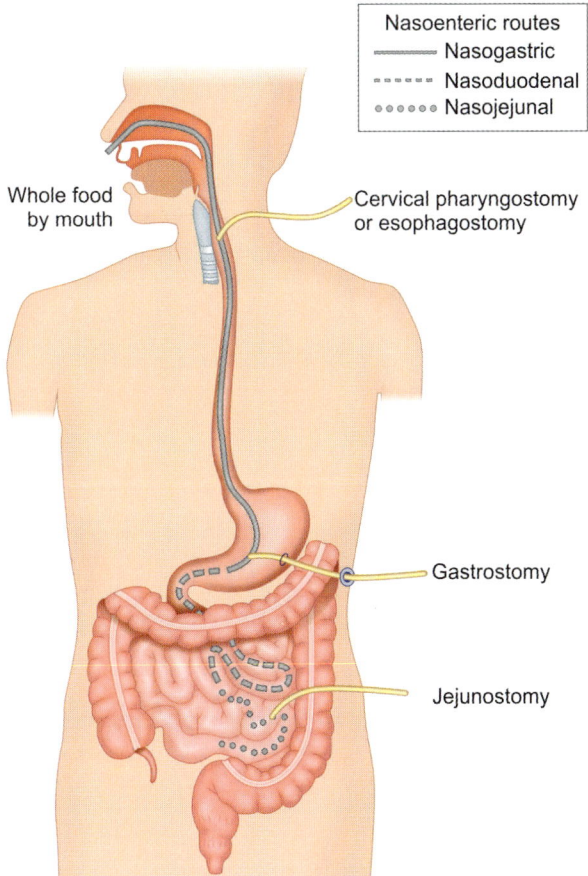

Fig. 2: Enteral routes for feeding.

Concept of a Nutrition Pyramid (Fig. 3)

The nutritional assessment starts at the first visit to OPD and supplements are started if inadequate oral intake as per PONS or <60–70% below the expected level. After reassessment (if possible weekly) shows <60% intake including supplements, tube feeding is to be started. Similarly, parenteral supplementation should be started if <60% intake on further assessment or inability to tolerate enteral diet. De-escalation down the nutrition pyramid done once >60% intake at every levels at fixed periods of assessment and slowly optimize on oral EN without any metabolic complications.

Refeeding Syndrome (Fig. 4 and Table 11)

Refeeding syndrome is defined as derangements in serum electrolytes (phosphate, potassium, and magnesium), vitamin deficiency, and fluid as well as sodium retention occurring in malnourished patients after initiation

Table 9: Types of enteral feeding along with their indications and disadvantages.

Types of feed	Indications and disadvantages
Bolus: • Infusion of up to 500 mL of enteral formula into the stomach over 5–20 minutes, usually by gravity or with a large-bore syringe • Initiate with full strength formula three to eight times per day with increase of 60–120 mL q 8–12 hours as tolerated up to goal volume; does not require dilution unless necessary to meet fluid requirements	*Indications:* • Recommended for gastric feedings • Requires intact gag reflex • Normal gastric function *Disadvantages:* • Increases risk for aspiration • Hypertonic, high fat, or high fiber formulas may delay gastric emptying or result in osmotic diarrhea
Continuous: • Administration into the gastrointestinal tract (GIT) via pump or gravity, usually over 8–24 h/day • Initiate at full strength at 10–40 mL/h and advance to goal rate in increments of 10–20 mL/h q 8–12 hours as tolerated	*Indications:* • Initiation of feedings in acutely ill patients • Promote tolerance, feeding into small bowel • Compromised gastric function (less aspiration) • Intolerance to other feeding techniques *Disadvantages:* • May reduce 24-hour infusion, may restrict ambulation • More expensive for home support • Pumps are more accurate; useful for small-bore tubes and viscous feedings
Intermittent: • Enteral formula administered at specified times throughout the day; generally in smaller volume and at slower rate than a bolus feeding but in larger volume and faster rate than continuous drip feeding • Typically 200–300 mL is given over 30–60 minutes q 4–6 hours. Precede and follow with 30 mL flush	*Indications:* • Intolerance to bolus administration • Initiation of support without pump • Preparation of patient for rehabilitation services or discharge to home or long-term care (LTC) facility (enhance quality-of-life) *Disadvantages:* • Increased risk for aspiration, gastric distension • Delayed gastric emptying

Cyclical:
• Administration of enteral formula via continuous drip over a defined period of 8–12 hours, usually nocturnally
	Indications:
	• Ensure optimal nutrient intake when:
	  – Transitioning from enteral support to oral nutrition (enhance appetite during the day)
	  – Supplement inadequate oral intake
	  – Free patient from enteral feedings during the day
	
	Disadvantages: May require high infusion rates—may promote intolerance

of nutritional therapy. This can occur after enteral feeding in prolonged starvation patients or after parenteral nutrition.

On refeeding with glucose-based nutritional regimens, however, inorganic phosphate is needed for phosphorylation of glucose which in this form enters

Table 10: Open versus closed system of feeding.

Open system	Closed system or ready-to-hang (RTH)
• Product is decanted into a feeding bag • Allows modulators such as protein and fiber to be added to feeding formulas • Less waste in unstable patients (may be) • Shortens hang time • Increases nursing time • Increased risk of contamination • Hang time 8 hours for decanted formula, 4 hours for formula mixtures	• Containers sterile until spiked for hanging • Can be used for continuous or bolus delivery • No flexibility in formula additives • Less nursing time • Increases safe hang time • Less risk of contamination • More expensive than canned formula • Hang time 24–48 hours based on manufacturer recommendations

Box 10: Complications of enteral feeding.

- *Aspiration pneumonia*—to avoid this—head end elevated 30–40°, 30–40 minutes after feed (no difference between nasojejunal or nasogastric tubes)
- *Diarrhea*—most common complication:
  - Definition: >500 mL every 8 hours or >three stool a day for at least two consecutive days. Relates more to stool consistency than frequency [causes—medications (high osmolar), altered bacterial flora, formula composition (increased osmolality and rate), hypoalbuminemia and bowel edema, and formula contamination]
- *Altered drug absorption, metabolism*
- *Tube clogging*
- *Complications while insertion*—always check position with X-ray of chest, tip subdiaphragmatically placed
- *Metabolic*—dyselectrolytemia, dehydration (high osmolar), and hyperglycemia
- *Refeeding syndrome*
- *Gastrointestinal complications*—diarrhea, constipation/fecal impaction, gastric distension/bloating, gastric residuals/delayed gastric emptying, and nausea/vomiting (sudden increase in gastric residual >200 mL—probable sepsis)
- *Hyperosmolar nonketotic coma*
- *Pneumatosis intestinalis with bowel necrosis and perforation*—with aggressive administration of hyperosmolar formulas

glycolysis. During glucose supply, endogenous insulin secretion is stimulated or insulin must be administered exogenously to maintain normoglycemia. Hyperinsulinism leads to protein synthesis accompanied by a transfer of glucose and phosphate into cells. The combined effects of phosphate loss during starvation and increased insulin-mediated transport of phosphate from the extracellular to the intracellular compartment during refeeding with glucose can lead to a dramatic drop in blood phosphate concentration.

The metabolic alterations noted are hypokalemia, hypomagnesemia, hypophosphatemia, and hypernatremia and water retention. A low serum phosphorus 48–72 hours after started feeding the patient is a definitive indication of refeeding syndrome. Insulin can cause sodium retention by acting in the renal tubules, especially when hyperglycemia causing extra insulin secretion with persisting insulin resistance situations.

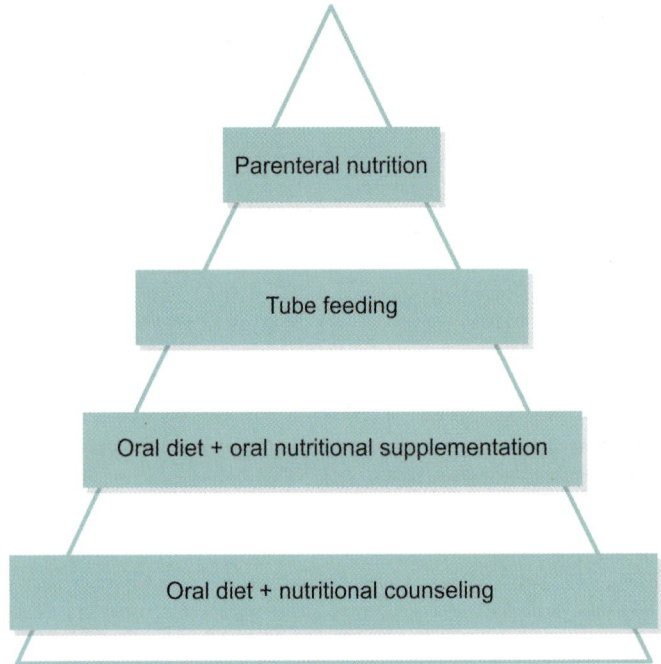

Fig. 3: Nutrition pyramid.

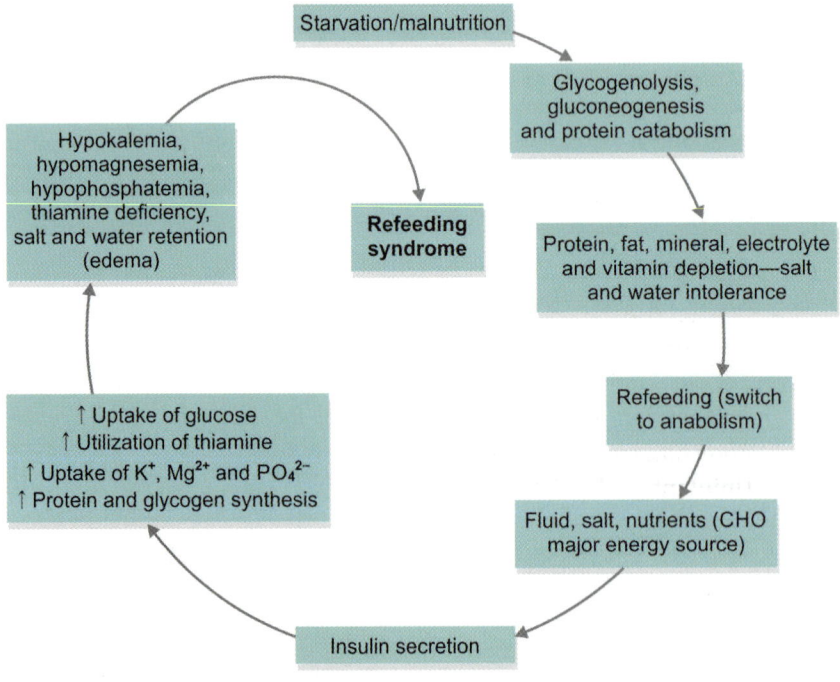

Fig. 4: Refeeding syndrome.
(CHO: carbohydrates)

Table 11: Systems involved in refeeding syndrome.

Systems involved	Clinical manifestations
Cardiac	• Hypo-/hypertension • Arrhythmia • Ventricular dysfunction, sudden death
Gastrointestinal	Ileus
Respiratory	• Respiratory failure/ventilator dependence • Pulmonary edema
Renal	• Prerenal failure • Osmotic diuresis
Neurological	• Paraesthesis/paralysis • Weakness/ataxia/tremor • Encephalopathy • Seizures
Hematological	• White blood cell (WBC), platelet dysfunction • Hemolysis
Musculoskeletal	• Osteomalacia • Rhabdomyolysis
Thiamine deficiency	Wernicke encephalopathy or Korsakoff syndrome, associated with: Ocular disturbance, confusion, ataxia, loss of ability to coordinate muscular movement, coma, short-term memory loss, and confabulation

Due to high complications in virtually all systems of the body, refeeding syndrome is very difficult to treat. Hence, it is crucial to prevent and identify early for successful outcomes.

The National Institute for Health and Care Excellence (NICE) has given level D recommendations to identify patients at high risk for refeeding syndrome:

- Patient with one or more of the following criteria:
    - Body mass index < 16 kg/m^2
    - Unintentional weight loss >15% in the last 3–6 months
    - Little or no nutritional intake for >10 days
    - Low levels of potassium, magnesium, and phosphate before feeding.
- Patient with two or more of the following:
    - Body mass index < 18.5 kg/m^2
    - Unintentional weight loss >10% in the past 3–6 months
    - Little or no nutritional intake for >5 days
    - History of alcohol miscues or drugs, including insulin, chemotherapy, antacids, or diuretics.

Management of patients identified to develop refeeding syndrome: The management of patients identified to develop refeeding syndrome are illustrated in **Flowchart 5**.

Flowchart 5: Management of patients identified to develop refeeding syndrome.

```
Patient at risk
      ↓
Check serum Ca²⁺, Mg²⁺, K⁺, and phosphorus
      ↓
Before feeding starts, administer thiamine 200–300 mg oral, vitamin B₁,
multivitamin, and trace elements supplementation
      ↓
Start slow calorie feeds at 10 kcal/kg/day—>gradually increase over 4–7 days
      ↓
Rehydrate and supplement K⁺, Ca²⁺, Mg²⁺, and PO₄²⁻ intravenous/oral
      ↓
Monitor electrolytes level for the first 2 weeks
```

> **Box 11:** Absolute and relative contraindications for EN.
>
> *Absolute contraindications for EN:*
> - Intestinal obstruction
> - Ischemic bowel
> - Acute peritonitis
>
> *Relative contraindications for EN (use PN if EN deemed to be not feasible):*
> - High output fistulas
> - Severe malabsorption
> - Septic shock with impaired splanchnic perfusion
> - Fulminant sepsis

Parenteral Nutrition

Though controversial data exists regarding routine use of PN in the past, emerging data shows promising results on supplemental PN in acute stress situation and perioperative period. Presence of malnutrition and its severity should be considered when making decisions regarding the type and timing of nutritional therapy. While most of the surgical patients can get advanced to oral diet in the postoperative period shortly after surgery, major surgery or postoperative complications can delay advancement to full oral diet. There are absolute and relative indications of PN where we cannot attain protein calorie requirements with enteral feed alone.

Parenteral nutrition indications in relation to feasibility of EN are described in **Box 11**.

In elective surgery, though there is limited data to support preoperative PN in severely malnourished patients, some evidence suggests that adequate feeding for at least 7–10 days prior to surgery and continued after surgery may decrease postsurgical complications. Nowadays, delay in elective surgery for preoperative prehabilitation has been recommended for patients with one or more of the following conditions:

- Lost > 10-15% of actual body weight within 3-6 months
- Body mass index < 18.5 kg/m²
- Subjective Global Assessment score grade C (severe malnutrition)
- Serum albumin < 30 g/L without hepatic or renal dysfunction or an IBW < 90%.

The current guidelines recommend starting nutrition therapy within 3-5 days of operation, if patients were nutritionally at risk preoperatively and are unlikely to achieve desired oral intake or EN. The ESPEN guidelines for clinical nutrition in surgery (recommendation 8) states that "if energy and nutrient requirements cannot be met by oral and enteral intake alone (<50% of calorie requirement) for >7 days, a combination of enteral and PN is recommended. The 2016 SCCM/ASPEN guidelines state that "we recommend that, in patients at either low or high nutritional risk, use of supplemental PN can be considered if unable to meet 60% of energy and protein requirements by enteral route alone. Though there is data on detrimental outcome on patients who are critically ill, who are on some form of EN, and commencement of PN prior to 7-10 days period, there is supportive evidence to start supplemental nutrition in carefully selected patients with less inflammatory surge after 3-5 days (i.e., safest period to start perioperatively is after 7-10 days)".

The indications of PN in setting of EN are:
- After major GI surgery when GIT is not accessible or not functioning (mechanical obstruction/ileus)
- After extensive small bowel resection with or without colonic resection
- With perforated small bowel
- With high output fistula (>600 mL) and/or proximal fistulas that necessitate bowel rest
- Other conditions leading to prolonged EN intolerance (like severe diarrhea, persistent emesis, significant abdominal distension, acute GI bleeding, hemodynamic instability, impaired gastric emptying, or paralytic ileus) preventing sufficient EN provision for 3-7 days.

Parenteral nutrition is contraindicated in (not fully evidence-based):
- Those with functional GIT and accessibility for EN
- Fluid-restricted patients who cannot tolerate the IV fluid load provided for PN
- Those with severe hyperglycemia or electrolyte abnormalities at day of PN initiation
- Parenteral nutrition therapy is unlikely to be given for >5-7 days
- If new access, line placement solely for PN causes unnecessary risks.

Parenteral nutritional solutions can be given through IV or centrally placed catheters. These centrally placed catheters can be placed peripherally (PICC line—peripherally inserted central line catheter) or in a no tunneled fashion percutaneously directly into a central vein. The types of PN vary—peripheral

PN (PPN) and central PN (CPN). PPN is preferred if nutritional supplement for <10–14 days and CPN is preferred if requirement up to 1 month exists (PICC line can be used in such scenario). For long-term PN (>30 days), a tunneled silicone-based cuffed catheter is preferred, though not much evidence-based. PPN is less osmolar (so safely given through peripheral IV access without getting much vascular complications like phlebitis) and large proportion of energy contents as lipid emulsions and CPN is hyperosmolar and more calories in the form of dextrose. A typical CPN provides 60–70% of nonprotein calories as dextrose and 30–40% of nonproteins as lipid emulsions. There are commercially available lipid emulsions and amino acid formulations providing all essential amino acids and several nonessential amino acids. Addition of glutamine once thought of benefit has not been demonstrated to provide no additional benefit in multiple randomized controlled trials (RCTs) in critically ill patients. The maximal recommended dose of lipid emulsions infusion is 1–1.3 g/kg/day, with TG monitoring (TG level to be maintained <400–500 mg/dL) to decrease risk of pancreatitis and respiratory diffusion abnormalities in COPD patients. Electrolyte and blood sugar corrections need to be optimized and refeeding syndrome should be prevented. The clinical practice guidelines recommend a glycemic goal range in hospitalized adult patients receiving nutrition support to be 140–180 mg/dL (7.8–10 mmol/L). The essential fatty acid requirement for a week is around ~ 100–200 g. 2–4% of daily requirements should be derived from linoleic acid and 0.5% from alpha-linolenic acid. Infusion of IV fat emulsion should be restricted to <30% of total calories or 1 g/kg/day and administered over a period of 8–10 hours. If infusion rates of LCT emulsions >0.15 g/kg/h, immunosuppressive effects may come. Endogenous glucose production is suppressed when glucose is infused at a rate of 1 mg/kg/min and maximally at 4 mg/kg/min. In pediatrics, 25% dextrose can be given maximally at 7 mg/kg/min. Studies have shown that delayed introduction of IV fat emulsions (>10 days) is associated with decreased complications in polytrauma patients. Most preparations contain soybean oil which has high content of omega-6 fatty acids, linolenic acid. Fish oils contain omega-3 fatty acids which are anti-inflammatory (eicosapentaenoic acid) and studies have shown decreased infectious complications and hospital stay with this. Nowadays, Soybean oil, MCT, Olive oil, and Fish oil (SMOF) combination is available. Nitrogen-to-calorie ratio of most feeding formulas prepared for surgical patients has been 1:150 (1 g nitrogen for every 150 kcal). For PN, a protein:fat:glucose calorie ratio has generally been approximated to 20:30:50.

Complications of Parenteral Nutrition

- Catheter-related bloodstream infections
- Mechanical complications associated with catheter insertion—hemo-/pneumothorax, thrombosis, and bleeding

- Metabolic complications—overfeeding and refeeding syndrome
- Liver dysfunction in long-term use during intestinal failure.

The concept of home PN was introduced as a treatment option for patients with long-term intestinal failure—in patients with Crohn's disease, mesenteric vascular disease, cancer, intestinal failure, and radiation enteritis who cannot meet their nutritional needs by EN and who cannot be treated outside the acute care setting. The goal of home PN is to prevent and/or correct malnutrition for a period of months or rest of one's life. The current practice guidelines do not recommend home PN for patients with a short life expectancy for at least 40–60 days. This is delivered through subcutaneously tunneled catheters or implanted ports. This itself is not without complications—thrombosis, catheter-related occlusion, infections, metabolic bone disease, and liver dysfunction which may require concurrent liver and intestinal transplantation.

MICRO-/MACRONUTRIENTS

Nutrient is a substance used by organism to survive, grow, and reproduce. Mainly, it includes carbohydrates, fats, proteins, minerals, and vitamins. It is classified into macro- or micronutrients based on the amount required for daily maintenance of bodily functions. Based on the location of absorption, deficiencies develop following surgical resection of those segments of GIT. The location of absorption, types of micro-/macronutrients, and their deficiencies have been briefly explained in **Table 12**.

Macronutrient Requirements

The major macronutrient requirements are depicted in **Table 13**.

Table 12: Location and nutrient absorption in gastrointestinal (GI) tract.

GI location	Nutrient absorption
Stomach	Water, ethyl alcohol, copper, iodide, molybdenum, and fluoride
Duodenum	Calcium, magnesium, phosphorus, copper, iron, selenium, thiamine, riboflavin, niacin, biotin, folate, and vitamins—A, D, E, and K
Jejunum	Lipids, monosaccharides, amino acids, small peptides, calcium, phosphorus, magnesium, iron, thiamine, riboflavin, niacin, pantothenate, biotin, folate, vitamin B_6, vitamin C, vitamins A, D, E, K, zinc, chromium, manganese, and molybdenum
Ileum	Amino acids, vitamin C, folate, vitamin B_{12}, vitamin D, vitamin K, magnesium, and bile salts
Colon	Water, sodium, chloride, potassium, vitamin D, biotin, and short-chain fatty acids

Table 13: Major macronutrient requirements.

Nutrients	European Association for the Study of Diabetes (EASD) (% energy)	American Diabetic Association (ADA) (% energy)
Protein	10–20	15–20
Fat	35	–
Saturated fatty acids (SFAs)	SFA + Trans-fat < 10	SFA < 7, limits trans-fat
Carbohydrates	45–60	At least 130 g/day

Table 14: Major minerals based on their daily requirement.

Macrominerals (>100 mg/day)	Microminerals (trace) (1–100 mg/day)	Microminerals (ultratrace) (<1 mg/day)
• Calcium • Chloride • Phosphorus • Potassium • Sodium	• Chromium • Copper • Fluorine • Iron • Manganese • Zinc	• Iodine • Molybdenum • Selenium

Minerals Requirements

Major minerals based on their daily requirement are shown in **Table 14**.

Major Significant Trace Minerals Requiring Supplementation in Perioperative Period

Zinc and selenium are very important during perioperative period and need to know their deficiency symptoms and need to supplement it at times of stress **(Table 15)**.

Vitamins and their Relevance

The vitamins and their relevance are described in **Table 16**.

FLUIDS AND ELECTROLYTES

Fluid intake is derived from both exogenous (consumed liquids) and endogenous (released during oxidation of solid food/energy transfers) fluids.

Average daily water balance of a 70 kg adult is shown in **Table 17**.

Minimum ~ 400 mL/day urine is required for excretion of end products of protein metabolism. Insensible loss from lungs is around 400 mL/day and from skin through sweating can be 600–1,000 mL/day. Simplest formula for daily maintenance of fluids is ~ 30–40 mL/kg. Jejunal mucosa is leaky and rapid sodium fluxes occur across it. If water or any solution with a sodium

Table 15: Major significant trace minerals requiring supplementation.

Trace minerals	Functions	Deficiency etiology	Deficiency symptoms
Zinc	• Protein, carbohydrate metabolism • Wound healing • Cellular immunity • Enzyme component • Anti-inflammation • Antioxidant	• Short bowel syndrome • Diarrhea • Short bowel syndrome • High output gastrointestinal (GI) fistula	• Hair loss • Altered taste • Altered smell • Diarrhea • Skin rash • Hepatic/respiratory dysfunction • Decreased muscle work capacity • Acrodermatitis enteropathica • Hepatic encephalopathy
Selenium	• Essential component glutathione peroxidase • Thyroxine production and conversion to thyronine • Reduce NF-KB expression and decrease of inflammation	• Unsupplemented parenteral nutrition/medical nutrition formula • Alcoholism • Trauma • Resection duodenum and proximal jejunum	• Affects muscles and heart • Arrhythmia • Congestive cardiac failure • Myositis • Weakness and muscle cramps

concentration <90 mEq/L is consumed, there is a net efflux of sodium from the plasma into the bowel lumen. This knowledge should be utilized during managing a small intestinal stoma or short bowel syndrome.

IMMUNONUTRITION

This consists of specific immune-modulating nutrients, thereby modifying host's immune response. Most of the benefits derive from reduced incidence of hyperglycemia and decreased production of proinflammatory cytokines like prostaglandin E2 and leukotrienes. The major nutrients are shown in **Table 18**.

Immunonutrition has shown clinical benefits in certain situations (recommendations) 7 days before and 7 days after surgery:
- Patients undergoing head and neck surgery.
- Severely malnourished patient (albumin < 2.8 g/dL) or patients undergoing major oncologic GI surgery (esophageal/gastric/pancreatic/duodenal/hepatobiliary).
- Patients with severe trauma ≥2 body systems (e.g., chest, abdomen, spinal cord, head, extremities) and severity score of ≥18 or an abdominal trauma index of ≥20 (which includes—grade 3 pancreaticoduodenal/grade 4 hepatic/grade 4 colonic/gastric injuries).

Table 16: Major vitamins, their functions, and deficiency disorders.

Vitamins	Functions	Deficiency
B_1—thiamine	Coenzymes in: • Pyruvate—acetyl-CoA • Alpha-ketoglutarate—succinyl-CoA • Ribose 5-phosphate + Xylulose 5-phosphate • Sedoheptulose 7-phosphate + Glyceraldehyde 3-phosphate • BCAA oxidation	• Beriberi • Wernicke-Korsakoff syndrome (in alcoholics) • Refeeding syndrome
B_2—riboflavin	• FMN/FAD supply—energy • Electron transfer	• Dermatitis • Angular stomatitis
B_3—niacin	• NAD/NADH supply—energy • Electron transfer	• Dermatitis, diarrhea, and dementia
B_5—pantothenic acid	CoA—acyl carrier	Rare
B_6—pyridoxine	Pyridoxal phosphate, coenzymes in amino acid metabolism	Glossitis, neuropathy
B_7—biotin	Carboxylation reactions	• Raw egg whites can cause deficiency • Dermatitis
B_9—folic acid	Tetrahydrofolate—one carbon unit, synthesis of serine/methionine/purines/thymidine monophosphate	Megaloblastic anemia, neural tube defects
B_{12}—cobalamin	Coenzymes for: • Homocysteine—methionine • Methylmalonyl-CoA—succinyl-CoA	Pernicious anemia, dementia, and spinal degeneration
C	• Antioxidant • Hydroxylation of proline/lysine—hydroxyl proline/lysine	• Scurvy • Sore, spongy gums • Loose teeth • Poor wound healing • Bleeding
A—retinoic acid	• Maintenance of reproduction • Vision, growth promotion • Differentiation and maintenance of epithelial tissues • Gene expression	• Night blindness • Xerophthalmia • Infertility • Growth retardation
D—cholecalciferol	• Calcium uptake • Gene expression • Modulate immune responses	• Rickets • Osteomalacia
E—α-tocopherol	Antioxidant	• RBC fragility • Hemolytic anemia
K—menadione	Gamma carboxylation of glutamate residues in clotting and other proteins	Bleeding

(BCAA: branched-chain amino acid; FAD: flavin adenine dinucleotide; FMN: flavin mononucleotide; NAD: nicotinamide adenine dinucleotide; RBC: red blood cell)

Table 17: Average daily water balance.

Output	Volume (mL)	Intake	Volume (mL)
Urine	1,500	Water from beverages	1,200
Insensible loss	900	Water from food	1,000
Feces	100	Water from oxidation	300

Table 18: Major nutrients.

Immune stimulating	Digestive tract health	Anti-inflammatory
Arginine—support T lymphocytes and substrate for nitric oxide	Glutamine—colonocyte fuel	Eicosapentaenoic acid (EPA)—omega-3 fatty acid (produce favorable prostaglandins)
Glutamine—fuel of immune system	Probiotic	Gamma-linolenic acid (GLA)
Iron	Prebiotic	• Antioxidants—vitamins C, E, and A • Selenium, zinc • Taurine • Copper • Manganese
Nucleotides	–	–

- Patients with mild sepsis [Acute Physiology and Chronic Health Evaluation II (APACHE II) score < 15], contraindicated in critically ill patients and in severe sepsis.
- Patients with acute respiratory distress syndrome.

MYTHS IN CLINICAL NUTRITION PRACTICE

- Do we need bowel sounds to initiate enteral feeding?
  After a GI surgery, small intestinal myoelectrical activity starts earlier at 4-8 hours, gastric myoelectrical activity starts at 24 hours, and colonic myoelectrical activity starts at 3-5 days. Delay in initiation of bowel sounds is commonly noted following the use of opioids and vasopressors in surgery. Onset of bowel sounds is a poor marker of GI function—it indicates only contractility, not mucosal integrity or absorptive function. Auscultation of bowel sounds and passage of flatus are not absolute necessities in clinical practice to start EN. "If you feed them, bowel sounds will follow".
- Do we need routine nasogastric decompression after major abdominal surgeries?
  Many clinical studies have proven that this clinical practice adds on to morbidity by increasing patient discomfort, gastroesophageal reflux, and

Table 19: Secretion of various digestive juices in the body.

Saliva	1.5 L
Gastric secretion	2.5 L
Pancreatic/biliary	2 L
Intestine	1 L

respiratory complications as atelectasis, pneumonia, and fever. Hence, routine nasogastric decompression should be avoided and practiced only as a therapeutic option.

- *Enteral feeding in hemodynamically unstable critically ill patients*: EN is not contraindicated in critically ill patients receiving IV vasopressor support. The ASPEN guidelines recommend initiation of enteral feeding within 24-48 hours of ICU admission, provided the patient is not on high catecholamine support. Clinical studies have proven safe tolerance of EN if the vasopressor requirement of noradrenaline equivalent of 12.5 µg/min or less and mean arterial pressure >60 mm Hg. Addition of dopamine or vasopressin adversely affects the enteral feeding tolerance by altering the mesenteric blood flow and gastroduodenal motility. EN can be safely administered keeping a careful watch on signs of intolerance as a rise in serum lactate and gastric residual volume >300 mL, emesis as well as signs of GI ischemia.
- *Routine gastric residual volume (GRV) measurement to withhold enteral feeding*: The secretion of digestive juices in the body is described in **Table 19**.

The residual volume aspirated contains not only the enteral feed given, but also these digestive juices, discarding which can lead to severe electrolyte imbalances. Many guidelines differ in the amount of GRV to slow down the enteral feeding protocol. Monitoring the GRV was thought to decrease the incidence of aspiration pneumonia, but studies have proven that even higher GRVs (400-500 mL) are not associated with increase in the incidence of aspiration. This in fact results in more enteral feed received by the patient without increasing the adverse effects. Sudden increase in GRV > 200 mL in a critically ill patient may be evidence of a new-onset sepsis.

CONCLUSION

Thorough knowledge of basic biochemical metabolism is essential for understanding surgical metabolism and evolution of complications. Optimal nutritional support at the earliest following a surgical insult or stress has to be started in order to reduce the inflammatory cascade and thereby morbidities. Body tries to conserve energy by utilizing ketone bodies in late fasting stage once glycogen stores got over in normal starvation. Stress starvation induces hypercatabolism and increased LBM degradation to maintain the energy expenditure of the body. Always EN is preferred whenever possible or the gut works. We need to follow the nutrition pyramid in escalating and de-escalating nutrition protocols. Supplemental or total PN is established when EN is contraindicated. Proper early nutritional support can attenuate the effects of neurohormonal responses associated with stress or sepsis. Nutritional optimization or prehabilitation should start from the OPD itself during the first visit and it should be continued in the perioperative period. Proper nutritional assessment should be undertaken early and executed adequately. Nutritional screening and assessment are a teamwork comprising of physicians, nurses, dieticians, pharmacists, and others which include social worker, research assistants, and administrative representatives/quality officers. With a proper teamwork, we can identify patients at nutritional risk, identify need for nutrition support, identify appropriate means of nutrition support, and identify and prevent complications of nutrition support.

30. Feeding Jejunostomy

Shafeek Shamsudeen

INTRODUCTION
- Jejunostomy is a surgical procedure by which a tube is inserted and secured into the lumen of the proximal jejunum, primarily to administer nutrients or sometimes medications and on rare occasions, to aspirate intestinal contents.
- The first to accomplish a jejunostomy for nutritional purposes was Bush in 1858 in a patient with inoperable carcinoma stomach. In 1891, Witzel described the most well-known technique for jejunostomy, and it has undergone diverse modifications to date.
- The procedure connects the intraluminal jejunum with the outside world through the abdominal wall using a flexible soft tube. The major goal of this procedure is long-term access to the proximal gastrointestinal (GI) tract for enteral nutrition when oral intake is impossible or inadequate.
- It can be performed as open or laparoscopic procedure.
- It provides benefit of early initiation of enteral nutrition after major GI surgeries.

PREOPERATIVE ASSESSMENT
- Detailed history and physical examination focusing on the following four aspects:
  1. Indication for enteral access
  2. Hemodynamic stability [if unstable, it should not undergo elective feeding jejunostomy (FJ)]
  3. Current functional status of GIT distal to ligament of Treitz (no obstruction/adynamic ileus/mesenteric ischemia/peritonitis)
  4. Details of previous surgeries [pre-existing tubes/drains/mesh/stoma, etc.]; also, previous history of laparotomy may preclude a laparoscopic approach.
- Radiologic studies are not generally indicated prior to FJ.

PREOPERATIVE PREPARATION
- Nil per oral (NPO) for minimum 6 hours prior to procedure.

- Antibiotic prophylaxis 30 minutes before incision (first generation cephalosporins).
- *General endotracheal anesthesia*—can be done under regional anesthesia (e.g., bilateral transversus abdominis plane block) also.
- Generally sited in LUQ (left upper quadrant).

Positioning
Supine.

Equipment
Most important is that tube should be soft, pliable, and not containing a balloon; enteral end should be free of sharp edges; adequate-sized holes (to allow feeds and minimize clogging) need to be present; usually, 12–18-Fr sized catheters are used *(at the author's institution, we use a 16-Fr Ryles tube)*.

Incision
- A site is chosen on the anterior abdominal wall so that it traverses the rectus abdominis muscle lateral to the epigastric vessels and inferior to the transverse colon **(Fig. 1)**.
- Supraumbilical vertical midline laparotomy incision (if done as a stand-alone procedure) of sufficient length to:
  - Locate the ligament of Treitz (LOT)
  - Mobilize 20–30 cm of jejunum from LOT
  - Allow fixation of jejunal segment to parietal peritoneum around tube exit site.
- The length can be limited to 5–7 cm, if there are minimal adhesions.

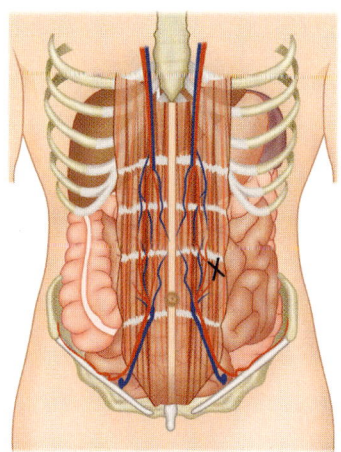

Fig. 1: Location of feeding jejunostomy (FJ) site on the anterior abdominal wall.

Jejunal Mobilization

- After gaining entry to peritoneal cavity, the omentum and transverse colon are retracted cephalad and LOT identified by tracing the small bowel proximally.
- The entire small bowel is then traced from LOT to ileocecal junction to rule out any occult pathology/obstruction or torsion.
- Choose a jejunal segment (20–30 cm from LOT) that will easily reach the tube insertion site without tension or torsion.
- The left cut edge of the abdominal wall is lifted up using Allis forceps to ensure exposure for tube placement.
- Adequate retraction is applied and a strong fine clamp is passed from inside abdomen and out through the point chosen on the abdominal wall (usually in left upper quadrant) by making a ~3 mm skin incision. The clamp is used to hold the tip of the tube and pull it inside the abdominal cavity. Both ends of the tube are then held together and further used to keep the left abdominal wall retracted.

Enterotomy

- A 4 mm purse string suture (3-0 nonabsorbable or absorbable suture) is placed on antimesenteric border of the chosen site on jejunum **(Fig. 2)** (double purse string can be used for added security).
- Note the proximal and distal end of jejunum and maintain orientation of small bowel.
- Make an enterotomy at the center of the purse string suture using cautery; cut the serosa and muscularis with cautery and use a fine mosquito artery forceps to pop into the lumen.

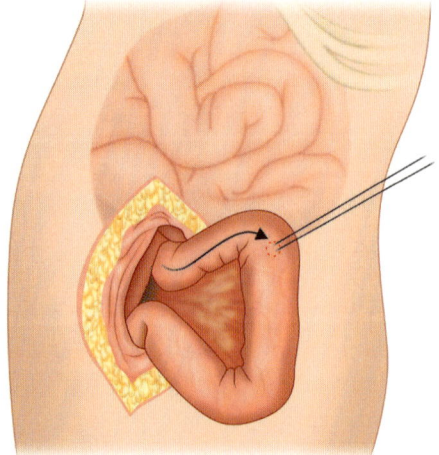

Fig. 2: Purse string suture at site of planned enterotomy.

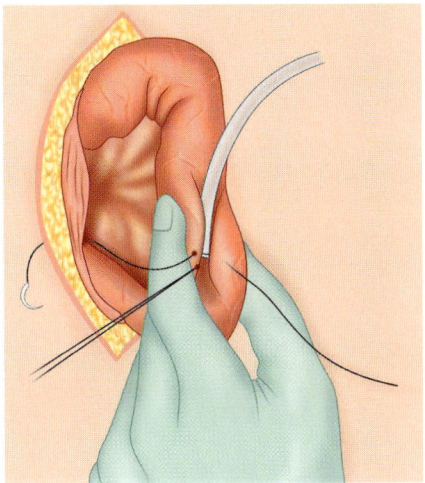

Fig. 3: Creating a Witzel tunnel.

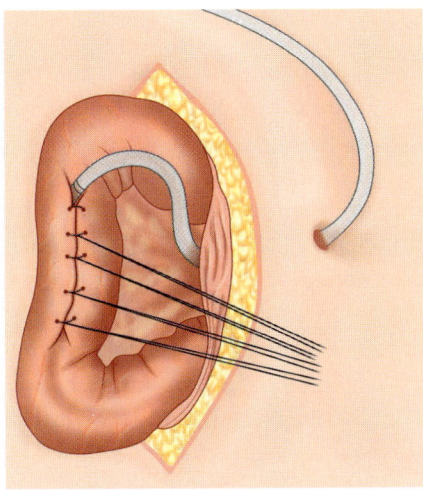

Fig. 4: Completed Witzel tunnel with intraluminal position of tube tip.

- Advance the distal end of the feeding tube through the enterotomy into the lumen and direct it distally for at least 10 cm.
- Tie down the purse string suture taking care not to occlude the tube and imbricate the tube entry site with a 3-point triangular stitch.
- A Witzel tunnel is then created **(Figs. 3 and 4)** by imbricating the small bowel over the feeding tube using interrupted 3-0 absorbable suture for a distance of 5 cm *proximally* [i.e., toward the LOT]; the bites should be seromuscular and spaced 5–10 mm apart (*Important caveat*: *Do not place the bites too far away from the tube because this will draw more bowels into the Witzel tunnel and narrow the jejunal lumen!*).

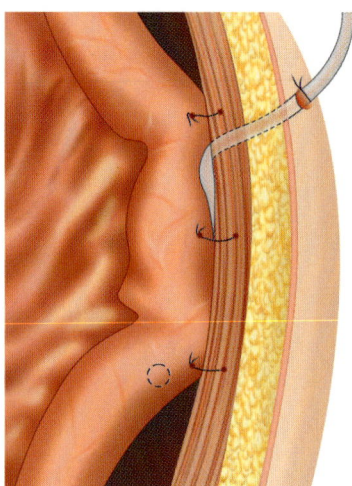

Fig. 5: The jejunal loop anchored to parietal peritoneum.

Fixing the Jejunal Segment to Abdominal Wall (Left Upper Quadrant)

- The aim is to allow a tract to form (with the bowel flush against abdominal wall) so that even if the tube gets dislodged inadvertently, it can be replaced as OPD procedure.
- Place four tacking sutures (3-0 absorbable) around the tube exit site—lateral, medial, superior, and inferior locations. This is accomplished by taking a seromuscular bite on bowel and another bite of parietal peritoneum at corresponding location on abdominal wall, starting with the lateral suture first (the one farthest away from operating surgeon).
- Once all the sutures have been placed, tie them in the order in which they were placed and place another tacking suture between small bowel and parietal peritoneum, 5–10 cm distal to the tube exit site (this ensures that a long enough segment is secured and guards against torsion around a single point) **(Fig. 5)**.
- The external part of the tube is then fixed to skin using 2-0 nonabsorbable suture **(Fig. 6)**.
- The laparotomy is then closed in layers.

POSTOPERATIVE CARE

- Feeding jejunostomy feeds can be started as early as 24–48 hours of the procedure at a low rate of 10 mL/h and if this is tolerated, the feeds can be advanced by 10 mL/hour every 4 hours until the nutritional goal is reached.
- Bolus feedings are delivered by gravity via a syringe over approximately 15 minutes. Intermittent feeding is usually via a feeding bag and administered over 30–45 minutes with or without an enteral feeding pump.

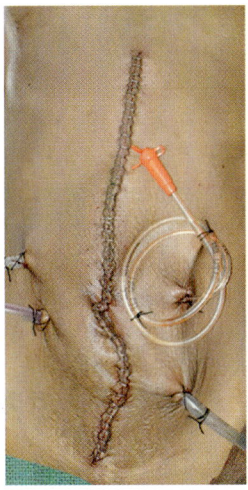

Fig. 6: Clinical photograph of a feeding jejunostomy (FJ) tube secured on abdominal wall.

- The calorie intake should be increased slowly because of the common complications of diarrhea and abdominal discomfort. Avoid enterostomy feedings during the night because of the possibility that distress and/or diarrhea may develop.
- Sterile water flushes (~30 mL) are recommended 4 to 6 hourly to maintain patency and should be done before and after each feeding session/administration of medicines.
- Flushing will be more effective with a "push–pause" technique.
- Aseptic technique should be ensured when cleaning for the first 48 hours postinsertion.
- Avoid immersion bathing for the first 2 weeks postinsertion. Showering is permitted.
- Check the length of external tubing daily.
- Ensure the security of the external fixator/sutures.
- Clean the site daily with water and dry thoroughly.
- Avoid the use of dressings unless exudate present.
- Do not rotate the tube.

COMPLICATIONS

- *Clogged tube*: It can be cleared by flushing with the smallest syringe that will fit into the tube opening. Carbonated beverages may also help to clear a clogged tube if allowed to stay within tube for an hour at least before attempting to flush it into the bowel using a syringe.
- *Dislodged tube*: Most important is that the caregiver/relative of the patient knows to reinsert the tube immediately so that the tract does not close (this should not be a problem if the tube has been in place for at least 1 month). However, if unable to reinsert, the patient should be taken

to an emergency department where reinsertion can be attempted with a smaller caliber catheter initially. If reinsertion is easy without any resistance and flushing causes no discomfort, then a proper-sized tube can be substituted and feeding restarted without need for radiologic confirmation of tube position.
- *Fractured tube*: It can be temporarily patched with waterproof occlusive tape till the tube can be exchanged for a new tube (over a guidewire) by a surgeon.
- *Abdominal wall abscess*: This happens very rarely as a sequela of tube site infection and it should be treated with incision and drainage and leaving the wound open and subsequent wound dressings till it heals.
- *Small bowel obstruction*: It is most frequently caused by torsion at tube insertion site. A computed tomography (CT) scan with oral contrast administered 2 hours prior to the study would help in assessing torsion of the bowel in this scenario. If torsion is confirmed, an operative exploration is required to relieve obstruction.

NEEDLE CATHETER JEJUNOSTOMY

- In 1973, Delany et al. reported a needle catheter technique with a thin tube that passed through a seromuscular tunnel in the intestinal wall before entering the intestinal lumen.
- This is used when the indication is temporary.
- A short midline incision to gain entry into peritoneal cavity and identify LOT and proximal jejunum.
- Another small incision is made at the proposed skin entry site.
- The needle catheter kit is used to enter the jejunum at a suitable point on the antimesenteric border approximately 20 cm from the ligament of Treitz.
- The catheter is passed and advanced distally into the jejunum.
- The intraluminal position of catheter tip is confirmed by free injection of saline.
- A purse-string suture of 3-0 silk is placed around the site where the catheter entered the jejunum.

31

Respiratory Complications after Surgery

Deepak Paul

INTRODUCTION

Respiratory complications are one of the most common postoperative complications a surgeon has to deal with. They account for significant amount of resources of a surgeon and his team. Respiratory complications account for 25% of postoperative deaths. They are also prime culprits of increasing intensive care stay and thereby driving up hospital bills. Therefore, it is of paramount importance to identify risk factors preoperatively and modify them. Early identification also play a big part in reducing morbidity and mortality.

CAUSES

There are multitude of causes that lead to an abnormal pulmonary physiology. Some of them are:
- Painful abdominal incisions
- Abdominal distension
- Obesity
- Use of narcotics
- Effect of anesthetic drugs
- Smoking
- Chronic obstructive pulmonary disease
- Fluid overload
- Patient being kept in the supine position for prolonged periods.

The common respiratory complications seen are:
- Atelectasis
- Pneumonia
- Aspiration pneumonia
- Acute respiratory distress syndrome (ARDS)
- Pulmonary edema
- Pulmonary embolism (PE).

Atelectasis

Atelectasis is the most common postoperative complication. The common culprits being upper abdominal and thoracic incisions. The use of narcotics and certain anesthetics also cause atelectasis. This leads to collapse of the alveoli in the periphery.

It is the most common cause for postoperative fever in the first 48 hours after surgery. It commonly affects the basal segments of the lung. Initially, it can be obscure that one needs to have a keen eye on the patient to pick it up early. If identified early, the use of incentive spirometry along with deep breathing and adequate analgesia can cause resolution without much difficulty. The patients who are left unidentified and untreated could have a grave prognosis.

Patients usually present with a low-grade fever, malaise, and decreased breath sounds in the lower lung fields. Usually, the patient would have fever with no overt pulmonary symptoms. The alveoli remains collapsed and there is buildup of secretions. Then, secondary bacterial infection results in pneumonia.

Pneumonia

Pneumonia is the most common nosocomial infection occurring in hospitalized patients. There are several factors associated with increased risk of pneumonia. They are depressed immune status, poor nutritional status, advanced age, smoking, long hospital stay, presence of endotracheal and nasogastric tubes, prior antibiotic therapy, proton pump inhibitors (PPIs), and concomitant disease:

- Hospital-acquired pneumonia—pneumonia occurring >48 hours after admission and without antecedent signs of infection.
- Ventilator-associated pneumonia—pneumonia occurring 48 hours after but within 72 hours of initial ventilation.

Common organisms causing pneumonia are *Streptococcus pneumoniae*, *Haemophilus influenzae*, *Escherichia coli*, *Klebsiella* spp., *Enterobacter* spp., *Staphylococcus aureus* [methicillin-resistant *Staphylococcus aureus* (MRSA)], *Pseudomonas aeruginosa*, and *Acinetobacter baumannii*. Patients with history of prior antibiotics exhibit multidrug resistance. With these superbugs causing havoc, it is very important to use antibiotics judiciously.

The patient presents with high fever-associated thick secretions while coughing and occasionally mental confusion. Investigations show leukocytosis and chest radiograph shows infiltrates. If not diagnosed and treated promptly it will rapidly deteriorate and progress to respiratory failure which would require intubation.

The patients are initiated on aggressive pulmonary toilet and sputum is sent for culture and sensitivity. Empirical antibiotics are started and switched over to appropriate antibiotics once the culture is available.

Prevention is better than cure is so true in the case of pneumonia. Smokers should be asked to stop smoking well in advance to an elective procedure. Adequate pain management goes a long way in preventing pneumonia. Incentive spirometry should be encouraged. Patients on ventilator should be kept in semi-recumbent position and endotracheal care should be given with frequent suctioning and prevents pooling of secretions. Sucralfate should be used instead of PPI as PPIs make the gastric environment alkaline and promote bacterial colonization which increases the risk of pneumonia.

Aspiration Pneumonia

Aspiration of oropharyngeal secretions into the respiratory tract leading to pneumonia is called aspiration pneumonia. It has an incidence of 0.03% and in the emergency setting has an incidence of 0.11%. It occurs when the mechanism of cough and glottic closure are compromised.

Aspiration pneumonitis (Mendelson syndrome) is acute lung injury that results from the inhalation of regurgitated gastric contents. The causes being an overdistended stomach, altered gastrointestinal mobility, and reduced sphincter tone due to anesthetic drugs or long-standing nasogastric tubes.

The patient may have altered level of consciousness. Patients usually have wheezing and labored breathing. A chest X-ray shows an infiltrate in the posterior segments of upper lobes and apical segments of lower lobes.

Preoperatively prevention of aspiration pneumonia can be achieved by keeping a patient nil per oral for 6 hours after a night meal or 4 hours after clear liquids. In case of emergency intubation, use of rapid sequence induction may be effective. Postoperatively reducing the use of narcotics, early ambulation, and cautious feeding of the patient can reduce the incidence of aspiration pneumonia.

Once a suspicion of aspiration is made, the patient needs to be placed on oxygen immediately and a chest X-ray is taken to confirm the diagnosis. Usually, bilateral fluffy infiltrates are seen. Close surveillance of the patient is very important. Antibiotic coverage of gram-negative organisms is started. If the patient deteriorates, the threshold for intubation should be low. Suctioning the bronchoalveolar tree confirms the diagnosis.

Aspiration pneumonia can have serious consequences hence, all precautions should be taken to prevent them.

Pulmonary Edema

Pulmonary edema is accumulation of fluid in the alveoli which leads to hypoxemia which results in increased work of breathing. It is usually caused by fluid overload, congestive cardiac failure, and acute myocardial infarction. It resolves quickly after diuresis and fluid restriction. Invasive monitoring in the form of Swan-Ganz catheter for evaluation of pulmonary capillary wedge pressure (PCWP) may be indicated. When there is elevated PCWP, aggressive diuresis and fluid restriction are to be followed.

Acute Lung Injury/Acute Respiratory Distress Syndrome

Acute lung injury (ALI)/ARDS is common manifestation of acute respiratory failure. The common conditions which lead to them are sepsis, massive blood transfusion, pulmonary contusion, aspiration, multiple rib fractures, ischemia reperfusion injury, and pancreatitis.

Preoperative Risk Factors

- Smoking
- General state of health
- Age
- Chronic lung disease
- Obesity
- Nutritional status
- Antecedent respiratory infection.

Intraoperative Risk Factors

- Type of anesthesia
- Duration of anesthesia
- Surgical site
- Type of surgical incision
- Intraoperative fluid management.

Postoperative Risk Factors

- *Inadequate analgesia*:
  - Pain inhibits coughing and deep breathing
  - Discourages early mobilization.
- *Immobilization*:
  - Reduction in functional residual capacity
  - Decreased secretion clearance.

Acute lung injury is associated with partial pressure of arterial oxygen (PaO_2)/fraction of inspired oxygen (FiO_2) ratio <300, bilateral infiltrates on chest X-ray, and PCWP < 18 mm Hg. It tends to have a shorter duration and is of less severity.

Acute respiratory distress syndrome is associated with PaO_2/FiO_2 ratio <200, bilateral infiltrates, and PCWP < 18 mm Hg. It tends to be more severe and longer in duration.

Patients experience tachycardia, dyspnea, and increased work of breathing.

Auscultation reveals reduced breath sounds associated with crackles. Arterial blood gas shows low PaO_2 and high partial pressure of arterial carbon dioxide ($PaCO_2$).

Patients with ALI/ARDS should be immediately intubated, there should be careful use of intravenous (IV) fluids, and invasive monitoring to assess

Respiratory Complications after Surgery

Table 1: Criteria for weaning from the ventilator.

Parameters	Weaning criteria
Respiratory rate	<25 breaths/min
PaO_2	>70 mm Hg
$PaCO_2$	<45 mm Hg
Minute ventilation	8–9 L/min
Tidal volume	5–6 mL/kg
Negative inspiratory force	25 cm of H_2O

($PaCO_2$: partial pressure of arterial carbon dioxide; PaO_2: partial pressure of arterial oxygen)

PCWP. The patient should be on ventilator with assisted breathing while the lung injury heals.

The ventilatory settings initially placed are:
- Fraction of inspired oxygen—100%
- Positive end-expiratory pressure should be set
- Tidal volume of 10–12 mL/kg of body weight
- Peak pressure at 35 cm of H_2O
- Respiratory rate should be chosen to produce $PaCO_2$ near 40 mm Hg and inspiratory to expiratory ratio is set to 1:2.

Careful monitoring of oxygenation, improvement of respiratory rate, and general alertness will guide extubation.

Criteria for Weaning from the Ventilator

The criteria for weaning from the ventilator are described in **Table 1**.

Pulmonary Embolism

Pulmonary embolism is a postoperative complication which if detected and treated can prevent morbidity and mortality. It accounts for 5–10% of all hospital deaths. If undiagnosed, hospital mortality rates are around 30% whereas with early detection and treatment, mortality rates fall to 8%. Pulmonary embolism is a sequel of venous thromboembolism (VTE). Most pulmonary emboli arise from deep vein thrombosis (DVT) of iliofemoral veins.

Risk factors for VTE can be summarized as:
- *General factors*:
  - Advanced age
  - Varicose veins
  - Prolonged immobilization.
- *Inherited factors*:
  - Protein C deficiency
  - Protein S deficiency

- Antithrombin III deficiency
- Factor V Leiden mutation
- Dysfibrinogenemia
- Hyperhomocysteinemia.
- *Acquired factors*:
  - Malignancy
  - Major surgery
  - Pelvic and orthopedic surgery
  - Trauma
  - Pregnancy
  - Previous history of VTE
  - Inflammatory bowel disease.

More than 50% of DVTs leads to silent pulmonary embolism that may be the first manifestation. The patient will be dyspneic, tachypneic, and will have tachycardia. The patient may have pleuritic chest pain, hemoptysis, and pain on palpation of leg.

Electrocardiogram will show S1Q3T3 pattern that may have features of a new right bundle branch block. Chest radiograph is of limited value. Lower extremity ultrasonography is a must if PE is suspected to rule out DVT. D-dimer, a fibrin degradation product, has high negative predictive value thereby if D-dimer is negative, DVT can be ruled out and hence PE can be ruled out, but the reverse cannot be true always if D-dimer is positive, DVT cannot be ruled out. Echocardiogram is a noninvasive bedside tool that provides quick results in critically ill patients. If leg symptoms are present, a venous Doppler should be done to rule out DVT. Pulmonary angiogram is the investigation of choice for PE. It has high specificity (92%) and sensitivity (86%). It is now the gold standard, as it visualizes the arterial tree and it detects intravascular filling defects.

Treatment

- *Anticoagulation*: The agents used are unfractionated heparin, low-molecular-weight heparin, and warfarin.

  Unfractionated heparin is given IV, a weight-adjusted bolus of 70 U/kg is followed by 1,000 U/h to achieve a partial thromboplastin time of 1.5–2 times the control.

  Low-molecular-weight heparin is given in once or twice daily subcutaneously depending on the weight.

  Warfarin is given orally to overlap heparin therapy until international normalized ratio (INR) is therapeutic. A target INR is 2.5–3.5.
- *Thrombolytics*: Examples are streptokinase, urokinase, and tissue plasminogen activator.
- Inferior vena cava filter.

CONCLUSION

Preventing respiratory complications after surgery are of paramount importance and the following are some points to remember:

- *Preoperatively*:
  - Stop smoking >8 weeks
  - Respiratory infection—intense preoperative respiratory therapy
  - Pulmonary function test—should be optimized
  - Obese—weight reduction
  - Patient education
  - Improve nutrition.
- *Postoperatively*:
  - Pain control
  - Early mobilization
  - Deep breathing exercises
  - Chest physiotherapy
  - Early weaning from mechanical ventilation
  - Early feeding and appropriate use of O_2.

Prophylaxis and Treatment of Deep Vein Thrombosis and Pulmonary Embolism

R Dayananda Babu

INTRODUCTION

Deep vein thrombosis (DVT) may be *provoked* or *unprovoked*.

The causes for provoked DVT are trauma, surgery, immobilization, pregnancy, dehydration, malignancy, etc.

In unprovoked DVT, the causes are unidentified.

The three factors described by Virchow, namely *Virchow's triad*, are still relevant in the development of DVT; they are:
- Endothelial damage
- Stasis (abnormal flow)
- Hypercoagulability (thrombophilia).

PROPHYLAXIS OF DEEP VEIN THROMBOSIS

They are common complications of surgery and they are often missed clinically. Sometimes, they are encountered in postmortem examination. Once patient develops DVT, it can lead on to fatal complication of pulmonary embolism (PE). Once DVT is established, it can cause significant morbidity in later years in the form of post-thrombotic syndrome (PTS) and varicose veins. Now, it is possible to prevent the occurrence of DVT in majority of the cases.

Important Risk Factors

- Age more than 60 years
- Obesity more than 30 BMI
- Smokers
- History of previous thromboembolism
- Oral contraceptive usage (stop 6 weeks before surgery)
- Pregnancy and postpartum period
- Hormone replacement therapy
- Economy class syndrome (patients on long haul flights)
- *E-thrombosis*: Those who are sitting in front of computer for hours.

Diseases and Surgical Procedures at Risk

- Patients with cancer
- Pelvic surgeries and orthopedic surgery like hip and knee replacement
- Trauma surgery
- Cardiac failure and recent myocardial infarction
- Paralysis of lower limbs
- Polycythemia
- Paraproteinemia
- Nephrotic syndrome
- Thrombophilia
- Immobilization
- Inflammatory bowel disease.

Hypercoagulable States

- Activated protein C/protein S deficiency
- Factor V Leiden gene defect
- Antithrombin III deficiency
- Dysfibrinogenemia
- Hyperhomocysteinemia
- Antiphospholipid antibody (lupus anticoagulant).

Hematologic Syndromes

- Myeloproliferative disorders
- Antiphospholipid antibody syndrome
- Disseminated intravascular coagulation (DIC)
- Heparin-induced thrombocytopenia (HIT)
- Thrombotic thrombocytopenic purpura (TTP).

Clinical Diagnosis of DVT

- Leg pain in 50% of patients
- Mild pitting edema of the ankle
- Stiff and tender calf muscle in 75% of patients (Homan's sign should not be elicited).

Modified Wells' Criteria for predicting Deep Vein Thrombosis

Modified Wells' criteria for predicting DVT are described in **Table 1**.

Confirmation

- *Duplex ultrasound examination*: Filling defects and lack of compressibility. It is not useful for diagnosis of DVT proximal to inguinal ligament. Incomplete compressibility suggests presence of clot.
- *Compression ultrasound*: This involves applying pressure with ultrasound probe over common femoral and popliteal vein. Normally, these veins

Table 1: Modified Wells' criteria for predicting deep vein thrombosis (DVT).

Variable	Score
Lower limb trauma or surgery or immobilization in plaster cast	1
Bedridden for more than 3 days or surgery in last 4 weeks	1
Tenderness along the line of femoral or popliteal vein	1
Entire limb swollen	1
Calf >3 cm larger circumference than the other side 10 cm below the tibial tuberosity	1
Pitting edema	1
Dilated collateral superficial veins (not varicose veins)	1
Previous DVT	1
Malignancy (including treatment up to 6 months ago)	1
Intravenous drug abuse	3
Alternative diagnosis more likely than DVT	−2

Note:
- (Score −2 to 0) low probability (5%) of DVT
- (Score 1–2) moderate probability (17%) of DVT
- (Score >2) high probability (17–53%) of DVT.

will compress tightly. In the presence of DVT, they will not fully compress. The problem with this method is that one is likely to miss calf vein thrombosis.
- *D-dimer*: It is a degradation product of circulating cross-linked fibrin [Normal is <0.5 μg/dL fibrinogen equivalent units (FEU)].
- Ascending venography (rarely done nowadays)—filling defects.
- MR venography—filling defects.
- Tc99m-apcitide scintigraphy.

Goals of DVT Prophylaxis

The goals are:
- Prevention of venous thromboembolism and sequelae
- Prevention of pulmonary embolism
- Prevention of PTS.

Types of DVT Prophylaxis

- *Mechanical*: Intermittent pneumatic compression, graduated compression stockings, and venous foot pump (avoid in peripheral occlusive vascular disease).
- *Pharmacological* **(Table 2)**: They are more effective than mechanical—
  - Unfractionated heparin—UFH (IV/SC)
  - Low-molecular weight heparin (LMWH)—subcutaneous; it does not require monitoring and the incidence of HIT is less. The injections are given once daily. LMWH is contraindicated in renal failure.

Table 2: Pharmacological deep vein thrombosis prophylaxis.
The unfractionated heparin and warfarin are not used for prophylaxis

LMWH	UFH
More expensive	Less expensive
Longer half-life	Shorter half-life
Less frequent dosing	Can be used in renal failure
Lower risk of HIT	Greater safety in patients with epidural catheters
	Higher risk of HIT

(HIT: heparin-induced thrombocytopenia; LMWH: low-molecular weight heparin; UFH: unfractionated heparin)

PROPHYLAXIS OF PULMONARY EMBOLISM

Diagnosis of Pulmonary Embolism

Clinical Diagnosis

Signs and symptoms of PE occur in about 10% of patients with confirmed DVT:
- Low-grade fever
- Dyspnea
- Hemoptysis
- Cyanosis
- Raised neck veins
- Fixed split second heart sound
- Pleural rub.

Differential Diagnosis
- Myocardial infarction (MI)
- Pneumonia
- Pleurisy
- Aortic dissection.

Modified Wells' Criteria for predicting Pulmonary Embolism

Modified Wells' criteria for predicting PE are described in **Table 3**.

Radiological Diagnosis

Computed tomography (CT) pulmonary angiography is the investigation of choice. This will demonstrate filling defect in the pulmonary arteries.

RISK STRATIFICATION—CAPRINI SCORING SYSTEM

A1—Each Risk Factor Represents 1 Point
- Age 40–59 years
- Minor surgery (planned)

Table 3: Modified Wells' criteria for predicting pulmonary embolism.

Variable	Score
Clinical signs and symptoms of DVT (minimum of leg swelling and pain on palpation of deep vein)	3
Alternative diagnosis less likely than pulmonary embolism	3
Heart rate more than 100 beats per min	1.5
Immobilization more than 3 days or surgery within 4 weeks	1.5
Previous DVT or PE	1.5
Hemoptysis	1
Malignancy (treatment or palliation within past 6 months)	1

(DVT: deep vein thrombosis; PE: pulmonary embolism)
Note:
- A score of less than 4—PE unlikely (12.4%)
- More than 4—suggestive of PE (37.1%).

- History of prior major surgery (<1 month)
- Varicose veins
- History of inflammatory bowel disease
- Swollen leg (current)
- Obesity (BMI >30)
- Acute myocardial infarction (<1 month)
- Congestive heart failure (<1 month)
- Sepsis (<1 month)
- Serious lung disease including pneumonia (<1 month)
- Abnormal pulmonary function (COPD)
- Medical patient currently at bed rest
- Leg plaster/cast or brace
- Central venous access
- Blood transfusion (<1 month)
- Other risk factors.

A2—For Women Only (Each Represents 1 Point)
- Oral contraceptives or hormone replacement therapy
- Pregnancy or postpartum (<1 month)
- History of unexplained stillborn infant, recurrent spontaneous abortion (more than or equal to 3), and premature birth with toxemia of pregnancy or growth restricted infant.

B—Each Risk Factor Represents 2 Points
- Age 60–74 years
- Arthroscopic surgery (>60 minutes)
- Major surgery (<60 minutes)
- Laparoscopic surgery (>60 minutes)

- Previous malignancy
- Morbid obesity (BMI >40).

C—Each Risk Factor Represents 3 Points

- Age 75 or more
- Major surgery lasting 2–3 hours
- BMI > 50
- History of superficial vein thrombosis (SVT), DVT/PE
- Family history of DVT/PE
- Present cancer or chemotherapy
- Positive factor V Leiden
- Positive prothrombin 20210A
- Elevated serum homocysteine
- Positive lupus anticoagulant
- Elevated anticardiolipin antibodies
- Heparin-induced thrombocytopenia (HIT)
- Other thrombophilia type.

D—Each Risk Factor Represents 5 Points

- Elective major lower extremity arthroplasty
- Hip, pelvis, or leg fracture (<1 month)
- Stroke (<1 month)
- Multiple trauma (<1 month)
- Acute spinal cord injury (paralysis) (<1 month)
- Major surgery lasting over 3 hours.

SUGGESTED GUIDE FOR THROMBOSIS PROPHYLAXIS

- All moderate- and high-risk patients should receive UFH, LMWH, or factor Xa inhibitor unless contraindicated by bleeding risk.
- *Scores of 2–3*: Intermittent pneumatic compression (IPC) perioperatively and during hospitalization.
- *Scores of 3–4*: UFH, LMWH, factor Xa inhibitor, foot pump, or IPC during hospitalization. Start anticoagulation 12–24 hours postoperatively.
- *Scores of 5–8*: Anticoagulation + IPC during hospitalization and 7–10 days UFH, LMWH, or Factor Xa inhibitor. Start anticoagulation 12 hours preoperatively.
- *Scores of >8*: Anticoagulation + IPC during hospitalization and 30 days UFH, LMWH, or Factor Xa inhibitor.

TREATMENT OF DEEP VEIN THROMBOSIS ONCE DIAGNOSED

- Immediate systemic anticoagulation is the standard therapy.
- *Therapeutic anticoagulation with LMWH (1 mg/kg BID) or UFH*: The LMWH is contraindicated in patients with significant renal impairment. In such patients, UFH is given.

- *Factor Xa inhibitor*: *Fondaparinux sodium*—a single daily *subcutaneous* dose of 7.5 mg to be given in patients with body weight 50–100 kg. In adults with bodyweight more than 100 kg, 10 mg is given. Patients having sensitivity to heparinoids and those with HIT, fondaparinux is the drug of choice. Oral anticoagulant warfarin is started at the same time as fondaparinux. Fondaparinux should be continued for at least 5 days until INR 2 hour more.
  (*For prophylaxis*, the adult dose of fondaparinux is 2.5 mg, which is to be given 6 hours after surgery and then 2.5 mg once daily).
- *Bivalirudin*: It is a direct thrombin inhibitor usually given for unstable angina. The dose is 100 µg/kg IV initially followed by 250 µg/kg/h for 72 hours.
- *Warfarin*: Start warfarin only after 48 hours because of the rebound hypercoagulation, which is likely to occur if you start from the beginning. It will take 5 days for the action of warfarin. Initially LMWH is started. The dose of warfarin is titrated against the INR to maintain at 2–3. Usually, a dose of 10 mg is given on day 1 and day 2 and 5 mg on day 3. The warfarin is continued for a minimum period of 3 months. If any other associated deficiencies are there, it should be continued lifelong.
- Thrombolysis with tissue plasminogen activator (TPA) or urokinase directly to the thrombus should be considered in patients with iliac vein thrombosis; either by popliteal vein or by direct puncture of the groin.
- Endovenous thrombectomy and stenting.
- *Inferior vena cava (IVC) filters*—when there is failure of anticoagulation or contraindication for anticoagulation and free-floating thrombus of >5 cm size. It is also for patients with high-risk for PE. The filter is placed below the level of *renal vein*. The filter is usually temporary until they are safe to be anticoagulated or the risk of embolization has subsided.

Novel Anticoagulants

These are oral agents either directly inhibit factor Xa (rivaroxaban and apixaban) or thrombin inhibitor like dabigatran:
- *Apixaban* is given orally as prophylaxis after hip replacement surgery and the dose is 2.5 mg twice daily for 10–14 days.
- *Rivaroxaban* is given orally for prophylaxis after knee replacement surgery. Dose is 10 mg once daily for 2 weeks. This should be started 6–10 hours after surgery.
- *Dabigatran etexilate* is a direct thrombin inhibitor with rapid onset of action, which is given orally. It is given for prophylaxis of total knee replacement and hip replacement. The adult dose for prophylaxis is 110 mg to be taken 1–4 hours after surgery followed by 220 mg once daily for 9 days. For hip replacement, it is continued for 27–34 days.
- *For deep vein thrombosis and PE*, 150 mg is taken twice daily following a 5-day treatment with parenteral anticoagulant. For adults over 80 years of

age, 110 mg twice daily is enough. The drug is also used for prophylaxis of recurrent DVT and PE.

Indications for Anticoagulation in Superficial Thrombophlebitis
- Long segment superficial thrombophlebitis of more than 5 cm length
- Superficial thrombophlebitis extending to the saphenofemoral or saphenopopliteal junction.

Indication for Lifelong Anticoagulation in DVT
- Recurrent unprovoked DVT
- Irreversible risk factor like thrombophilia
- Deep vein thrombosis with congestive cardiac failure (CCF)
- Active metastatic malignancy.

Indication for Prolonged Anticoagulation (3–12 months)
- Recurrent provoked DVT
- Recurrent provoked DVT with risk factors
- Unprovoked proximal DVT
- History of symptomatic PE.

Prothrombotic Workup
It can be carried out initially before anticoagulation or after 1 month of stopping the warfarin.

TREATMENT OF PULMONARY EMBOLISM
Depending upon the severity, the following options are available:
- Anticoagulation
- Fibrinolytic treatment
- Radiologically guided catheter embolectomy
- Surgical pulmonary embolectomy.

33. Burst Abdomen (Wound Dehiscence) and Tension Sutures

R Dayananda Babu

INTRODUCTION

It is also called *acute wound failure*.

What are the causes for burst abdomen (Fig. 1)?
- Technical error in fascial closure
- Emergency surgery
- Intra-abdominal infection/hypertension
- Advanced age
- Wound infection, hematoma, and seroma
- Elevated intra-abdominal pressure
- Obesity
- Corticosteroids
- Previous wound dehiscence
- Malnutrition/hypoproteinemia
- Radiation therapy/chemotherapy
- Diabetes mellitus/immunosuppression.

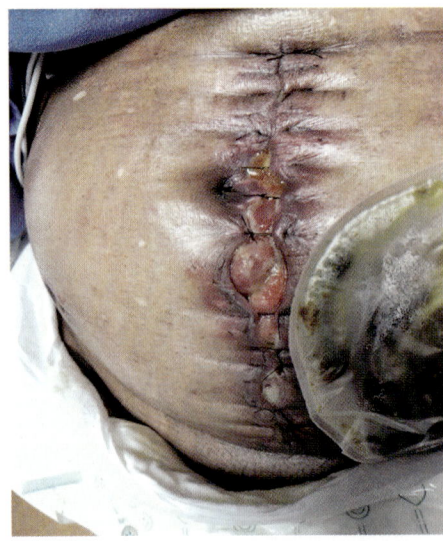

Fig. 1: Burst abdomen with colostomy.

What are the premonitory signs of burst abdomen?
- Unexplained serosanguineous pink discharge (25%) due to exudation from visceral peritoneum
- A ripping sensation for the patient
- Gut lying extraperitoneally
- Half of all disruptions occur without warning
- It is usually seen in 7–10 days, postoperatively 1–20 days.

PREVENTION

The most important cause for burst abdomen is technical error in fascial closure. The aponeurosis and deep fascia are considered to be the strongest structures of the abdominal wall. Therefore, after laparotomy secure and close apposition of the cut edges of these structures are made with nonabsorbable monofilament sutures (slowly absorbable is currently recommended), in order to prevent postoperative hernia. Usually, a single layer aponeurotic closure is recommended. In high-risk patients, single layer interrupted sutures are recommended. There is no need for a separate peritoneal closure.

Careful attention is given to the technique of fascial closure. The standard technique was the *Jenkins formula*, i.e., 1:1 (1 cm wide and 1 cm apart) with suture to wound length of 4:1. Currently, the "small bite" approach is recommended, in which sutures are taken 5 mm apart and 5 mm deep. The proper spacing of the suture and adequate depth of the bite of the fascia are important. For high-risk patient, interrupted closure is better.

Hughes technique—here interrupted double near and far horizontal mattress sutures are put.

What are the options available when there is difficulty in abdominal closure?

Postlaparotomy closure of abdomen in the presence of sepsis or intestinal edema will lead onto intra-abdominal hypertension with subsequent respiratory embarrassment and cardiorespiratory complications:

- *Laparostomy*: There is little to be lost and sometimes much to be gained by leaving the abdomen open temporarily. The abdomen is closed later by a delayed primary technique (laparostomy by Sir Miles Irving in 1980). Geoffrey Baggott, an Irish anesthesiologist from Illinois, has been trying for over >45 years persuading surgeons not to close the abdomen when there is tension. This will avoid abdominal hypertension. When there are edematous loops of bowel, especially in case of intestinal obstruction, it will compound the problem of abdominal hypertension.

  Suggested method: In cases of extensive intra-abdominal sepsis and where further explorations are required, a mesh is sutured to the fascial edges of the wound after positioning the omentum beneath the mesh to prevent loops of intestine becoming adherent to it. The wound wall sometimes epithelializes over the mesh. The mesh is best removed when the patient is well. Alternatively, the granulating surface can be covered with a split skin graft after a later date. The subsequent incisional hernia may be repaired at later stage.

- *Bogota bag*: It is a sterile plastic bag used for closure of temporary closure of abdominal wounds. Generally, a 3 L sterilized genitourinary irrigation bag is cut open and used. This is sewn to the skin or fascia of the abdominal wall. This was first described by Oswaldo Borraez, Bogota, Colombia **(Fig. 2)**.
- *Negative pressure wound therapy (vacuum pack closure)*: A fenestrated nonadherent polyethylene sheet is applied on the bowel omentum, moist surgical towel or gauze with drains placed on top of it. An iodophor impregnated adhesive dressing is placed over the moist surgical gauze and tubes. A continuous section is then applied. If the fascia cannot be closed in 7-10 days, the wound is allowed to granulate and then covered with a skin graft. The most important complication is intestinal fistula. The advantages are—increased wound contraction and improved drainage of infectious material and peritoneal fluid containing the damaging cytokines.
- *Use of prophylactic mesh*: It is preferable not to use mesh in the presence of sepsis.
- Conventional tension sutures (it is condemned nowadays).

Why tension suture is because of the fear of a burst abdomen?
A heavy reinforcing suture placed deep within the muscles and fascia of the abdominal wall to relieve tension on the primary suture line.

The tension sutures were popular in yesteryears. Through and through mattress sutures of strong nylon/Prolene/black silk are taken as shown in **Figure 3**. Stitches are made to pass through all layers of the abdominal wall about 2.5 cm from the wound edge (sometimes excepting the peritoneum). They are passed through pieces of rubber tubing (cushion tube) to prevent

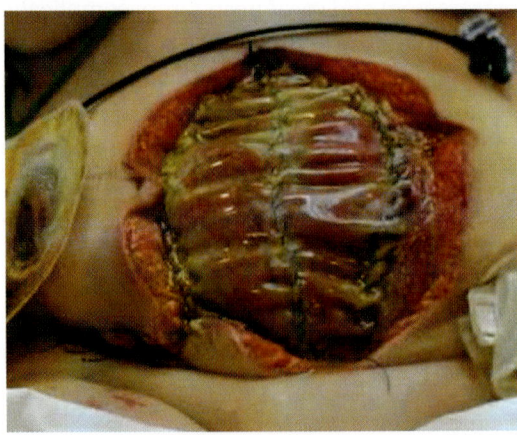

Fig. 2: Bogota bag.

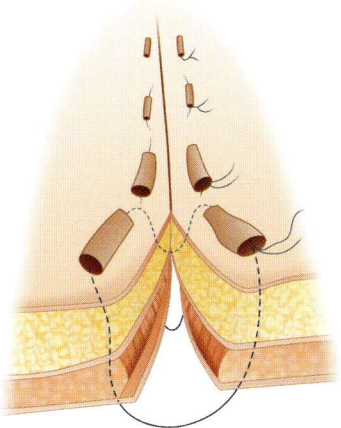

Fig. 3: Closer view of the suturing.

them from cutting into the skin. A few additional stitches are inserted to coapt aponeurosis and skin.

Complications of conventional tension sutures are:
- Abdominal hypertension
- Cardiorespiratory complications
- Increased postoperative pain
- Skin necrosis
- Ugly wound
- Suture may cut through the intestine.

Therefore, the conventional tension sutures are not recommended at present when there is difficulty in closure.

Methicillin-resistant *Staphylococcus aureus* (MRSA)*

R Dayananda Babu

INTRODUCTION

- Methicillin-resistant *Staphylococcus aureus* (MRSA) is a major reason for litigation in the West.
- MRSA infection increases mortality and length of hospital stay at least threefold.
- MRSA is more invasive and difficult to treat than other *S. aureus*.
- The spread of MRSA is predominantly through unwashed hands of doctors and nurses.
- MRSA tends to colonize patients exposed to broad-spectrum antibiotics.
- Colonization means the presence of MRSA at superficial sites in the absence of symptoms.
- Nose and throat are common initial sites (through contact or inhalation of aerosol).
- Many wound infections develop in the ward due to contamination in the early postoperative period rather than events in the theater.
- MRSA can survive on a surface for up to 80 days.
- Clothing or wrist watches of staff are common sources.
- MRSA can spread throughout a ward within a few hours of cleaning.
- Staff, patients, and their relatives disseminate MRSA throughout a ward.

MANIFESTATIONS OF MRSA INFECTION

- It causes purulent infection of surgical wounds.
- Usually, it is associated with erythema, serous discharge and dehiscence of the wound.
- Abscess formation will occur and it can lead on to deep invasion, especially if a prosthesis is present.
- The number of organisms required to develop infection is reduced to 100-fold in the presence of foreign material.

PREVENTION OF MRSA INFECTION IS BY HAND HYGIENE

- Senior staff and doctors have lower hand hygiene compliance.
- Surgeons pay great attention to hand hygiene in the theater but practice poor hygiene in the ward.

Source: Recent Advances in Surgery 30; 2007.

- MRSA colonized patients are isolated in a single room.
- Practice hand hygiene on entering and leaving the room.
- Plastic apron is worn within the room.
- Pool together all MRSA patients in a ward (cohort nursing).
- Sleeves should be rolled above the elbow before any ward procedure.
- Wrist watches must be removed before doing any ward procedure.
- Wash hands and apply disinfectant (read hand hygiene).
- Topical decontamination for MRSA carrier sites—mupirocin applied to the anterior nerves three times a day for 5 days and chlorhexidine used daily on a sponge to apply to the skin before showering (chlorhexidine is used as a shampoo for 2-3 days).
- Antibiotics for MRSA—teicoplanin, vancomycin, and linezolid (for 7-14 days). Linezolid has excellent penetration into all tissues whether given orally or IV. It can cause thrombocytopenia and peripheral neuropathy. For teicoplanin, high doses should be used. The minimum dose should be 6 mg/kg/day. When vancomycin is used, the dose should be determined by serum levels through 5-10 mg/L.
- Irrigate the wound with normal saline (vacuum dressing, if available, may be used).
- Dressings are essential to cover the wound to prevent dissemination.
- Hydrocolloids are useful.

MRSA PROPHYLAXIS AT THE TIME OF SURGERY

- Conventional surgical prophylaxis is ineffective.
- Teicoplanin 6-12 mg/kg or vancomycin 1 g administered intravenously at the time of induction.
- Vancomycin is to be infused over 1 hour to avoid hypotension.

35 Ingrowing Toe Nail

R Dayananda Babu

ZADIK'S OPERATION

It is a procedure of avulsion of nail with complete excision of the nail bed along with excision of germinal matrix of fingers or toes.

Indication
- Ingrowing toe nail
- Onychogryphosis.

In case of infection and where there is a risk of spreading infection into the bone joint, only avulsion of nail is done and excision of nail bed is delayed for around 6 weeks for the infection to get settled.

Anesthesia
- Either a general anesthetic or digital block
- Tourniquet is used to get a bloodless field.

Procedure
It can be done by two ways:
1. Either wedge excision of the nail of the lateral or medial side along with nail bed removal with granulation tissue and wedge of nail fold.

   Or

2. Complete avulsion of the nail followed by incisions over the skin overlying the matrix of the nail on either side making a flap and drawing it up to expose the matrix. The matrix is completely excised and the skin flaps are loosely sutured back with interrupted sutures.

Avulsion of the Nail (Fig. 1)

One blade of a heavy artery forceps is introduced under the nail either in medial or lateral third.

Rotation of the closed forceps lifts the medial or lateral nail edge out of the basal corner and the nail fold.

The maneuver is repeated on the other side and the whole nail is avulsed.

Ingrowing Toe Nail

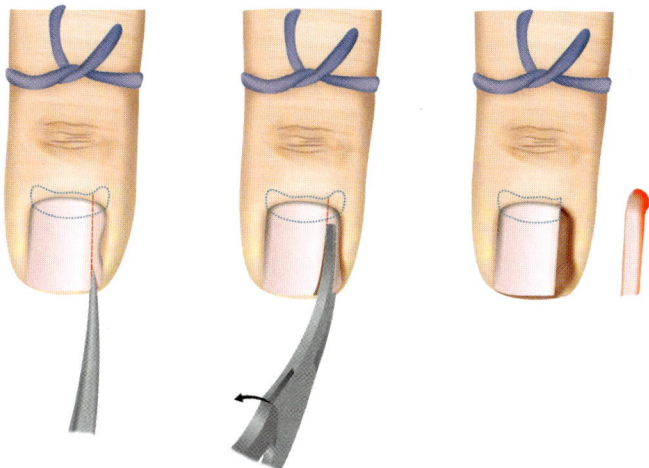

Fig. 1: Removing a nail segment.

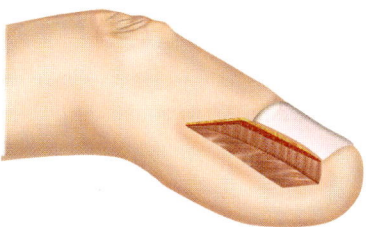

Fig. 2: Wedge excision of the nail bed.

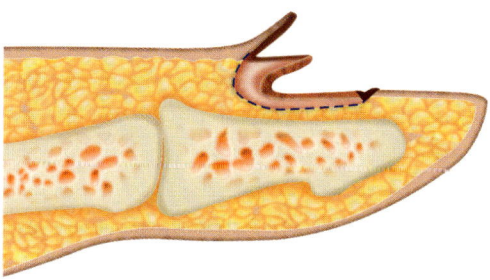

Fig. 3: Total nail bed excision.

The tissue overgrowth and proud granulations are curetted or excised from the nail fold.

Excision of Nail Bed (Figs. 2 to 5)

Two incisions are made out from the basal corners and the flap of skin overlying the base of the nail is elevated.

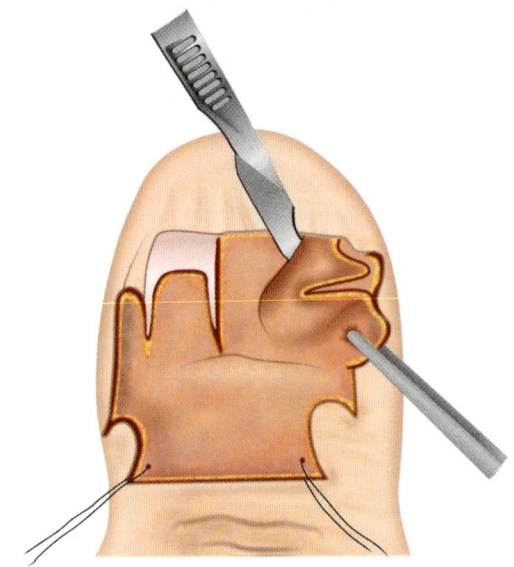

Fig. 4: Removal of germinal matrix after total nail bed excision.

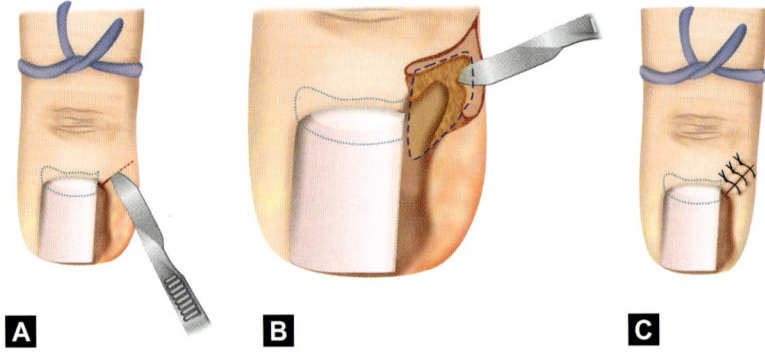

Figs. 5A to C: Segmental nail bed excision.

The germinal matrix area of nail bed situated at the proximal third of the nail bed is excised.

The germinal area has medial and lateral extensions which are loosely attached to the bony expansions at the base of the proximal phalanx. These extensions are also excised.

At the end of a Zadik excision, the medial and lateral corner extensions of germinal matrix should be checked for completeness.

Incomplete Removal Leads to Recurrence

Two incisions made from the base of the nail bed are sutured and the raw tissue of the nail bed is dressed with absorbent dressings.

Nasogastric Intubation (Ryle's Tube)

R Dayananda Babu

INTRODUCTION

A nasogastric intubation is a medical process involving the insertion of a nasogastric tube through the nose, past the throat, and down the stomach. The original tube for nasogastric aspiration was designed by an English physician, Ryle of Guy's Hospital Medical School. The original Ryle's tube was made up of rubber. The modern nasogastric tubes are made up of polyvinyl chloride (PVC)/Portex. These tubes are presterilized with ethylene oxide and usually 1 m long.

PARTS OF A NASOGASTRIC TUBE

It has a tip, body, and base. Near the rounded tip, there are rounded lead shots, to make the tip radiopaque **(Fig. 1)**.

MARKINGS ON THE NASOGASTRIC TUBE

- *First marking (single line)*: It is situated 40 cm from the tip. When the tube is inserted up to this mark, the tip lies in gastroesophageal junction.
- *Second marking (two lines)*: This is situated 50 cm from the tip and when inserted, the tip will be at the body of the stomach.

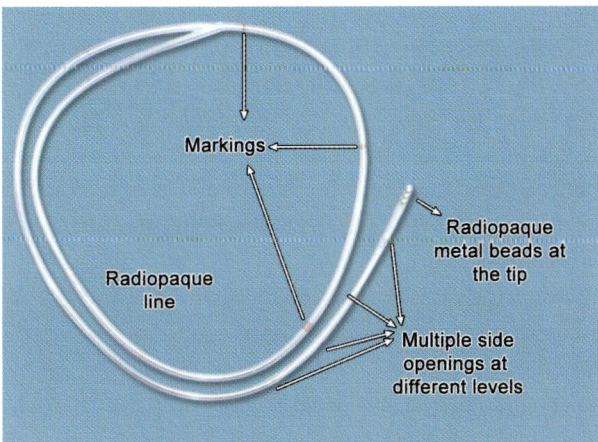

Fig. 1: Parts of nasogastric tube.

- *Third marking (three lines)*: This is situated 60 cm from the tip and when inserted, it will be at pyloric region.
- *Fourth marking (four lines)*: This is situated 70 cm from the tip and when inserted, the tip will be at duodenum.

INDICATIONS

The indications may be classified as diagnostic and therapeutic.

Therapeutic

- For nasogastric decompression in cases of intestinal obstruction, acute abdomen, peritonitis, and acute dilatation of stomach
- In cases of established paralytic ileus
- For decompression of intestine after surgical procedures like intestinal anastomosis
- To decompress stomach and give rest until the return of peristalsis after laparotomy
- To prevent distension of abdomen
- In conservative management of subacute intestinal obstruction
- In multisystem trauma to decompress the stomach and prevent aspiration
- *For feeding*: Nasogastric feeding is used in unconscious patients and in those who are not taking oral feeds
- For gastric lavage in cases of noncorrosive poisoning, gastric outlet obstruction, and upper gastrointestinal (GI) bleeding.

Diagnostic

- To diagnose gastric outlet obstruction by doing saline load test—700 mL of normal saline at room temperature is infused through the nasogastric tube over 3–5 minutes and then the tube is clamped. After 30 minutes, the stomach is aspirated and the residual volume of saline is recorded. If more than 350 mL is recovered, it indicates obstruction
- To diagnose upper GI source in cases of melena
- To diagnose tracheoesophageal fistula
- To diagnose pseudocyst of pancreas by taking a lateral view after putting a nasogastric tube—the stomach will be pushed forward and the Ryle's tube tip will be seen anteriorly
- For performing gastric function tests for the assessment of acid production in olden days
- For doing pentagastrin test in suspected Zollinger–Ellison syndrome.

Other Uses

- It can be used as a tourniquet
- It can be used as a sling during surgery
- It is used as a catheter in cystostomy, nephrostomy, etc.

CONTRAINDICATIONS

- Acute corrosive poisoning (absolute)
- Fracture of the cribriform plate in trauma (absolute)
- Kerosene poisoning
- Aortic aneurysm
- Patients with respiratory diseases, cardiac patients, and esophageal varices.

PROCEDURE

Equipment Required (Fig. 2)

- 16–18 French nasogastric tube
- Lignocaine jelly
- 10-cc syringe
- A small cup with water for the patient to swallow
- Adhesive tape to secure the tube
- Sterile gloves
- Suction apparatus.

Inserting the Ryle's Tube

- Take the consent of the patient.
- Explain the procedure to the patient that a tube needs to be inserted through the nose and that he has to swallow it.
- *Position of the patient*: Preferably propped up position with slight flexion at the neck.
- Choose the nostril which is wider (the nostril is cleansed with a cotton swab in antiseptic).
- In nervous and noncooperative patients, 4% lignocaine is sprayed to the nasopharynx. If required, sedation may be used.

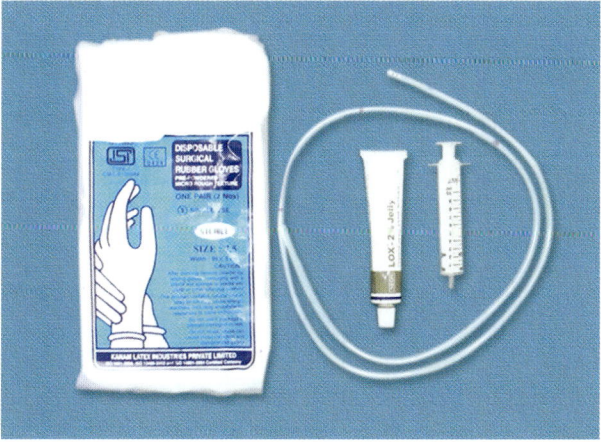

Fig. 2: Equipment required for nasogastric tube insertion.

- The tip of the tube is lubricated with lignocaine jelly and is gently passed through the bigger nostril. Ask the patient to swallow when it reaches the posterior pharyngeal wall.
- Patient may be given water at this stage and is asked to swallow.
- Keep on pushing till it is between the second and third marking.
- When the tip has passed beyond the cricoids, the procedure is easy.
- Confirm that the tube is in stomach by aspiration which will reveal gastric contents.
- Secure the tube to the nose with adhesive tapes.

Danger: See that the tube is not in the air passage before injecting any solution. This can be confirmed by keeping the outer end of the tube under water in a kidney tray. If bubble is appearing, then it is in the air passage.

How to confirm that it is in stomach?
Inject about 5–10 mL of air through the tube and then listen with a stethoscope over the epigastrium. Audible gurgling sound will be heard, if it is in the stomach.

Unconscious Patients

They do not have swallowing reflux and therefore nasogastric tube insertion is difficult. In this situation, a Magill's endotracheal tube is passed transnasally beyond the pharyngeal sphincter and then the nasogastric tube is passed through this tube. The Magill's tube is withdrawn when the nasogastric tube reaches the stomach.

Complications

- Reflux esophagitis
- Aspiration pneumonia—in unconscious patients
- Epistaxis
- Sinusitis
- Bleeding from esophageal varices
- Esophageal perforation.

PROBLEMS OF NASOGASTRIC TUBE

- Blocked tube
- Dislodged tube.

Blocked Tube

Causes for Blockage

- Debris within the tube lumen—this may be food or medications (it is important to irrigate the tube routinely)
- Clotted blood
- *Kinked tube*: A tube that is folded within the esophagus.

The important complication of blocked tube is aspiration pneumonia. The nonfunctioning tube does not adequately empty the stomach and hence aspiration.

Management of Blocked Tube

Flush the tube with 30–40 mL of sterile saline. Listen over the epigastrium to hear the audible entry sound of the fluid. Remove the tape and reposition the tube a few centimeters in or out. If this is not working, replace the tube.

Dislodged Nasogastric Tube

Causes for Dislodgement

- Failure to secure the tube
- Inadvertent traction.

Complication of dislodged tube: Aspiration pneumonia.

Management: Remove the tape and reposition the tube. Flush the tube with 30–40 mL of saline. If required, the tube may be replaced.

Removal of the Nasogastric Tube

Inject 5–10 cc of air in to the tube so that the tube will remain empty of secretions. The outer end of tube is shut by folding. Then it is pulled out gently. When the tip is brought out, it is covered with a gauze piece so as to prevent spillage.

37 Urethral Catheterization

R Dayananda Babu

INTRODUCTION

"Catheter" comes from the Greek word "katheter", which means "let down". A catheter is a tube inserted into body cavity, duct, or blood vessel that provides a channel for fluid passage. The process of inserting catheter is called catheterization. Urethral catheterization is a procedure for direct drainage of urinary bladder.

INDICATIONS

- *Therapeutic*:
    - To relieve urinary retention
    - To provide bladder irrigation
    - To instill medications
    - For neurogenic bladder—intermittent decompression.
- *Diagnostic*:
    - To determine the etiology of genitourinary conditions
    - To monitor urine output
    - For imaging urinary tract.

CONTRAINDICATIONS

- *Absolute contraindication*: Suspected urethral trauma (indicated by blood at the meatus, perineal swelling, and high-riding prostate).
- *Relative contraindications*:
    - Previous difficult catheterization
    - Recent urethral surgery
    - Congenital malformations
    - Allergy to latex.

CATHETER MATERIALS

- Latex
- Silastic (silicone or silicone-coated. It is least irritant and can be left for longer duration)
- Antibiotic impregnated
- Silver alloy.

Urethral Catheterization

Catheterization may be for one time drainage purpose or left indwelling with a self-retaining device for short-term drainage (during surgery), or indwelling for long-term drainage.

TYPES OF CATHETER (FIG. 1)
- One way—one lumen for drainage
- Two way—two lumens (one for drainage and one for the inflation of the balloon for retaining)
- Three way—three lumens (one for drainage, one for balloon inflation, and one for bladder irrigation).

Types of Catheter Available in the Market
- Red rubber catheter (irritant to urethra) **(Fig. 2)**.
- Foley's catheter **(Fig. 3)**.

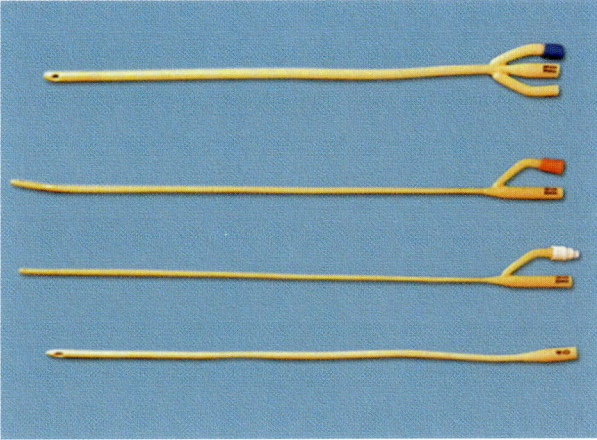

Fig. 1: Types of catheter.

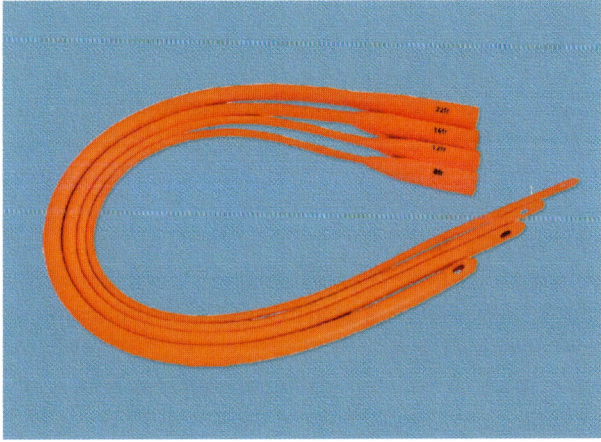

Fig. 2: Red rubber catheters.

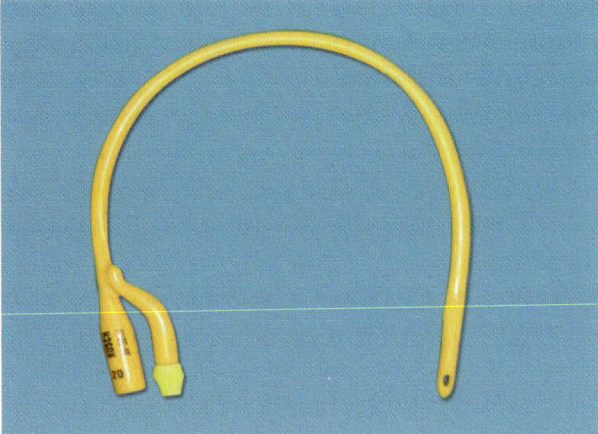

Fig. 3: Foley's catheter.

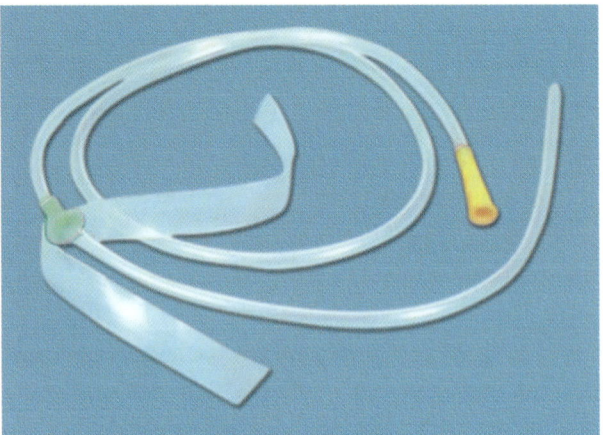

Fig. 4: Gibbon catheter.

- *Gibbon catheter*: It is made of polyvinyl chloride and is relatively small. It causes minimal irritation. It has a wide bore, in relation to the external diameter. It is used for relief of long-standing urinary retention. The catheter is stiffened by a plastic stylet. It has two flaps attached to the tubing about 20 cm from its tip **(Fig. 4)**. These flaps are secured to the shaft of the penis by strapping (to the inner side of the thigh in females).
- Plastic catheter **(Fig. 5)**.
- *Tiemann neoplex catheter (Coudé catheter)*: It is relatively rigid. It has a slightly curved extremity. It is used to negotiate a urethra rendered narrow by prostatic disease **(Fig. 6)**.
- *Condom catheter*: It is used for incontinent males. The condom is inserted on the penis and the tip of the condom is cut and connected to a drainage system. It carries low risk of infection than the indwelling catheter **(Fig. 7)**.

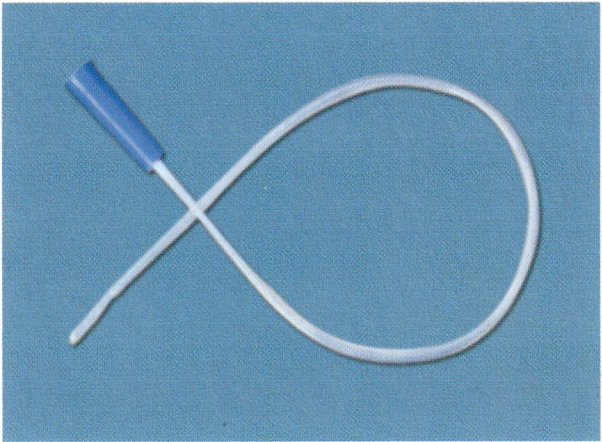

Fig. 5: Plastic catheter.

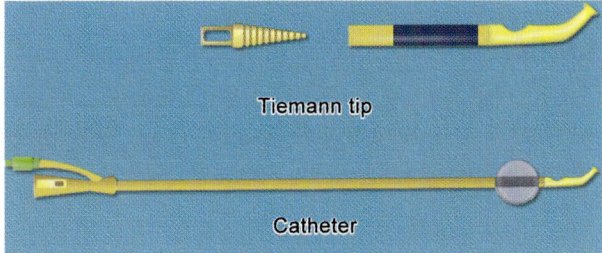

Fig. 6: Tiemann catheter.

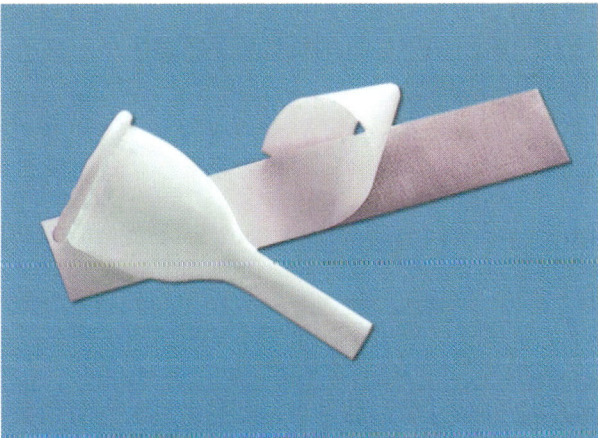

Fig. 7: Condom catheter.

Foley's Catheter

It is the most commonly used indwelling catheter. It is made of latex, which is soft. It has an inflatable bulb near the tip, which is distended with water, so that it will remain in position within the bladder **(Fig. 8)**. The capacity of the bulb varies from 30 to 50 mL, which will be written on the catheter. The disadvantage of this catheter is that it cannot overcome urethral obstructions.

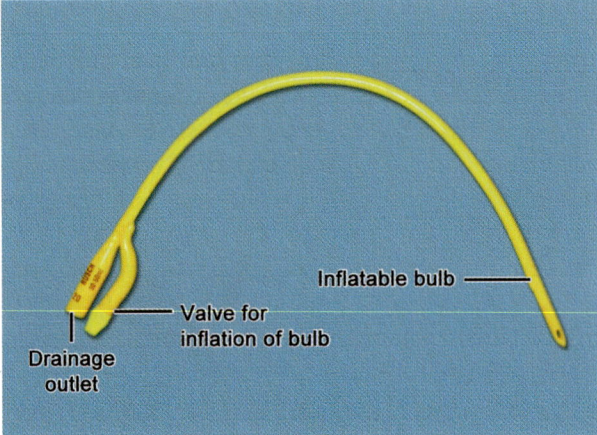

Fig. 8: Parts of a Foley's catheter.

SIZES OF CATHETER

The catheter diameter is sized in Charrières or French catheter scale (F). It indicates the external circumference of the catheter in millimeters:
- 1 F = 1/3 mm diameter
- 10 F = 3.3 mm diameter
- 28 F = 9.3 mm diameter.

The selection is done by seeing the diameter of the external urethral meatus.

TECHNIQUE OF URETHRAL CATHETERIZATION (NO-TOUCH TECHNIQUE)

Catheterization must be an aseptic procedure and a "no-touch technique" reduces the risk of infection of the bladder.

Other Requirements for Urethral Catheterization (Fig. 9)
- Sterile cotton balls
- Povidone iodine
- Sterile drapes
- Sterile gloves
- Lubrication gel
- Syringe
- Distilled water
- Collection bag **(Figs. 10 and 11)** system.

Male Catheterization Procedure

Explain the procedure and risks of the procedure to the patient. Patient is kept in supine position. In case of acute retention, intravenous diazepam sedation may be used. Use the nondominant hand to hold the penis throughout the

Urethral Catheterization

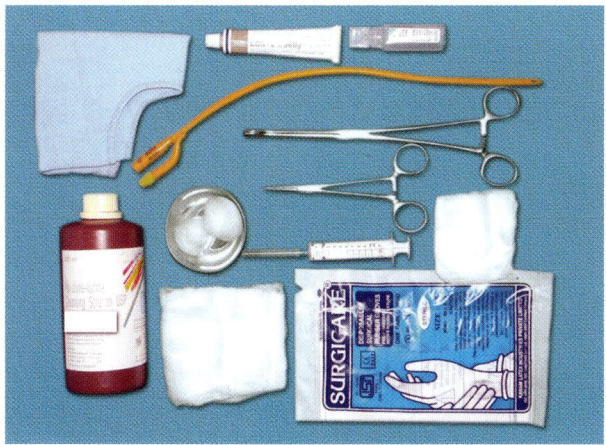

Fig. 9: Materials required for male catheterization.

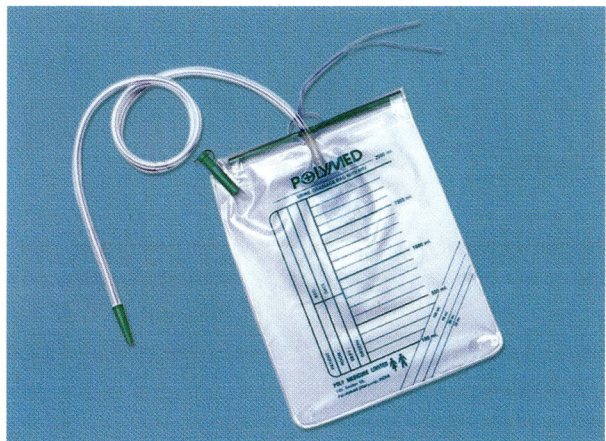

Fig. 10: Collecting bag.

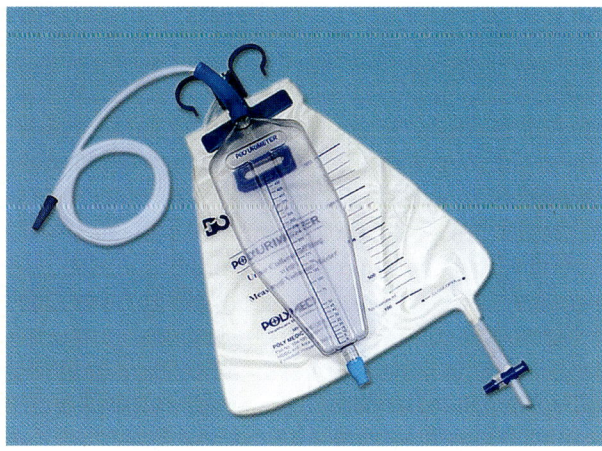

Fig. 11: Collecting bag polyurimeter.

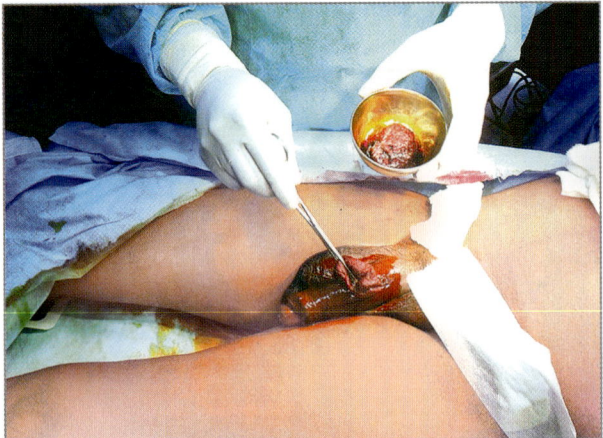

Fig. 12: Cleaning the genitalia.

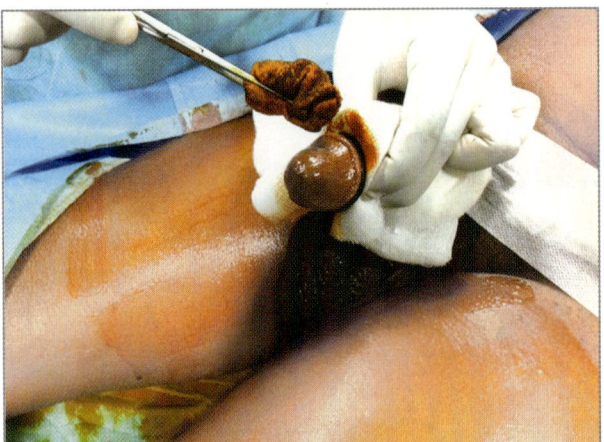

Fig. 13: Cleaning after retraction of prepuce.

procedure. Retract the prepuce and clean the glans using the dominant sterile hand **(Figs. 12 and 13)**. Sterile drapes are used to create a sterile field around the penis. Keep the penis straight and stretch it slightly upwards to overcome the first curve of the urethra. Insert 10–20 mL lignocaine gel 2% into the urethra using a single-use insertion device **(Fig. 14)**. Allow some spillover of the gel to the surrounding glans. Allow 2–3 minutes for getting the anesthetic action. Hold the catheter with sterile hands and allow it to slip into the urethra **(Fig. 15)**. During the second urethral curve, a soft resistance will be encountered. Straighten the stretched penis further while pushing the catheter gently **(Fig. 16)**. Once the catheter is inside, the bladder urine flow is achieved **(Fig. 17)**. Push the catheter further until the fork of the catheter. This will prevent the inflation of the balloon while the catheter is in the urethra. Inflate the balloon with appropriate amount of water **(Fig. 18)**.

Urethral Catheterization

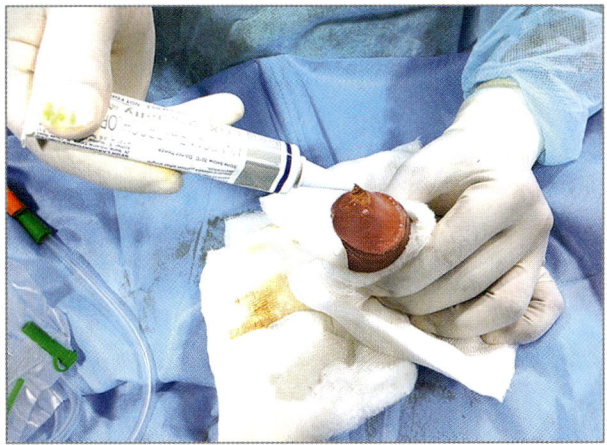

Fig. 14: Introducing the lignocaine jelly.

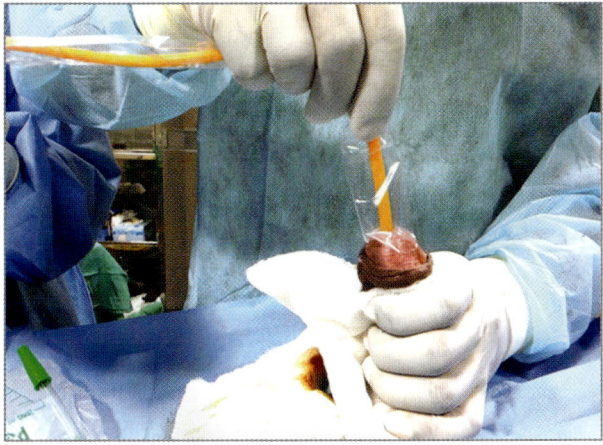

Fig. 15: Introducing catheter by non-touch technique.

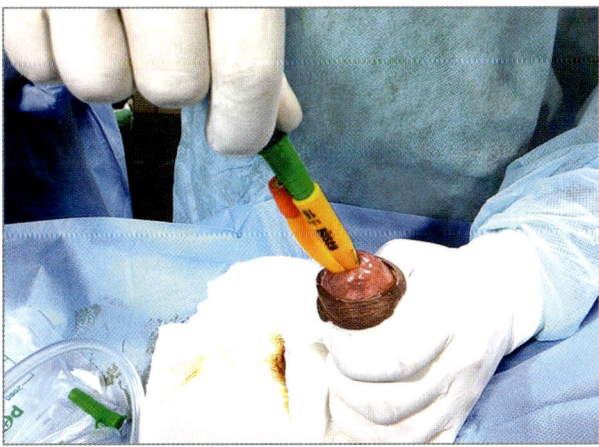

Fig. 16: Introducing catheter fully.

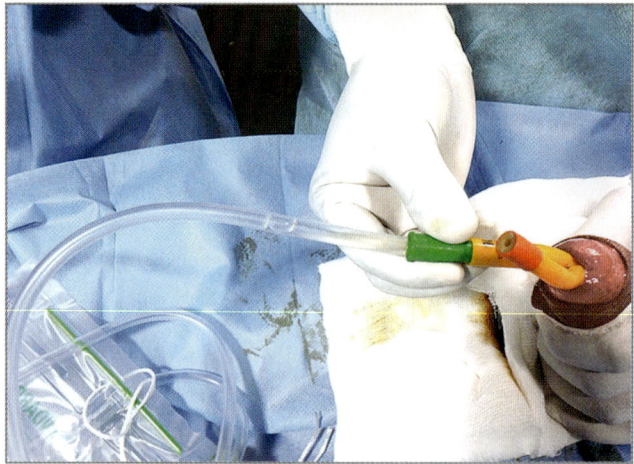

Fig. 17: Urine outflow seen in drainage tube.

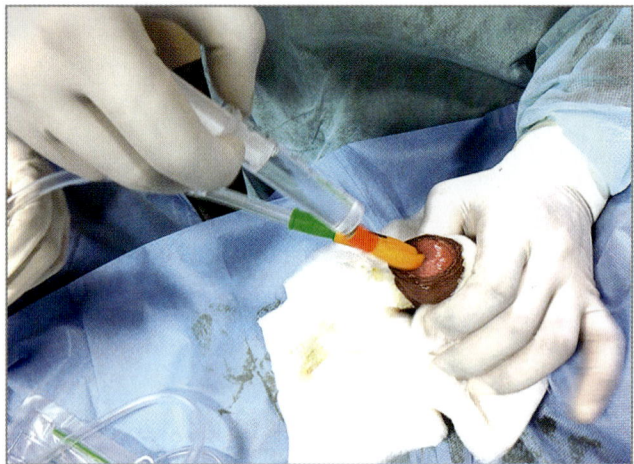

Fig. 18: Inflating the balloon.

Withdraw the catheter gently until there is a tug to indicate that the balloon is resting against the bladder neck **(Fig. 19)**. The urine should flow freely this time. Once the catheter is inside the bladder, it is connected to the drainage bag. Bring back the prepuce to the normal position, otherwise paraphimosis will result **(Fig. 20)**.

Female Catheterization
- Patient is positioned in lithotomy position
- Wipe the labia around the urethra with antiseptic
- Lubricate the catheter tip with lignocaine gel
- Open the labia and allow the catheter to slide in
- Push the catheter into the bladder till urine flows freely
- Inflate the balloon with water

Urethral Catheterization

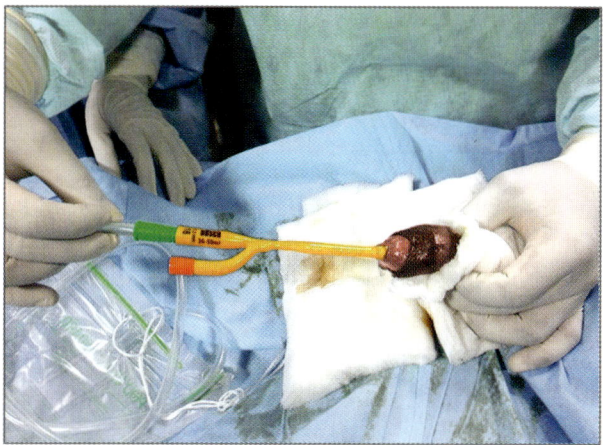

Fig. 19: Withdrawing the catheter.

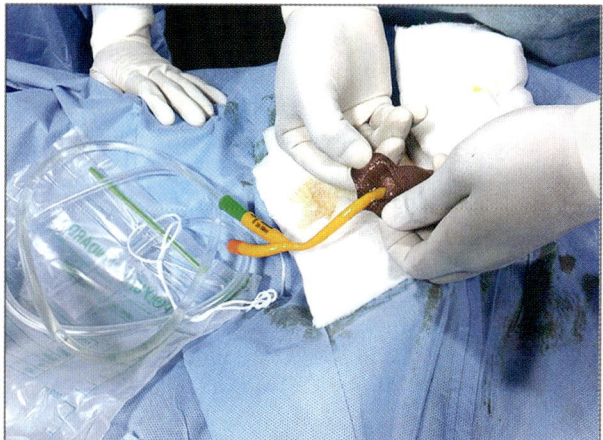

Fig. 20: Bringing back prepuce to normal position.

- Connect the catheter to the drainage bag
- Withdraw the catheter gently until there is a slight tug indicating that the balloon is against the bladder neck.

Collecting Apparatus

This is usually a transparent plastic tube. This is directly connected to the catheter. Some are provided with trap at its distal end to avoid bacterial contamination. The sterile disposable collecting bags are usually transparent so that the quality and quantity of drainage can be assessed. Some bags are incorporated with a printed scale for measurement of the amount. For hourly accurate measurement of urine output, polyurimeter is used (*see* **Fig. 11**).

Problems during Catheterization

- Difficulty to pass the prostatic urethra—try a large diameter catheter or a silicone catheter

- Phimosis—if the phimosis is tight, try dilatation
- Difficulty to pass bladder neck—try smaller size.

Note: In case of difficulty, avoid making a false passage.

MANAGEMENT OF CATHETER

- *Encrustation*: Precipitation of minerals, mucus, protein, and bacteria can occur on the surface of catheter and this will be exacerbated by infection with proteus and the resultant alkaline urinary pH. Treat the infection in the presence of infection and also increase the fluid intake.
- *Leak along the side of the catheter*: Use a larger gauge catheter.
- *Catheter block*: This requires a bladder wash or a change of catheter.
- *Foreign body reaction and inflammation*: Try a different type of catheter.

Removal of the Catheter

Using a syringe, draw back the water in the balloon and pull the catheter out gently. It is preferable to remove the catheter during morning hours so that if patient is not able to micturate, which will be apparent during daytime, recatheterization can be done.

Retained Catheter

If the side channel is blocked and the water cannot be withdrawn (failure to deflate which may be due to malfunctioning of the inflation valve due to clamping or crushing or by obstruction of valve by crystallization when nonsterile fluid is used to inflate the balloon), a sono-guided puncture of the balloon by transabdominal approach is recommended. Following this, a thorough bladder wash and cystoscopy should be done to ensure that there are no bits of the balloon within the bladder. Another option is to cut the balloon port proximal to inflation valve. This removes the valve and allows the water to get drained.

COMPLICATIONS

- Paraphimosis in males as a result of failure to reduce the foreskin
- *Infections*: Any instrumentation will introduce the microorganisms from outside in—
  - Urethritis
  - Cystitis
  - Pyelonephritis
- Creation of false passages
- Urethral strictures
- Bleeding.

Caution: In chronic retention, the bladder evacuation must be gradual. This will prevent intravesical hemorrhage, shock, and reflux anuria.

DAILY CARE OF THE CATHETER TO PREVENT INFECTION

- Cleansing the urethral area and catheter itself using antiseptic solution
- Disconnecting the drainage bags with clean hands and as seldom as possible
- Drinking lots of fluids.

FAILED CATHETERIZATION

In such situations, as a temporary measure, suprapubic aspiration may be performed. Later on, a fine catheter can be introduced by the SupraCath.

38. Resuscitation in Trauma

R Dayananda Babu

INTRODUCTION

Trauma is called the "neglected disease" of the modern society. It is also called the "unsolved epidemic of the future". It is the principal cause of death between 15 and 44 years of age, the most productive group of population. As per the Royal College of Surgeons data, 20% of the deaths are preventable. If the neurosurgical cases are excluded, up to 40% of the deaths are preventable. It is not the lack of hi-tech care, but ordinary surgical care in the form of identifying and managing the internal hemorrhage and treatment of hypoxia. It was not the fractures that killed, but internal hemorrhage according to the American series. It is important to note that some of the patients died while being transported to the computed tomography (CT) room. An estimated 5 million people die from injuries worldwide, forming the third leading cause of death. The economic impact of trauma is huge and the social cost is still higher.

PREVENTION

Prevention is better than cure. The trauma prevention consists of:
- Primary prevention—consisting of anti-drink driving, speed limit, etc. 10% increase in impact speed translates into 40% rise in the case fatality risk.
- *Secondary prevention*:
  - *Active secondary prevention*—helmets for two wheelers and seat belts for four wheelers. All vehicle occupants should wear seat belts. There is 45% reduction of mortality if front passengers are wearing seat belt. If the rear passenger is wearing seat belt, the risk of death of the belted front passenger will be reduced by 80%. Ejection from a vehicle is associated with a significantly greater severity of injury. The seats should be moved as far back as possible from the steering wheel or dashboard. Children younger than 12 years should be properly restrained in the back seat. Infants less than 1 year must be seated in a rear facing child safety seats and they should never be seated in the front seat of a vehicle fitted with air bags.

The two-wheeler death rate is 35 times greater than the occupants of a car. Helmets decrease the mortality rate by one-third and decrease the risk of facial injury by two-third.
- Passive secondary prevention—ABS brakes and air bags.
- Tertiary prevention—minimizing the effects of injury by improving the healthcare delivery system.

PREHOSPITAL CARE

There is ongoing controversy regarding basic life support versus advanced life support at the scene. Now, there is evidence to say that additional 12 minutes are taken for advanced life support measures and this increases the risk of death, therefore, a "scoop and run" policy is recommended.

TRAUMA TEAM IN TRAUMA CENTERS

Trauma team consists of one or more anesthetists, one or more nurses, one or more surgeons, and a radiographer. Whenever there is a team, there must be a captain and it is preferable to have a general surgeon with sufficient experience as the captain of the team.

RESUSCITATION AREA IN TRAUMA CENTER

Resuscitation area should have an adequate room, so that the team members can move freely unhindered by others. There should be adequate storage spaces for keeping venous cannulae, resuscitation fluid, chest drains, drainage bottles, and drugs. There should be at least 10 electricity sockets for each resuscitation couch.

UNIVERSAL PRECAUTIONS AND MIST

It is imperative to take universal precautions while dealing with trauma victims. The mnemonic MIST is for ascertaining:
- *M*—for Mechanism of injury
- *I*—for Injuries identified
- *S*—for vital Signs at scene
- *T*—for Treatment administered.

TRIAGE

It is a French term; triage means "to sort". It is the principle of "best for most". In a mass casualty, the patients are categorized into following groups:
- *Immediate*—life-threatening injuries
- *Delayed*—treatment required within 6 hours
- *Minimal*—walking, wounded, and psychiatric
- *Expectant*—severe injuries, unlikely to survive with current resources
- Dead.

Trimodal Distribution of Death by Donald Trunkey

- Immediate death—50% (within first few minutes)
- Early death—30% (within first few hours); first hour after trauma is called "golden hour"
- Late death—20% (days or weeks after trauma).

ADVANCED TRAUMA LIFE SUPPORT

The Advanced Trauma Life Support (ATLS) was initially devised by James Styner, an orthopedic surgeon in 1970. He was involved in an air crash and found that there is no structured way of trauma management, and hence devised ATLS. This was later on adapted by the American College of Surgeons Committee on Trauma. This is a four-stage continuous approach:

1. Primary survey
2. Resuscitation
3. Secondary survey
4. Definitive care (+ 5—tertiary survey).

Primary Survey

It is a 60-second head-to-toe examination looking for ABCDE:
- A—Airway with cervical spine protection
- B—Breathing and ventilation
- C—Circulation and hemorrhage control
- D—Disability and neurological status
- E—Exposure/environmental control.

Airway

The simplest method of checking the airway is to ask the patient "what is your name? and what hurts?" A correct answer shows that patient has got a patent airway. In addition, it also shows that the patient has got sufficient cerebral function to process the stimulus and sufficient ventilation to phonate the answer. Complete obstruction will produce aphonia. Partial obstruction will produce snoring/stridor.

*Airway control (**Figs. 1 to 4**):* There are basic airway techniques and advanced airway techniques. But, however, it should be instituted while protecting the cervical spine. Clear the mouth and airway with a large bore sucker. If foreign bodies are there, finger sweep will be enough. If the Glasgow Coma Scale (GCS) is less than 8, consider definitive airway.

The basic airway techniques include:
- Modified jaw thrust maneuver
- Oral/nasopharyngeal airway **(Fig. 5)**.

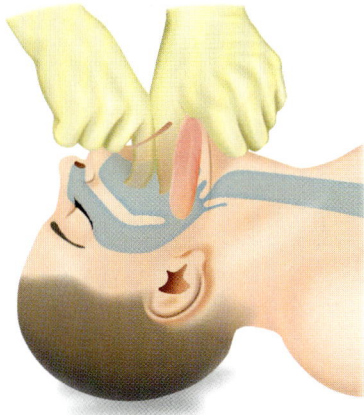

Fig. 1: Finger sweep method of clearing the oral cavity.

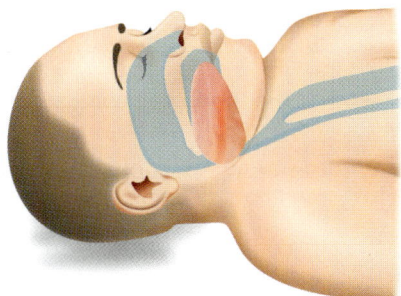

Fig. 2: Compromised airway.

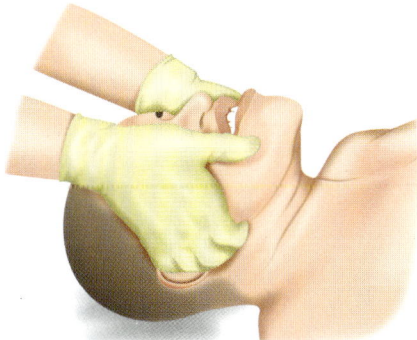

Fig. 3: Jaw thrust maneuver.

The advanced airway techniques consist of:
- Oral/nasal intubation **(Figs. 6 and 7)**
- Surgical/needle (13G) cricothyroidotomy. It is preferable to avoid tracheostomy
- Drug-assisted intubation is done nowadays.

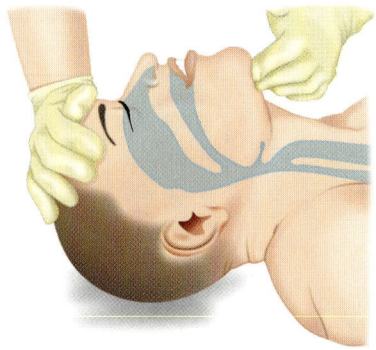

Fig. 4: Chin lift.

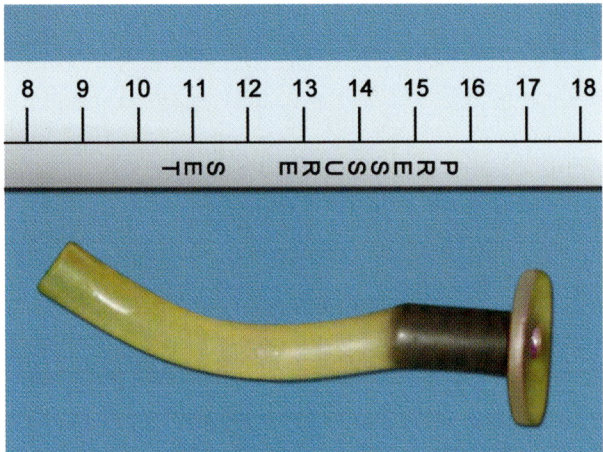

Fig. 5: Oropharyngeal airway.

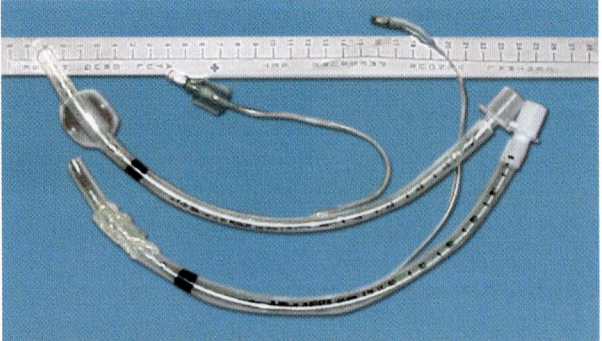

Fig. 6: Endotracheal tubes.

Glasgow Coma Scale less than 8 is an indication for definitive airway placement. Altered level of consciousness may also be due to hypoglycemia, alcohol, narcotics, and other drugs. Therefore, it is important to get a proper history.

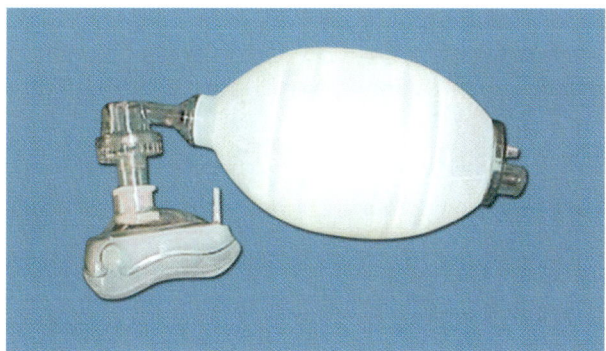

Fig. 7: Ambu bag.

Breathing and Ventilation

It is important to identify hypoxia, tension pneumothorax, flail chest, hemothorax, and other life-threatening injuries. They are not radiological diagnosis but clinical diagnosis by observation or the absence of chest movements and percussion and auscultation findings.

Open chest wounds: Open chest wounds are called sucking wounds and they should be managed by occluding it with a three-sided dressing followed by tube thoracostomy through a separate incision.

First aid management of flail chest: It is by turning the patient to the side of paradoxical movement, so that segment will be immobilized.

Tension pneumothorax: It is identified by tracheal shift and mediastinal shift in a patient with acute dyspnea and absent air entry on one side with hyper-resonance on percussion. It is important to treat tension pneumothorax without waiting for X-ray chest by either tube thoracostomy (in safe triangle—read tube thoracostomy) using 28–32-Fr size tube (for hemothorax) or needle thoracostomy at 5th intercostal space slightly anterior to the mid axillary line. In pediatric trauma victims, the needle thoracocentesis site is unchanged (i.e., 2nd intercostal space anteriorly). When ultrasound is available, tension pneumothorax can be diagnosed using an extended FAST (eFAST).

Administration of oxygen: 100% oxygen must be administered to all trauma patients at a high flow rate.

Hemothorax: Massive hemothorax is rapid accumulation of more than 1,500 mL of blood or one-third or more of the patients' blood volume in the chest cavity. Continuous bleeding of 200 mL/h of blood for 2–4 hours may also be considered as massive hemothorax. The neck veins will be usually flat. If the neck veins are distended, consider tension pneumothorax in addition.

Indications for mechanical ventilation:
- Tachypnea above 40
- PaO_2 below 60 mm Hg or less

- $PaCO_2$ above 45 mm Hg
- Progressive fall in PaO_2
- Extensive pulmonary contusion or diffused infiltrative changes on X-ray
- Severe flail chest (>8 U/L or >4 B/L rib fractures).

Life-threatening chest injuries during primary survey:
- Airway obstruction
- Trachea bronchial tree injury
- Tension pneumothorax
- Open pneumothorax
- Massive hemothorax (>1,500 mL of blood)
- Flail chest
- Cardiac tamponade
- Traumatic circulatory arrest.

Circulation

Rough estimation of the BP is possible by palpating the pulse. If the radial pulse is palpable, the BP will be 80 mm Hg. If the radial pulse is not felt, feel the femoral. If femoral alone is palpable, the BP will be 70 mm Hg. If both radial and femoral are not felt, feel the carotids. The carotid pulse is felt with a BP of 60 mm Hg.

The pulse will be rapid and thready in case of hemorrhagic shock. The skin color will be pale, ashen, and gray looking in hypovolemia. Assessment of the conscious level is also important.

Look for evidence of internal and external bleeding. "Blood on the floor and four more places" externally—chest, abdomen, retroperitoneum and pelvis, and muscle compartment.

Table 1 lists the modified "Tennis score" classification of hemorrhage amended with base excess as per ATLS.

Primary hemorrhage control of a bleeding wound is by pressure bandaging (not by tourniquet).

Medical Antishock Trousers (MAST) (Pneumatic Antishock Garment)

It was extensively used in Vietnam War. It consists of inflatable sections for each leg and abdomen and it is radiolucent. There is access for per-rectal examination and urinary catheter. When it is inflated, it will reduce hemorrhage, reduce the total functioning volume of the vascular compartment, and give autotransfusion effect of 0.5–1 liter of blood. In addition, it will splint the lower limb and pelvic fractures.

Indications:
- Splinting and control of pelvic fractures
- Abdominal trauma with hypovolemia.

Table 1: Modified "Tennis score" classification of hemorrhage amended with base excess as per Advanced Trauma Life Support (ATLS).

Hemorrhage	% loss	Volume loss (mL)	Pulse rate	BP	Pulse pressure	Respiratory rate	Glasgow Coma Scale	Base deficit	Need for blood products	Urine output
Class I	15	750	<100	NL	Normal/more	14–20	—	0 to -2 mEq/L	Monitor	—
Class II	15–30	750–1,500	>100	NL	Decreased	20–30	—	-2 to -6 mEq/L	Possible	—
Class III	30–40	1,500–2,000	>120	Decreased	Decreased	30–40	Decreased	-6 to -10 mEq/L	Yes	Decreased
Class IV	>40	>2,000	>140	Decreased	Decreased	>40	Decreased	-10 mEq/L or less	Massive transfusion	Decreased

Contraindications:
- Pulmonary edema
- Diaphragmatic rupture
- Thoracic and upper limb hemorrhage.

Blunt cardiac injury: This will manifest as unexplained tachycardia, atrial fibrillation, premature ventricular contraction, and ST segment changes.

Pulseless electrical activity (PEA): PEA indicates cardiac tamponade, tension pneumothorax, and/or profound hypovolemia.

Disability:
- GSC—Glasgow Coma Scale or AVPU score
- AVPU: A—alert; V—response to vocal stimuli; P—response to painful stimuli; U—unresponsive.

Glasgow Coma Scale: Neurological assessment in trauma is done by Glasgow Coma Scale **(Table 2)** (for details of head injury, read Chapter 32: Head injury).

Resuscitation Phase

The role of conventional aggressive resuscitation is slowly going out of vogue in favor of a controlled infusion of fluid (graded resuscitation), especially in penetrating injury.

Conventional Aggressive Resuscitation

- Secure large bore IV access for shock therapy
- Continuous ECG monitoring
- Blood samples for complete blood count (CBC), electrolytes, glucose, coagulation studies, arterial blood gas (ABG), and cross-matching
- Nasogastric tube is introduced in all multisystem trauma cases
- Foley's catheter (if not contraindicated).

Table 2: Glasgow Coma Scale.

Eye opening	Spontaneously	4
	To verbal command	3
	To painful stimulus	2
	Do not open	1
Verbal response	Normal oriented conversation	5
	Confused	4
	Inappropriate/words only	3
	Sounds only	2
	No sounds	1
	Intubated patient	T
Motor response	Obeys commands	6
	Localizes to pain	5
	Withdraws/flexion	4
	Abnormal flexion	3
	Extension	2
	No motor response	1

Contraindications for Nasogastric Tube and Foley's Catheter

- Nasogastric tube is contraindicated when there is fracture of cribriform plate (cerebrospinal fluid rhinorrhea).
- Foley's catheter is contraindicated when urethral trauma is suspected (blood per urethral meatus).
- *Peripheral IV lines central line*: It is preferable to put two 14-G peripheral IV lines rather than a 16-G, 8-inch length central cannula. As per Poiseuille's law, the flow is proportional to the fourth power of radius of the cannula and inversely related to its length. A 14-G cannula with 2¼ inch length will give a flow of 200 cc/minute compared to 150 cc for a 16-G, 8-inch length central cannula. Therefore, peripheral lines are recommended for resuscitation.

Intravenous cannula:
- Avoid injured or paralyzed limb.
- Avoid femoral vein in pelvic and abdominal injuries.
- A great saphenous vein cut down 6 cm below the inguinal ligament may be useful at times.
- A No 12-Fr pediatric feeding tube can be introduced to the level of IVC through this cut down.

Crystalloid versus Colloid Debate

Crystalloid is preferred over colloid. The crystalloid solutions of choice are Ringer's lactate and normal saline. The replacement to loss ratio should be 3:1 when crystalloids are used. This is because of the large distribution space of crystalloid. There is no place for dextrose in resuscitation of trauma. Theoretical problems of colloid are concerns about transmission of diseases and transudation of fluid into the pulmonary interstitium.

Hypertonic Saline

The current trend is to use hypertonic saline (3-7.5% formulation) with or without added colloid. This will effectively improve hemodynamics, oxygen transport, microcirculation, and immunological protection.

Controlled Infusion of Fluid/Graded Resuscitation: The New Trend

Fluid administration before surgical control of hemorrhage may actually worsen bleeding and increase mortality. Therefore, the current aggressive resuscitation is potentially harmful and at best experimental. Permissive hypotension is recommended in penetrating injury.

One liter of crystalloid fluid is given judiciously as isotonic solution for adults and 20 mL/kg for pediatric patients of less than 40 kg. If a patient is unresponsive to initial crystalloid therapy, the patient should receive blood transfusion and definitive control of hemorrhage.

Problems of IV Fluids in Aggressive Resuscitation

- Inhibit platelet aggregation
- Dilute clotting factors
- Modulate the physical properties of thrombus
- Mechanical disruption of clot by increased BP.

Aggressive resuscitation before control of bleeding has been demonstrated to increase mortality and morbidity.

After giving 1 liter of isotonic solution, patients are categorized into the following groups:
- *Rapid responders*: Patients become hemodynamically normal without signs of inadequate tissue perfusion and oxygenation. They have less than 15% loss of blood. No further fluid bolus or immediate blood administration is required; however, blood should be kept available. Surgical consultation and evaluation by the surgeon is recommended. Operative intervention could still be necessary.
- *Transient response*: After the initial response to the fluid bolus, they begin to show deterioration of perfusion. This indicates ongoing blood loss or inadequate resuscitation. This is seen in blood loss of 15-40%. Patient needs blood and blood products followed by operation to control bleeding or angiographic control. If the patient sill bleeding, initiate massive transfusion protocol (MTP).
- *Minimal or no response*: This is seen in class-4 hemorrhage and such patients will fail to respond to crystalloid and blood administration.

Immediate definitive intervention in the form of operation or angioembolization may be required.

It may also be due to cardiac injury, cardiac tamponade, or tension pneumothorax, resulting in pump failure.

Damage Control Resuscitation

The controlled infusion of fluid with permissive hypotension until surgical hemostasis is called damage control resuscitation. Other components are:
- Minimize crystalloid use
- Use 5% hypertonic saline
- Use blood products early
- Use of r-factor VIIa and factor IX
- Avoid hypothermia.

Early use of blood and blood products: Early use of blood and blood products must be considered in patients with evidence of class-3 and class-4 hemorrhage.

Blood transfusion and hemoglobin-based oxygen carriers—Packed red cells (PRCs): It has immunosuppressive potential. A second indication must be present in addition to a decreased hemoglobin concentration. Young trauma patients can tolerate a hemoglobin level of 7 g/dL.

New generation hemoglobin-based oxygen carriers provide volume expansion and oxygen carrying capacity.

Role of recombinant activated factor VII (rFVIIa): Massively bleeding multitransfused coagulopathic trauma patients benefit from this.

Resuscitation with whole blood: "Walking blood bank" concept is there in war situations. However, aggressive use of fresh frozen plasma (FFP) is recommended nowadays. FFP, packed red cell (PRC), and platelets are used in ratio of 1:1:1.

Massive transfusion: Transfusion of more than 10 units of pRBC within the first 24 hours is called massive transfusion or more than 4 units in 1st hour. Early administration of pRBCs, plasma, and platelets in a balanced ratio as mentioned above to minimize the excessive crystalloid administration may improve the patient survival. This is called balanced, hemostatic, or damage control resuscitation.

Monitor coagulation with thromboelastography (TEG) or rotational thromboelastometry (ROTEM). Consider administering platelet transfusion even with normal platelet count.

Monitoring progress and treatment: This is done by monitoring the following—
- Urinary output
- Pulse rate
- Pulse pressure
- Temperature

- Mental state
- Arterial pressure
- Central venous pressure/Swan–Ganz catheter
- Oxygen saturation.

Tranexamic acid (TXA): The European and American military studies demonstrated improved survival when 1 g TXA is administered over 10 minutes within 3 hours of injury in bleeding patients. If bolus injection is given in the field, infusion of TXA 1 g over 8 hours is repeated in the hospital.

Avoid hypothermia:
- All fluids for transfusion must be stored at 39°C in a fluid warmer
- Packed red cells reconstituted by warm saline
- Irrigating fluid should be warm
- Use warm blankets
- Hypothermia will lead onto cardiac irritability, coagulopathy, and enzyme impairment.

Bloody vicious cycle: It is formed by hypothermia, metabolic acidosis, and coagulopathy.

Management of coagulopathy: Uncontrolled bleeding can occur in patients taking antiplatelet medication. Obtain the medication list from the patient or relatives as early as possible and administer the reversal agents **(Table 3)**. Monitor the coagulation profile and administer platelet transfusion even if the platelet count is normal.

Secondary Survey

A detailed head-to-toe examination is done by "look, listen, and feel technique". Get three high yield X-rays, the three most important X-rays in multisystem trauma:
1. *Cervical lateral (swimmer's view)—visualizing all the 7 cervical vertebrae*: Plain radiograph is not adequate to rule out cervical spine fracture and the investigation of choice is multidetector computed tomography (MDCT) from occiput to T1 with sagittal and coronal reconstruction, as per the Canadian cervical spine rule (remember never shift an unstable patient for CT scan). If MDCT facility is not there, then in addition to lateral view,

Table 3: Anticoagulation reversal.

Anticoagulants	Treatment
Aspirin	Platelet
Warfarin	FFP, vitamin K, and factor VIIa
Heparin	Protamine sulfate
Low-molecular weight heparin (enoxaparin)	Protamine sulfate
Direct thrombin inhibitors (dabigatran etexilate)	Idarucizumab (praxbind)

take AP and open mouth odontoid views, which will visualize the entire odontoid process, and right and left c1 and c2 articulation. The AP view will also reveal unilateral facet dislocation.

Do not remove cervical collar until neurological assessment is completed and evaluation of the cervical spine including palpation is done. Look for voluntary movements of neck in all planes. If MDCT or plain X-ray is normal and patient continues to have pain, MRI is recommended. 10% of cervical fracture will have vertebral column fracture in another site.

Canadian cervical spine rule: If the following factors are there, then consider radiography:
- Age more than 65 years
- Dangerous mechanisms.

Fall from more than 1 meter or 5 stairs:
- An axial load to the head
- A motor vehicle collision with high speed (more than 100 km/h), roll over, and ejection of a victim
- Motorized recreational vehicle collision
- A bicycle collision.

Paresthesia in extremities: In the absence of the above factors and if the patient is able to rotate the neck actively (45° to right and left) then there is no need for radiography.

NEXUS is a mnemonic for the indications for radiography of the cervical spine (ATLS, 10th edition):
- N—Neurological deficit
- E—EtOH intoxication
- X—eXtreme distracting injury
- U—Unable to provide history, altered level of consciousness
- S—Spinal tenderness (midline).

2. Upright chest.
3. Pelvis.

Rule out intra-abdominal bleeding: Rule out intra-abdominal bleeding in all cases of multisystem trauma by Focused Assessment Sonography for Trauma (FAST) and eFAST. FAST is 90–95% accurate. If FAST and CT scan are not available, do a diagnostic peritoneal lavage (DPL). If more than 10 mL of blood, GI contents, vegetable fibers, or bile is obtained in DPL, it is considered as positive. DPL is done usually after putting a nasogastric tube and urinary catheter. The method adopted may be either a closed, open, or semiopen method. The site selected for incision is infraumbilical. A supraumbilical site may be selected in pregnant patient. Intra-abdominal addition is a contraindication for DPL. If the patient is stable, patient is sent for CT scan of the abdomen and other suspected areas.

Serial hematocrit and repeated physical examinations are done in the secondary survey.

In the history, "AMPLE" is important (A—allergy, M—medication, P—past medical history and pregnancy, L—last meal, E—events of the incident).

Assume cervical spine injury until proven otherwise. Four people are required for transfer of a trauma victim—one for spinal in-line traction (anesthesiologist), one for the torso, one for pelvis, and one for lower limbs. The turning of the patient, if required, is by the spinal log roll.

Dangerous Mechanisms of Injury
- Fall from height of 20 feet or more
- Crash greater than 20 miles per hour
- 20-inch impingement on the passenger compartment
- Ejection of the passenger
- Roll over of the vehicle
- Death of another person.

Definitive Care
Coordinate consultations and all planned operations in definitive care.

Tertiary Survey (When the Dust is Settled)
Another detailed examination is conducted for identification of missed injuries. Missed injuries are called "the nemesis of the trauma surgeon". 15% incidence of clinically significant injuries is diagnosed after initial resuscitation. The tertiary survey is by a physical examination and review of results. Early detection of all clinically significant injuries is important to save the life of the patient.

Quaternary Survey
This is a preparation for transfer of the patient to the next higher center, by checking the following things:
- Stability for transfer
- Transport needs
- Receiving facility
- Critical care needs
- Evacuation delays
- Ongoing resuscitation.

Zero Survey
This is a new terminology used for prearrival preparation in the trauma center.

39 Intercostal Drainage Tube

John S Kurien

INTRODUCTION

Tube thoracostomy is in existence from the time Hippocrates used metallic tubes to drain empyemas and necessity being the mother of invention, with every grim event in human history (World War-2, influenza epidemic 1917), the standard of care with chest tubes kept improving. Finally, by the time, the Vietnam War ended, tube thoracostomy had become a standard procedure in the trauma setting.

Closed water-seal drainage for empyema had been used by a German internist, Gotthard Bülau, as early as 1875. Hence, we, sometimes, still call the intercostal drain (ICD) a Bülau Drain.

INDICATIONS

- *Pneumothorax*:
    - Primary spontaneous pneumothorax (persistent or recurrent, after simple aspiration)
    - Secondary spontaneous pneumothorax
    - Tension pneumothorax (after initial needle aspiration)
    - In any ventilated patient
- Malignant pleural effusion, empyema, and complicated parapneumonic pleural effusion
- Traumatic hemopneumothorax
- Postoperative, e.g., after esophageal, cardiac, pulmonary, mediastinal, or pleural surgery
- Treatment with sclerosing agents or pleurodesis
- Post-pneumonectomy bronchopleural fistula
- Patients with penetrating chest wall injury who are intubated or about to be intubated.

CONTRAINDICATIONS

Some surgeons are of the view that when a chest drain is needed for any of the indications listed above, no absolute contraindications exist for chest drain insertion. But relative contraindications are:

- Coagulopathy
- Pulmonary bullae
- Pulmonary, pleural, or thoracic adhesions
- Loculated pleural effusion or empyema
- Skin infection over the chest tube insertion site.

PRINCIPLE

One should remember that inspiration is not mainly an active process. Simply put, the lungs expand during inspiration because of the negative intrathoracic pressure we create during our inspiratory effort. This negative pressure is best maintained in the pleural space, which is the potential space between the parietal and visceral layers of the pleura. Collections of air, fluid, or blood in the pleural space not only compress the lung tissue but also cause the pleural pressures to become positive, causing inappropriate ventilation.

Chest drains are inserted to remove pathological collections of air or fluid in the pleural space, to allow the recreation of the essential negative pressures in the chest, and to permit complete expansion of the lung, thereby, restoring normal ventilation **(Fig. 1)**.

Intercostal drains drain by three mechanisms—the gravitational force, patients own expiratory effort, and occasionally suctioning. The size of the ICD varies according to the age of the patient:
- *Adult*: 28–32 F
- *Child*: 12–28 F
- *Infant*: 12–16 F
- *Neonate*: 10–12 F

Preparing the Patient

Elevating the patient to 45° in supine position lessens the risk of diaphragm elevation and consequent misplacement of the chest tube into the abdominal space. The ipsilateral arm should be placed behind patient's head so as to expose the axillary area. After maintaining sterile precautions and making sure that all the equipment are ready at stand by, especially the chest tube and the underwater seal bag/bottle. Never forget to take an informed consent, even in the trauma setting. After seeing all the relevant radiological images, two members of the team should decide the side of ICD insertion and mark it.

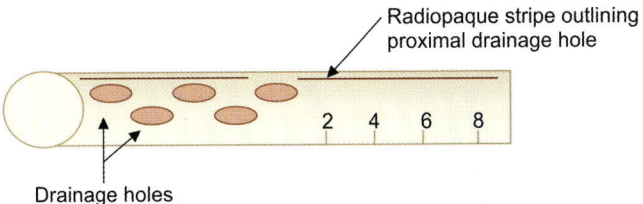

Fig. 1: Tip of the drainage tube showing the side holes.

SITE OF INSERTION

The next step is to choose the site of insertion. The exact site depends on the location of the abnormality.

The *"Triangle of Safety"* **(Fig. 2)**, an area bordered by the mid-axillary line, the lateral border of the pectoralis major anteriorly, and the upper border of the 5th rib are the usual sites, which correspond to the fourth space in the midaxillary line. The dome of the diaphragm extends up to the 5th rib and so if we insert an ICD any lower than the 5th rib, there is a chance of entering the abdomen and injuring the subdiaphragmatic organs **(Fig. 3)**.

Follow strict aseptic precautions or else there is a chance that a pleural effusion may turn into an empyema after chest tube insertion.

Inject 1 mL each of 2% lignocaine solution into the skin and subcutaneous tissue just under the upper rib in the 4th, 5th, and 6th spaces, so as to block the intercostal nerves.

Using a surgical blade, make a skin incision approximately 4 cm long overlying the 5th rib **(Fig. 4)**. The skin incision should be in the same direction as the rib itself.

Use an artery forceps or Bailey forceps to bluntly dissect a tract in the subcutaneous tissue by intermittently advancing the closed instrument and opening it **(Figs. 5 and 6)**. Make sure that the tract ends at the upper border of the 5th rib.

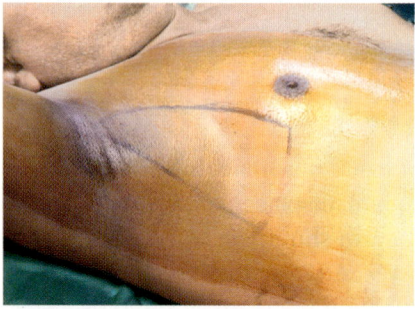

Fig. 2: Triangle of safety marked for the tube insertion.

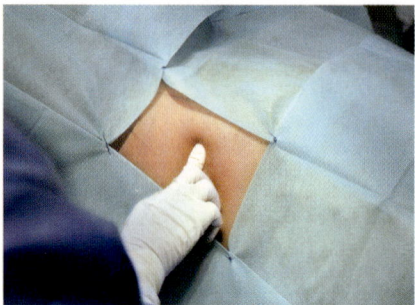

Fig. 3: Site of incision above the 5th rib in the triangle.

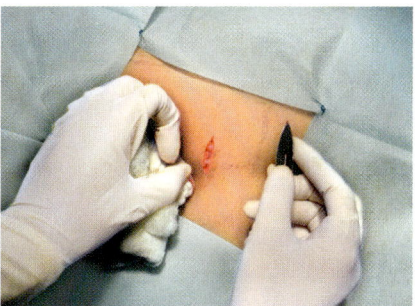

Fig. 4: Incision.

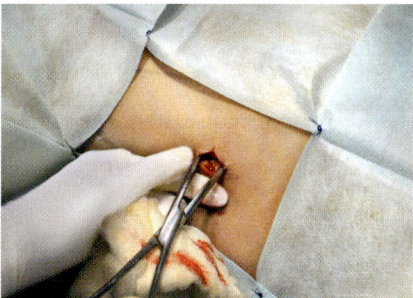

Fig. 5: Artery forceps enlarging the incision.

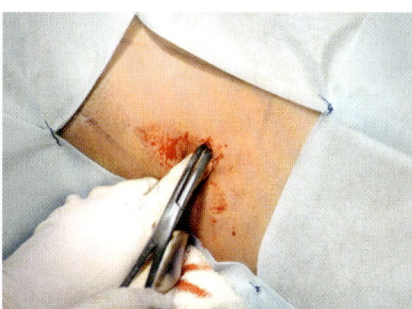

Fig. 6: Inserting the artery forceps.

Insertion of the chest tube as close as possible to the upper border of the rib will minimize the risk of injury to the nerve and blood vessels that follow the lower border of each rib.

Adding more local anesthetic to the intercostal muscles and pleura at this time is a good idea.

Use a closed large Bailey forceps to pass through the intercostal muscles and parietal pleura and enter into the pleural space. This maneuver requires some force and twisting motion of the tip of the closed Kelly clamp.

This motion should be done in a controlled manner, so that the instrument does not enter too far into the chest, which could injure the lung or diaphragm. Therefore, it is imperative to guard the Bailey forceps with the

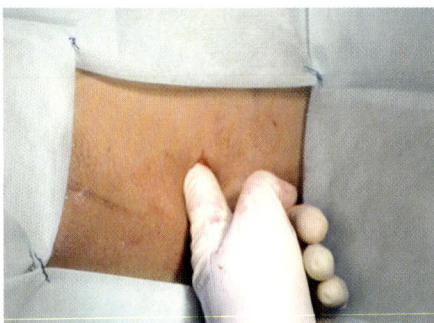

Fig. 7: Gloved finger separating the adhesions of the pleura.

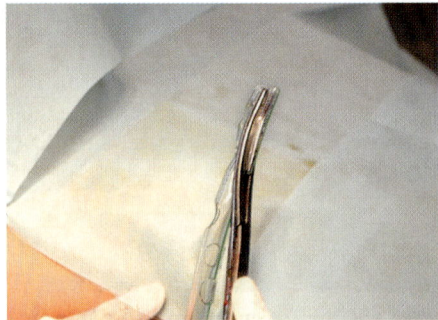

Fig. 8: Holding the tip of the tube with artery forceps.

left hand to prevent sudden entry into the pleural cavity. Upon entry into the pleural space, a rush of air or fluid should occur. The surgeon knows that he has entered the pleura when the clamp suddenly gives away.

The Kelly clamp should be opened (while still inside the pleural space) and then withdrawn so that its jaws enlarge the dissected tract through all layers of the chest wall. This will facilitate the passage of the chest tube when it is inserted.

Use a sterile, gloved finger to appreciate the size of the tract and to feel for lung tissue and possible adhesions. Rotate the finger 360° to appreciate the presence of dense adhesions that cannot be broken and require placement of the chest tube in a different site **(Fig. 7)**.

Measure the length between the skin incision and the apex of the lung to estimate how far the chest tube should be inserted. Grasp the proximal end of the chest tube with the large Kelly clamp and introduce it through the tract and into the thoracic cavity posteriorly and superiorly **(Fig. 8)**.

Release the Bailey forceps and continue to advance the chest tube posteriorly and superiorly. Make sure that all of the fenestrated holes in the chest tube are inside the thoracic cavity **(Fig. 9)**.

Connect the chest tube to the drainage device after cutting the distal end of the chest tube to facilitate its connection to the drainage device tubing.

Release the cross-clamp that is on the chest tube only after the chest tube is connected to the drainage device.

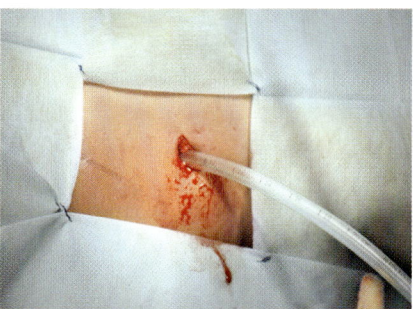

Fig. 9: Tube inserted into the pleural cavity.

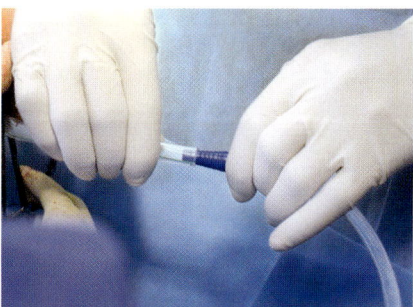

Fig. 10: Chest tube connected to the underwater seal.

Before securing the tube with stitches, look for a respiration-related swing in the fluid level of the water seal device to confirm correct intrathoracic placement. Secure the chest tube to the skin using 0 or 1-0 silk or nylon stitches **(Fig. 10)**.

Securing Sutures

Two separate through-and-through, simple, and interrupted stitches on each side of the chest tube are recommended. This technique ensures tight closure of the skin incision and prevents routine patient movements from dislodging the chest tube. Each stitch should, in turn, be tightly tied to the skin, then wrapped tightly around the chest tube several times to cause slight indentation, and then tied again **(Fig. 11)**.

Sealing Suture

An optional central vertical mattress/purse string stitch with ends left long and knotted together only once and then wrapped several times around the chest tube before tying the final knot causing as light indentation around the tube allows for sealing of the tract once the chest tube is removed.

Press hard with a gauze piece around the tube to prevent peritubal leak of pleural fluid or air entering into the pleural space while the patient is breathing. Create an occlusive dressing to place over the chest tube by turning regular gauze squares (4 × 4 inch^2) into Y-shaped fenestrated gauze squares and using 4-inch adhesive tape to secure them to the chest wall,

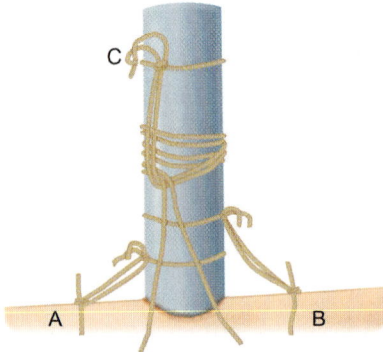

Fig. 11: Fixing the tube. Sutures A and B are tied to close the wound and then tied around the tube to ensure it in place preventing a dislodgment that may lead to a pneumothorax. Stitch C is knotted only once, albeit tied very snugly to prevent peritubal.

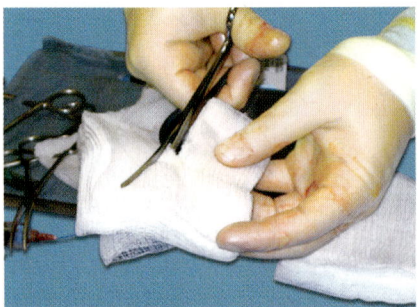

Fig. 12: Dressing pad application.

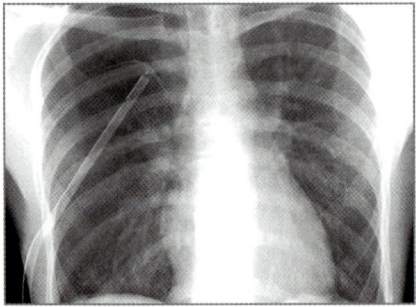

Fig. 13: Chest tube in position (the tube should be directed upwards and posteriorly).

as shown here. Make sure to provide enough padding between the chest tube and the chest wall **(Fig. 12)**. Obtain a chest radiograph, shown here, to ensure correct placement of the chest tube.

Some prefer a chest tube directed inferiorly to drain fluid and superiorly to drain a pneumothorax. But ideally, any position of the tube is effective for draining air or fluid, since the patient is in the supine position most of the time, and one should remember that an effectively functioning tube should not be repositioned solely because of its position in the postprocedure chest X-ray **(Fig. 13)**.

COMPLICATIONS

Minor complications of thoracostomy tube placement such as unresolved/reaccumulation of pneumothorax or misplacement of the tube (too deep/kinked) are common:

- *Improper placement*:
  - Horizontal (over the diaphragm)—acceptable for hemothorax; should be repositioned for pneumothorax
  - Subcutaneous—must be repositioned: Subcutaneous emphysema can occur due to slippage of the chest tube, with the holes lying in the subcutaneous tissue. The chest tube then needs to be repositioned
  - Placed too far into the chest (against the apical pleura)—should be retracted
  - Placed into the abdominal space—should be removed.
- *Bleeding*:
  - Local—usually responds to direct pressure
  - Hemothorax (lung vs. intercostal artery injury)—might require thoracotomy, if it does not resolve spontaneously
  - Hemoperitoneum (liver or spleen injury)—requires emergent laparotomy.
- *Organ penetration (usually requires surgical repair)*:
  - Stomach, colon, or diaphragm—occurs as a result of unrecognized diaphragmatic hernia
  - Lung—occurs as a result of pleural adhesions or use of a thoracostomy tube trocar
  - Liver or spleen—hemoperitoneum warrants emergency laparotomy.
- Tube dislodgement.
- Empyema—chest tube (foreign object) could introduce bacteria into the pleural space.
- Retained pneumothorax or hemothorax—might require insertion of a second chest tube.
- Re-expansion pulmonary edema is a rare and potentially fatal complication that can occur after treatment of pneumothorax or a pleural effusion. It is more common in patient with diabetes and in patients with tension or larger-size pneumothoraces and in patients with large pleural effusions. It is seen when large effusions are drained in a short period of time. It is best prevented by gradual decompression. Not more than 1 liter should be drained in the first go, after which the tube should be clamped for a few hours. The fluid can then be drained at intervals of a few hours, about 500 mL at a time, with the tube clamped in-between.
- *Blocked tube due to poor positioning*: Sometimes, the tube gets trapped in the major fissure of the lung. If this occurs, the tube needs to be withdrawn and reinserted.
- *Cardiac dysrhythmia*—the tube may ABUT the mediastinum and occasionally cause cardiac irregularities. First, try withdrawing the tube

2–3 cm. If this does not resolve the problem, the tube may need to be reinserted at a separate location. Medical management of the arrhythmia is also needed.
- Persistent pneumothorax—if a pneumothorax persists, check for obstructions or leaks. Clear any obstructions and seal any leaks in the drainage system. If no leak or obstruction is found, apply suction of up to 20 cm of water to the drainage system.
- Failure of the lung to fully re-expand—this is rarely due to blockage of the tubes, and change of tubes seldom helps. The common causes of nonexpansion of the lung are as follows:
    - Bronchial blockage leading to collapse, usually by retained sputum [fiberoptic bronchoscopy helps clear secretions and rule out other causes of bronchial obstruction (e.g., tumor)]
    - The presence of a fibrinous "peel" (cortex) over the lung (this is the thickened visceral pleura over the collapsed lung tissue and is usual in cases of delayed treatment of an empyema. A decortication is the best way to deal with this problem).

MANAGEMENT POSTPROCEDURE

It is important to provide adequate pain relief to patients to get their maximum cooperation with respect to deep breathing. On the 1st day, injectable analgesics should be given (diclofenac sodium or tramadol) and thereafter, oral analgesics can be started. *Pain relief is very important and should not be neglected.* A thoracic epidural catheter with epidural analgesia is the best.

Breathing exercises and chest physiotherapy are the mainstays for the quick expansion of the lung. All three balls of the incentive spirometer should rise and be held there for a second **(Fig. 14)**.

Upper limb movements, especially at the shoulder, help to restore the movements of the chest wall. Steam inhalations and nebulized bronchodilators also encourage quick lung expansion **(Fig. 15)**. Keep the patient in a propped-up position (i.e., 45–90°).

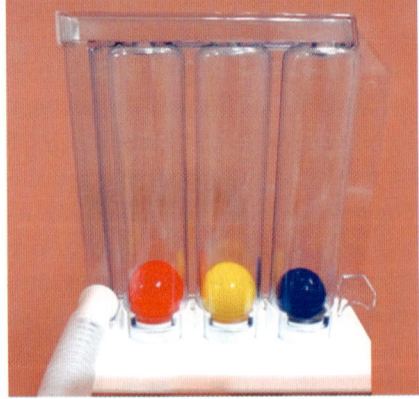

Fig. 14: Incentive spirometer.

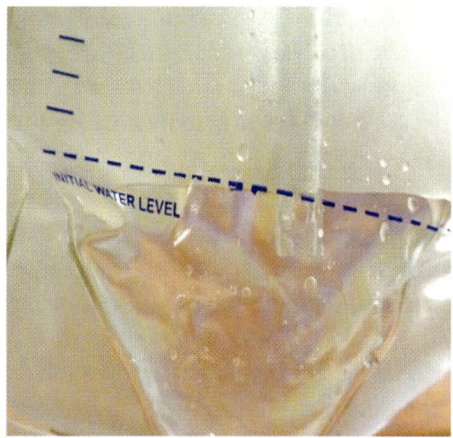

Fig. 15: Underwater seal of the collecting bag showing water level.

Always ensure the correct position of the underwater seal bottle **(Fig. 15)**. The bottle should be erect and at least 100 cm below the level of the patient's chest. The tip of the tube that connects to the chest drain should be at least 2 cm below the fluid level in the bottle (and not more than 7 cm below the fluid level).

In addition to vital signs, the following items need to be monitored every 4 hours:
- Swinging or oscillation of the column of water in the glass tube connected to the chest drain.
- Blowing or air bubbling in drainage bottle with quiet respiration and on coughing (bubbling of air indicates that the lung is still leaking air. The cessation of bubbling during both quiet respiration and coughing indicates that the air leak in the lung has closed).
- Type and quantity of drainage (inform practitioner, if drainage is >70 mL/h or if quality of the drainage changes to frank blood).

Never lift the drainage bottle above the level of the patient's chest, as fluid from the bottle may siphon off into the patient's chest.

Do not clamp a bubbling chest drain. All nursing procedures, patient movement, and physiotherapy are permitted without clamping the drain. Clamp tubes only for procedures related to the tube or bottle (e.g., to change the tube or bottle, to empty the bottle, to reconnect an accidental disconnection of the tube at any of the joints).

Avoid kinks in the tubes. Teach the patient to look for kinks and to avoid sitting or lying on the tubes.

"Milk" the tubes frequently to avoid blockage by fibrin plugs or clots.

SUCTION

When suction is needed, it should be a constant low-pressure suction to fully remove the pleural contents without causing pain to the patient. The recommended level of suction is −5 to −20 cm of water. Higher negative pressure can increase the flow rate out of the chest, but it can also damage tissue. Suction can improve the speed at which air and fluid are pulled from the chest. Serial chest radiographs are needed to monitor and confirm the expansion of the lung.

TUBE REMOVAL

The timing of tube removal depends on clinical and radiological evidence of complete expulsion of all contents of the pleural cavity with complete expansion of the lung. Minimal drainage should have occurred over the previous 24 hours. Level 1 recommendations state that this should be less than 2 mL/kg/day. When the patient coughs or performs the Valsalva maneuver, no air leak should ensue. The chest radiograph should confirm complete expansion of the lung.

The swing in the fluid level in the tube in the underwater seal bottle should be minimal, relating to the normal negative pressures in the chest during the phases of respiration.

Generally, for pneumothorax, a trial period of tube clamping for 24 hours is done. A repeat chest radiograph is then taken. If this shows complete expansion of the lung, it confirms that the lung leak has sealed and that a proper adhesion between the layers of the pleura has occurred. The tube may be safely removed at that time.

Tube thoracostomy removal is a sterile procedure that requires a practitioner and an assistant. Cut loose the securing stitch while the tube is being supported. If a sealing stitch was previously applied, free the mattress (sealing) stitch that was inserted and kept long at the time of tube insertion. If this stitch is not in position, place a vertical mattress stitch with strong suture material across the center of the incision.

Hold the ends of the mattress suture ready to tie a knot. Instruct the patient to cease respiration in either expiration or inspiration. Gently ease out the tube while simultaneously tying the knot to close the track.

Apply a soft dressing. If the stitch breaks or cuts through, simply compress the oblique track and apply an occlusive dressing. If such a stitch was not put, simply pull out the tube, while the patient holds his breath, preferably in full inspiration, and seal the wound with an occlusive dressing for 24 hours.

A chest radiograph is repeated 24 hours after the removal of the tube thoracostomy. The results of this radiograph should confirm that no air has entered the chest and that the lung continues to remain fully expanded. If the patient is afebrile, patient can be discharged.

Cardiopulmonary Resuscitation

PG Venugopalan

INTRODUCTION

First artificial mouth-to-mouth resuscitation dates back to 5,000–3,000 BC. First attempt of newborn resuscitation by blowing was done in 1780. The year 1874 records first experimental direct cardiac massage. First successful direct cardiac massage in man was reported in 1901. 1980 records the development of cardiopulmonary resuscitation (CPR) due to the works of Peter Safar.

CARDIAC ARREST (FLOWCHARTS 1 TO 4)

Definition

It is loss of cardiac function, breathing, and loss of consciousness.

Diagnosis: By TRIAD
- Loss of consciousness
- Loss of apical and central pulsations (carotid and femoral)
- Apnea.

Types of Cardiac Arrest
- Asystole (isoelectric line)
- Ventricular fibrillation
- Pulseless ventricular tachycardia
- Pulseless electrical activity (PEA).

Causes of Cardiac Arrest: 6H and 4T
- Hypoxia
- Hypotension
- Hypothermia
- Hydrogen ion (acidosis)
- Hypo/hyperkalemia (electrolyte disturbances)
- Tamponade cardiac
- Tension pneumothorax

Flowchart 1: Management of adult cardiac arrest and postcardiac arrest care.

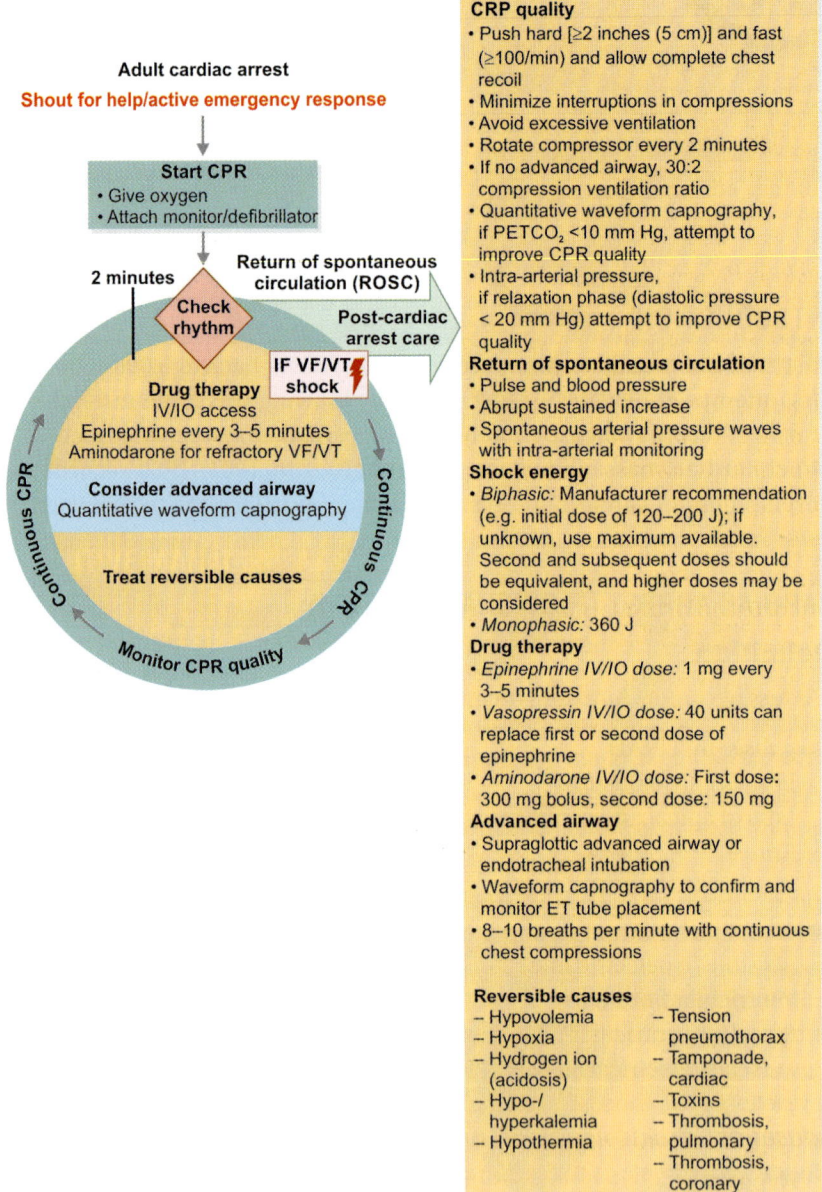

(CPR: cardiopulmonary resuscitation; IV: intravenous; VF: ventricular fibrillation; VT: ventricular tachycardia; IO: intraosseous; ET: endotracheal)

- Thromboembolism (pulmonary and coronary)
- Toxicity [e.g., digoxin, local anesthetics, tricyclic antidepressant (TCA), and insecticides].

Cardiopulmonary Resuscitation

Flowchart 2: Adult immediate postcardiac arrest care algorithm.

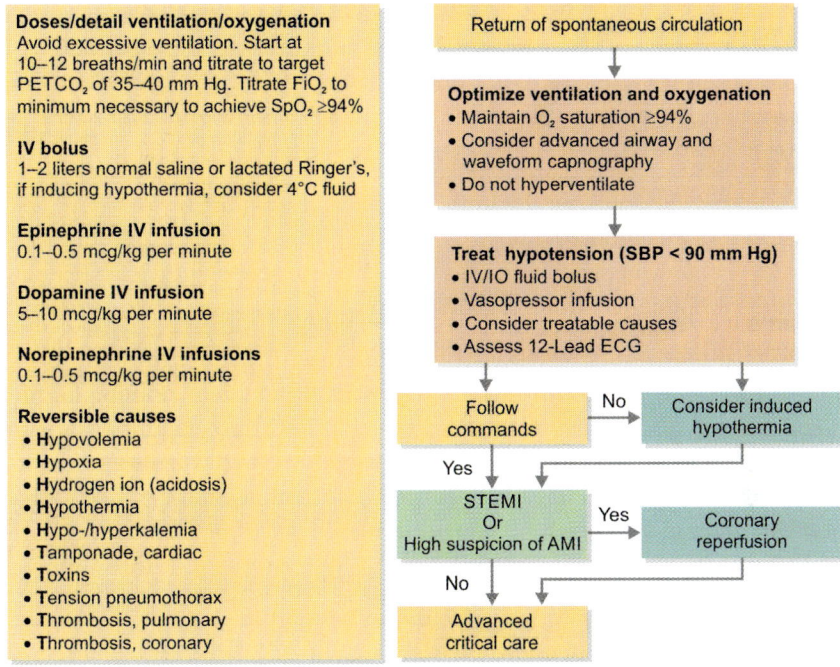

(ECG: electrocardiography; IV: intravenous; SBP: systolic blood pressure; IO: intraosseous)

Flowchart 3: Management of adult bradycardia (with pulse).

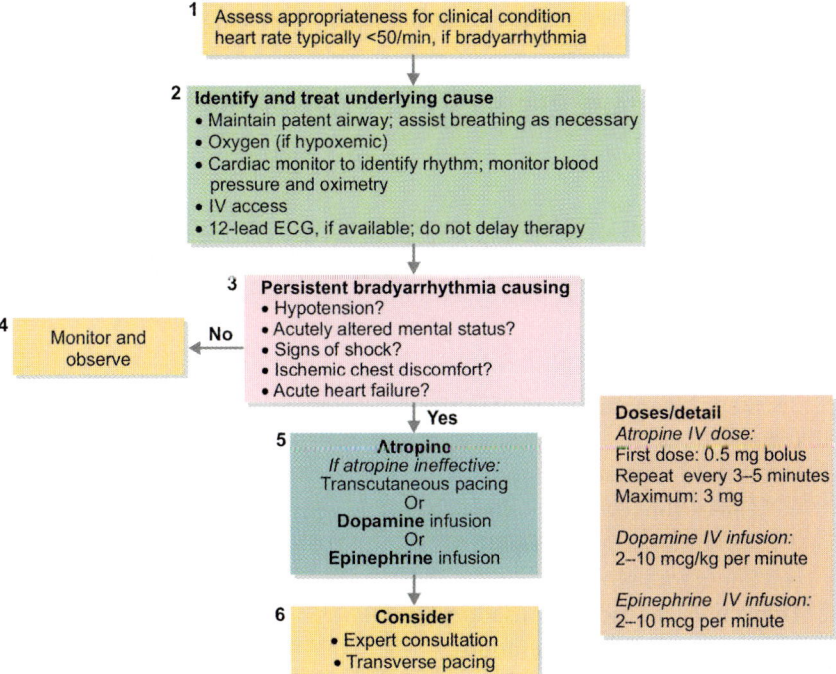

(ECG: electrocardiography; IV: intravenous)

Flowchart 4: Management of adult tachycardia (with pulse).

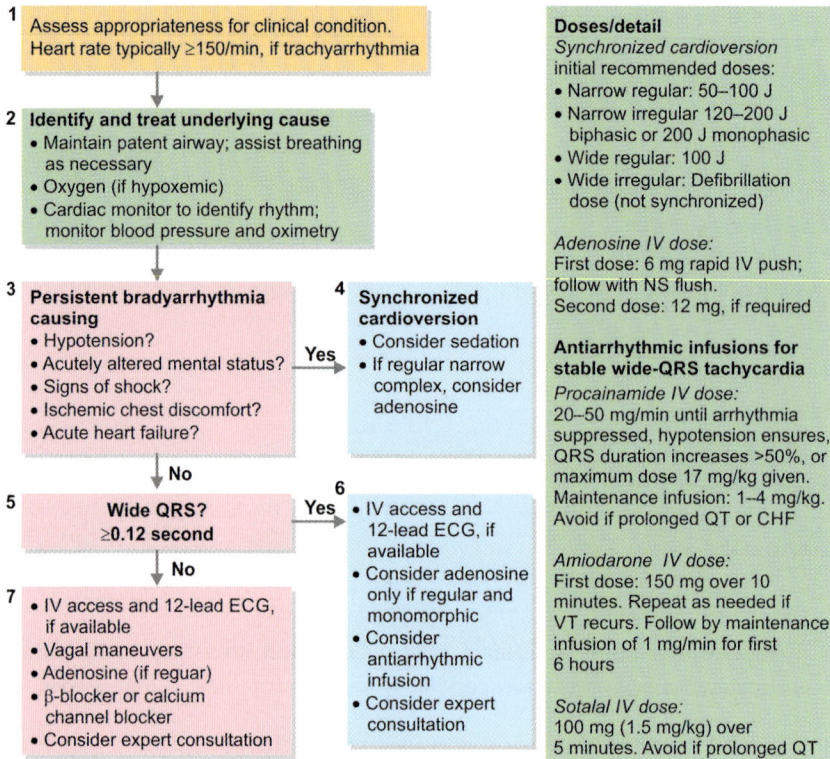

(CHF: congestive heart failure; ECG: electrocardiography; IV: intravenous; VT: ventricular tachycardia; NS: normal saline)

CARDIOPULMONARY RESUSCITATION DEFINITION

It is an emergency medical procedure for a victim of cardiac arrest or respiratory arrest.

Basic life support (BLS): It is life support without use of special equipment.

Advanced cardiovascular life support (ACLS): It is life support with the use of special equipment (e.g., airway, endotracheal tube, and defibrillator).

Basic Life Support

- 3 S: Steps before initiation of resuscitation for management of a collapsed patient:
    - Ensure your own safety
    - Check the level of responsiveness by gently shaking the patient and shouting/Are you alright?
    - Shout for help.
- Then check for carotid pulsation.
- Apnea (cessation of respiration):
    - *Look*: To see chest wall movement, seesaw (paradoxical) movement of chest wall indicates airway obstruction

- Listen to breath sounds from mouth
- *Feel*: Airflow for at least 10 seconds.

CHAIN OF SURVIVAL

There are four cornerstones for optimizing the outcome following cardiac arrest:
1. *Early recognition and call for help*: To prevent cardiac arrest.
2. Early CPR (with minimal interruptions) to buy time.
3. Early defibrillation to restart the heart.
4. Postresuscitation care to rest or equality of life and to minimize neurological insult.

GOLDEN HOUR

Refers to the period of time immediately following trauma during which approximately 50% of the deaths occur. The cause of death is usually preventable provided adequate resuscitation, diagnosis, and surgical intervention.

Cardiopulmonary resuscitation revised guidelines **(Figs. 1A to C)**: Think C-A-B:
- *Compressions*: Push on at least 2 inches on adult breast bone, 100 times per minute, to move oxygenated blood to vital organs.

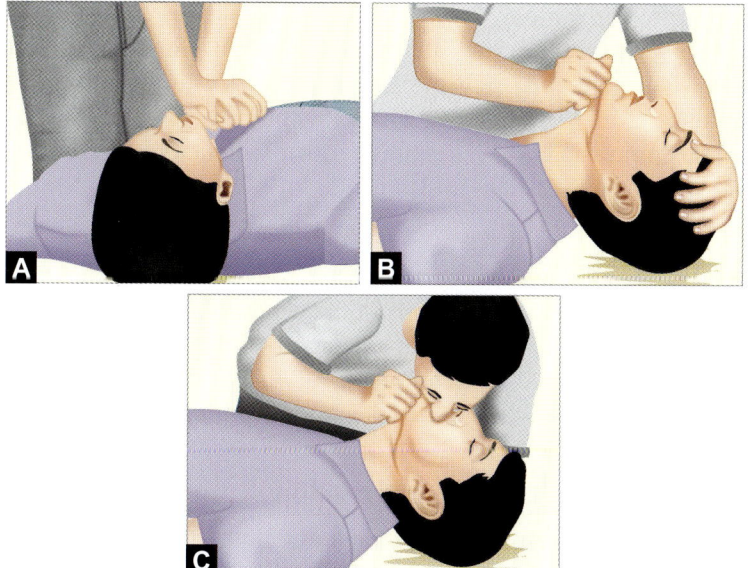

Figs. 1A to C: Cardiopulmonary resuscitation revised guidelines: Think C-A-B: (A) Compressions: Push at least 2 inches on adult breast bone, 100 times per minute, to move oxygenated blood to vital organs; (B) Airway: Open the airway and check for breathing or blockage; watch for rise of chest and listen for air movement; (C) Breathing: Tilt chin back for the unobstructed passing of air; give two breathes and resume chest compressions.

- *Airway*: Open the airway and check for breathing/blockage. Watch for rise of chest and listen for air movements.
- *Breathing*: Tilt chin back for the unobstructed passing of air; give two breaths and resume chest compression.

Those untrained in CPR can simply do chest compression until help arrives.

CARDIOPULMONARY RESUSCITATION/AUTOMATED EXTERNAL DEFIBRILLATION

Chest compressions and breaths are the same for adults, child, and infant if you are alone.

Compressions

Push hard and fast. Rate should be at least 100 per minute. Provide 30 compressions then 2 breaths. Make sure to allow the chest to re-expand completely at the end of each compression.

Adult CPR/AED

Open the airway with head tilt-chin lift. Place mask on patient's face. Use the E-C clamp technique. Deliver each breath over 1 second.

Pediatric CPR/AED

Make sure that the scene is safe. Check responsiveness and breathing. If alone, call at emergency number and get an automated external defibrillation (AED). Check for CPR and if no pulse, begin CPR. Always start CPR with compression first. If despite adequate ventilation and oxygenation, pulse is <60, begin chest compression.

Performing CPR on a Child

Place the heel of one or both hands in the center of the chest, in between nipples, avoiding the xiphoid process. Compress the chest at a rate of at least 100 times/minute. Coordinate compressions with ventilations in a 30:2 ratio (one rescuer) or 15:2 (two rescuers), pausing for ventilations.

Performing Infant Chest Compressions

Position infant on a firm surface while maintaining the airway. Place two fingers on the middle of sternum just below a line between nipples. Use the two fingers to compress the chest one-third to one-half its depth at a rate of at least 100 per minute. Allow the sternum to return to its normal position between compressions.

Automated External Defibrillation on Children (1–8 years of age)

There are some safety considerations with the use of an AED on children:
- If the AED has child pads, use these on children between 1–8 years of age.
- A manual defibrillator is preferred for defibrillation of infants.
- Some AEDs have a key or a switch that will deliver a child shock dose.
- If the AED does not have child pad/key/switch, adult pads may be used. Use of adult dose is better than no attempts at defibrillation.

Adult CPR/AED

The AED should be applied as soon as possible to the patient's bare chest. Make sure that the pads adhere to the skin. Remove all clothing from the area where the pads need to be placed. Remove any medication patches from the area. Shave any chest hair. The pads need to be on as much bare skin as possible. If the patient has an implanted pacemaker, place the pad at least 1 inch away.

CPR/AED

All styles of AEDs work the same. The first step is to turn the unit on and follow the voice prompts. Assess compression effectiveness if CPR is in progress. If the patient is unresponsive and CPR has not been started, begin providing chest compressions and rescue breaths at a ratio of 30 compressions to 2 breaths, continuing until an AED arrives and is ready to use.

Turn on AED. Apply the AED pads to the chest and attach the pads to the AED. Stop CPR. Verbally and visually clear the patient. Push the analyze button, if there is one. Wait for the AED to analyze the cardiac rhythm. If no shock is advised, perform five cycles (2 minutes) of CPR and then reanalyze the cardiac rhythm. If a shock is advised, recheck that all are clear and push the shock button. After the shock is delivered immediately, resume CPR beginning with chest compression. After five cycles (2 minutes) of CPR, reanalyze the cardiac rhythm. Do not interrupt chest compressions for >10 seconds. If shock is advised, clear the patient, push the shock button, and immediately resume CPR. If no shock is advised, immediately resume CPR. Transport and contact medical control as needed.

If after AED, patient breathing independently, administer oxygen and check pulse. If breathing inadequate with pulse, assist ventilations.

ADVANCED TECHNIQUES FOR AIRWAY PATENCY

- *Face mask*: Signs of successful seal and ventilation include foggy mask and rising chest. It is easy and do not require skilled personnel. Stomach inflation is a disadvantage and also it is not protective against regurgitation and aspiration of gastric contents.

- *Oropharyngeal airway*: It is easy and does not require skilled personnel. It can be used by paramedics. Disadvantages are: (1) Not protective against regurgitation and aspiration of gastric contents; (2) Poorly tolerated by conscious patients due to gag.
- *Nasopharyngeal airway*: Airway is lubricated and inserted through the nose. Better tolerated in conscious patients. Contraindicated in fractured skull base and in anticoagulated patients. It is also not protective against regurgitation and aspiration of gastric contents.
- *Laryngeal mask airway (LMA)*: Available in a variety of pediatric and adult sizes. It is easy to use and does not require highly skilled personnel. Stomach inflation is a disadvantage. It is not protective against regurgitation and aspiration of gastric contents.
- *Endotracheal tube*: It ensures proper lung ventilation without gastric inflation. There is no regurgitation or aspiration of gastric contents. Disadvantage is that it requires insertion by highly skilled personnel.
- *Combitube*: It is easy to use and does not require highly skilled personnel.
- *Cricothyrotomy (surgical airway)*: It is done either by a commercially available cannula in a specialized cricothyrotomy set or a large bore IV cannula 12–14 gauge. It is done in case of difficult endotracheal intubation. Nu-Trake cannula is especially designed to allow ventilation by a self-inflating bag (AMBU). An IV cannula needs a special connection to a high pressure source to generate sufficient gas flow (transtracheal jet ventilation).
- Tracheostomy (surgical airway).

Head Injury

Ganesh Divakar

INTRODUCTION

Traumatic brain injury (TBI) remains the leading cause of death and long-term disability in people younger than 40 years worldwide. Population-based studies have shown that the single most cost-effective surgical operation is removal of an acute extradural hematoma, given the severe consequences of that hematoma in terms of death or vegetative survival. The definition of TBI is unclear and a matter of debate. TBI refers to injury to the intracranial structures following physical trauma to the head. The term *head injury* is preferred when addressing injuries that encompass both intracranial and extracranial structures, including the face, scalp, and skull. Unless otherwise specified, the consensus and guidelines as published by the Brain Trauma Foundation (BTF), New York (4th edition, 2016) are followed in this discussion. The 2019 guidelines for management of severe TBI in pediatric population are not discussed in this chapter and can be accessed from the BTF website.

CLINICAL CLASSIFICATION OF TRAUMATIC BRAIN INJURY

The clinical severity of intracranial injuries is commonly assessed according to the degree of depression of the level of consciousness as assessed by the Glasgow Coma Scale (GCS), devised by Teasdale and Jennett (1974). The GCS consists of the sum score (range: 3–15) of three components (best eye response, best motor response, and best verbal response), each assessing different aspects of reactivity. The motor component provides more discrimination in patients with severe injuries, whereas the eye and verbal scales are more discriminative in patients with moderate and mild injuries. For assessment of severity in individual patients, the three components should be reported separately. For purposes of classification, however, calculation of the sum score is useful. Severe TBI is defined as a GCS score of 3–8, moderate TBI as a GCS score of 9–12, and mild TBI as a GCS score of 13–15.[1]

---

[1]Adapted from World Health Organization Collaborating Centre Task Force on Mild Traumatic Brain Injury (2004). Some authors define mild TBI as GCS of 14–15 and a patient with GCS 13 is included under moderate head injury.

Glasgow Coma Scale[2]

Eye Opening Response

- Spontaneous—open with blinking at baseline: *4 points*
- To verbal stimuli, command, speech: *3 points*
- To pain only (not applied to face): *2 points*
- No response: *1 point.*

Verbal Response

- Oriented: *5 points*
- Confused conversation, but able to answer questions: *4 points*
- Inappropriate words: *3 points*
- Incomprehensible speech: *2 points*
- No response: *1 point.*

Motor Response

- Obeys commands for movement: *6 points*
- Purposeful movement to painful stimulus: *5 points*
- Withdraws in response to pain: *4 points*
- Flexion in response to pain (decorticate posturing): *3 points*
- Extension response in response to pain (decerebrate posturing): *2 points*
- No response: *1 point.*

Limitations of GCS

- Prehospital use of sedation or paralysis can change the GCS.
- Bilateral periorbital edema can affect eye response.
- Absent motor response in a quadriplegic patient (e.g., with coexisting cervical spine trauma) significantly lowers GCS.
- In an intubated or tracheotomized patient verbal response cannot be assessed and is written VT. Here, the total score is written as sum of E and V scores followed by a T. For example, a patient with E3M5VT has a GCS of 8T.

EVALUATION OF A PATIENT WITH TBI

History

The exact mechanism causing the injury should be asked for as this alerts the physician toward a potential underlying major traumatic intracranial injury in a seemingly alert patient who had had a high-velocity impact.

---

[2]Teasdale G, Jennett B. Assessment of coma and impaired consciousness. Lancet. 1974;2(7872):81-4.

Teasdale G, Jennett B. Assessment and prognosis of coma after head injury. Acta Neurochir (Wien). 1976;34(1-4):45-55.

Head Injury

History of alcohol use prior to the event should be correlated with a poor GCS in a patient with normal brain radiology. Remote or active drug or alcohol use may raise the risk of intracranial bleeding and cloud the mental status assessment.

Mild TBI (mTBI) or cerebral concussion, in a patient with normal GCS and mechanical injury to the head, is diagnosed from history by one or more of the following features:
- Headache
- Loss of consciousness
- Retrograde amnesia (forgetting events that happened before the concussion)
- Anterograde or post-traumatic amnesia (forgetting events happening after the concussion)
- Confusion about injury events or details
- Balance problems
- Fatigue
- Visual changes (double or blurry vision most common)
- Emotional or sleep disturbances
- Attentional dysfunction
- Short-term memory and learning problems
- Behavior or personality problems
- Phonophobia or photophobia
- Bradyphrenia (slowness of thought)
- Feeling mentally "foggy".

Lucid interval is a temporary improvement in a patient's condition after a traumatic brain injury, after which the condition deteriorates. A lucid interval is especially indicative of an epidural hematoma (EDH), but is seen in only 20% of patients with EDH.

Present anticoagulant and antiplatelet therapy carries a higher risk of intracranial bleed following head trauma.

Physical Examination

Vital Signs

Physical examination of a patient with head injury begins with assessment of vital signs. Cushing's reflex of hypertension, bradycardia, and irregular respiration should prompt one to suspect elevated intracranial pressure (ICP).

Isolated head injury usually causes hypertension as part of Cushing's response. In a patient with TBI, hypotension occurs in the following situations:
- Brain death and brainstem failure
- Hypovolemia secondary to blood loss from vascular injury, other visceral, pelvic, or long bone injuries

- Myocardial contusion or tension pneumothorax
- Cervical spinal cord injury.

Rule out other injuries: In a conscious and alert person, physical examination is rather straightforward. Ask for the patient's name and a correct answer without delay should give considerable confidence to the treating doctor. In a drowsy patient with telltale evidences of head injury, one should not overlook life-threatening injuries to the spine, chest, abdomen, pelvis, or long bone fractures requiring urgent intervention.

Glasgow Coma Scale: In a head injury patient, periodic assessment of the GCS is mandatory and should be more frequent in patients with poor GCS. Rather than the absolute total score value, a drop in GCS of 2 or more points on serial assessment should alert the clinician toward follow-up imaging or urgent neurosurgical referral.

Pupils: Pupillary examination is an integral part in the evaluation of patients with TBI. The size, reaction, and symmetry should be carefully tested and documented. Pupillary asymmetry (anisocoria) is defined as a size difference greater than 1 mm. A fixed pupil is defined as one that has a response to light of less than 1 mm. Progressive increase in size of the pupil or reduction in the reactivity on serial examination in a drowsy patient should be viewed seriously. When examining the pupils, it should be borne in mind that local trauma can cause traumatic mydriasis in the absence of TBI. Past history of ocular surgeries can lead to irregularity of the pupils rendering further assessment difficult. Also, local application of mydriatics can interfere with pupillary assessment.

Hutchinson's pupil: Hutchinson's pupil is a clinical sign in which the pupil on the side of an intracranial mass lesion (like a post-traumatic intracranial hematoma) is dilated and unreactive to light due to compression of the oculomotor nerve on that side by the herniating uncus of the temporal lobe (**Fig. 1**). The parasympathetic fibers to the pupil being carried by the oculomotor nerve are responsible for pupillary constriction. These fibers pass through the periphery of the oculomotor nerve and, hence, are the first to be affected in case of compression of the nerve. In stage 1, the parasympathetic fibers on the side of the lesion are irritated, leading to constriction of pupil on that side. In stage 2, the parasympathetic fibers on the side of the lesion are paralyzed, leading to dilatation of pupil. With increasing mass effect and rise in ICP, the fibers on the opposite oculomotor nerve are irritated, leading to constriction of contralateral pupil. In stage 3, the parasympathetic fibers on both sides are paralyzed, leading to bilateral pupillary dilatation and later on to bilateral fixed pupils. This indicates grave prognosis.

Focal neurological deficits: Examination of the cranial nerves is important in head injury. The olfactory nerve is liable to be damaged in anterior skull base and cribriform plate fractures. Moreover, contusions of the frontal

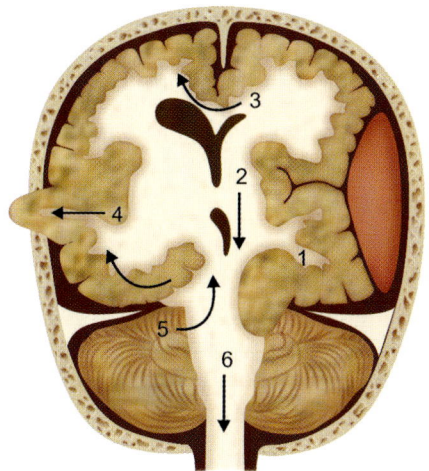

Fig. 1: Types of brain herniation in raised intracranial pressure as is caused by a left temporal epidural hematoma here. (1) Transtentorial/uncal; (2) Central; (3) Subfalcine/cingulate; (4) Transcalvarial—through a bony defect in skull (if any); (5) Upward transtentorial herniation; (6) Tonsillar herniation.

lobe are notorious to cause anosmia. Traumatic optic neuropathy (TON) can be caused either directly or indirectly and visual loss may be partial or complete. An indirect injury to the optic nerve typically occurs from the transmission of forces to the optic canal from blunt head trauma. This is in contrast to direct TON, which results from an anatomical disruption of the optic nerve fibers from penetrating orbital trauma, bone fragments within the optic canal, or nerve sheath hematomas. Extraocular and eyelid movements should be tested to look for the involvement of 3, 4, and 6 cranial nerves of which oculomotor lesions are the most common. Temporal bone fractures can cause facial nerve injury and especially in patients with ear bleed, ENT examination to assess the integrity of tympanic membrane and audiometry to assess hearing loss due to otic capsule involving temporal bone fractures are mandatory. Lower cranial nerve paresis is rarely seen in trauma.

Hemiplegia is often a localizing sign in patients with moderate-to-severe head injury. The relative paucity of limb movements on one side associated with anisocoria is an indication for urgent surgical intervention in a patient with intracranial hematoma or depressed fracture contralateral to the side of hemiplegia. In this context, one has to be aware of Kernohan's notch phenomenon, which is a false localizing sign in head injury. When an increase of pressure in a hemisphere of the brain occurs, the cerebral peduncle on the opposite side is pushed up against the tentorium (producing a visible "notch" in the peduncle) leading to hemiparesis ipsilateral to the side of the intracranial mass lesion.

Horner's syndrome: It may be seen in patients with associated trauma to the neck or cervical spine.

Open depressed fractures: Thorough physical examination of a scalp injury is important to check for an underlying depressed fracture. Open depressed fractures require neurosurgical intervention.

Cerebrospinal fluid (CSF) otorrhea and rhinorrhea: It is discussed later in this chapter.

Subconjunctival hemorrhage: Local orbital trauma as well as basilar skull fractures can cause subconjunctival hemorrhage. This is usually benign and clears spontaneously in a matter of days to weeks unless the patient is on anticoagulants or antiplatelets. But, it is always prudent to check for vision and ocular movements to rule out associated cranial nerve palsies due to local trauma. The appearance of hemorrhage after 24 hours or more after a head injury is pathognomonic for basilar fractures.

Battle's sign or mastoid ecchymosis: It is an indication of fracture of posterior cranial fossa of the skull, and may suggest underlying brain trauma. It consists of bruising over the mastoid process, as a result of extravasation of blood along the path of the posterior auricular artery.

Raccoon eyes or periorbital ecchymosis: It is a sign of anterior skull base fracture. If bilateral, it is highly suggestive of basilar skull fracture, with a positive predictive value of 85%. In the event of local signs of orbital trauma, it is always mandatory to check vision (to rule out optic neuropathy), extraocular movements, eye closure, and pupillary reaction (to rule out traumatic third cranial nerve palsy).

MANAGEMENT OF HEAD-INJURED PATIENT

Mild TBI

In a patient with GCS 15, mTBI is diagnosed from history as mentioned above.

Indications for CT Head in Mild TBI

Numerous guidelines have been published by various authors in this field and the points given below are an abstract from these studies:
- Older than 60 years
- Focal neurologic deficit(s)
- Headache or vomiting
- Memory deficits
- Loss of consciousness of 5 minutes or more
- Bleeding diathesis or history of anticoagulation/antiplatelet therapy
- Physical evidence of trauma above the clavicle
- Drug or alcohol intoxication
- Seizure
- Suspected open or depressed skull fracture/basal skull fracture[3]
- GCS of 13 or 14.

---

[3]As evidenced by hemotympanum, raccoon eyes, Battle's sign, or CSF rhinorrhea/otorrhea.

Revised Scandinavian Guidelines (2013) for Admission and Discharge in Mild TBI

Adult patients after mild head injury with GCS 15 and without risk factors (loss of consciousness, two or more episodes of vomiting, anticoagulation therapy or coagulation disorders, post-traumatic seizures, clinical signs of depressed or basal skull fracture, and focal neurological deficits) can be discharged from the hospital without a computed tomography (CT) scan, with advice to review immediately in case of any symptoms as described above.

S100B is a brain biomarker that has been recently introduced for screening mTBI patients as per Scandinavian guidelines. Adult patients after mild head injury with GCS 14 and without risk factors, or GCS 15 with loss of consciousness or two or more episodes of vomiting and no other risk factors, shall be sampled for analysis of S100B, if less than 6 hours have elapsed following trauma. If S100B is less than 0.10 µg/L, the patient may be discharged without a CT. Using a low cutoff of 0.10 µg/L, the biomarker has shown considerable ability to predict the absence of CT pathology and neurosurgical intervention. However it is clinically nonspecific with a short half-life and its routine use as a guideline is yet to be validated with clinical trials.

As a general rule, any symptomatic patient in whom CT scan is indicated shall be admitted to hospital for observation irrespective of the scan findings, especially if the imaging is done within 6 hours of the injury.

Follow-up CT Scans in Mild TBI

There are no standard guidelines for follow-up CT head in mild TBI. It is to be borne in mind that urgent follow-up CT scan should be done in any patient with a drop in GCS after admission. CT scan has to be repeated, if the patient develops fresh or worsening symptoms suggestive of raised ICP, despite symptomatic therapy. Bradycardia, anisocoria, focal neurological deficits, or seizures seen after admission that cannot be correlated clinically or radiologically mandates follow-up scan. Moreover, patients with initial scan showing TBI not necessitating neurosurgical intervention have to be followed up with at least one more scan, preferably between 24–48 hours of the first scan and prior to discharge from hospital. In the present scenario of ever increasing medicolegal cases, the threshold for follow-up scan should be very low, especially if the first imaging was done before 6 hours post-injury or in patients using antiplatelets/anticoagulants. In mild head injury without significant radiological lesions, a third CT scan is very rarely indicated.

Indications for Neurosurgical Referral

Any patient with moderate or severe head injury should be managed only in a specialized neurosurgical center. If encountered in a primary care center, such a patient shall be urgently referred to the nearest neurosurgical unit after following the guidelines mentioned in the next section. The following patients with mTBI also need neurosurgical care:

- CSF rhinorrhea or otorrhea
- Open fractures of the skull
- Focal neurological deficits, especially hemiparesis or hemiplegia
- Recurrent seizures
- CT scan showing intracranial bleed, cerebral edema, parenchymal contusions, or significant pneumocephalus
- Drop in GCS of two or more points while under observation
- Mild TBI patients with GCS 13 or 14 and not improving over 12–24 hours, despite normal CT head
- In infants and children, the threshold for neurosurgical referral should be low.

Transport of Patients with Head Injury

Primary care physicians dealing with head injured patients should refer patients with severe head injury to a neurosurgical center only after the following aspects are dealt with.

Airway, breathing, chest compressions (ABC) of resuscitation is of prime importance in patients with severe head injury. The details of resuscitation in polytrauma are discussed in Chapter 26. All patients with severe head injury require endotracheal intubation for airway protection and mechanical ventilation, if required. In this context, one has to be careful about the pitfalls of GCS. For example, a patient with GCS E1M6V1 due to bilateral periorbital edema, Broca's aphasia and no upper airway injuries do not require endotracheal intubation merely because of the poor GCS. Additionally, patients with fractures of the facial bones, especially those involving the mandible, bleeding wounds of the throat or not so easily accessible areas of the oral cavity should be carefully assessed for airway compromise due to blood clots and subsequent laryngeal edema. Endotracheal intubation is mandatory in this subset of patients even with a good GCS.

Likewise, breathing and circulation has to be maintained in any patient who needs transport to alternate center. In a patient who is drowsy or with clinical evidence of spine injury, it is mandatory that the spine (especially cervical spine) is immobilized till a spine injury is ruled out radiographically **(Fig. 2)**. Any bleeding external injury of the scalp has to be sutured till hemostasis is achieved. As discussed below, hypoxia and hypotension are independent predictors of poor prognosis in patients with TBI. Hence, all measures are to be taken to ensure adequate oxygen saturation and blood pressure in a head-injured patient prior to transport.

Emergency measures to lower ICP including hyperosmolar therapy, use of analgesia and sedation, general measures as outlined in the ensuing section, etc. should be instituted at the primary care facility as and when required. If there is facility for CT scan, it should be done within few minutes so that precious time can be saved at the referral hospital.

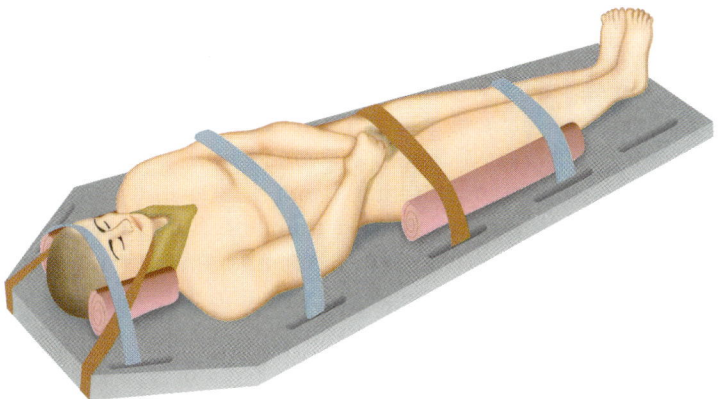

Fig. 2: Transport of a patient with head injury and suspected spine trauma. The cervical spine should be immobilized with a Philadelphia collar and the patient should be transported on a spine board held with fasteners and adequate padding to restrict mobility.

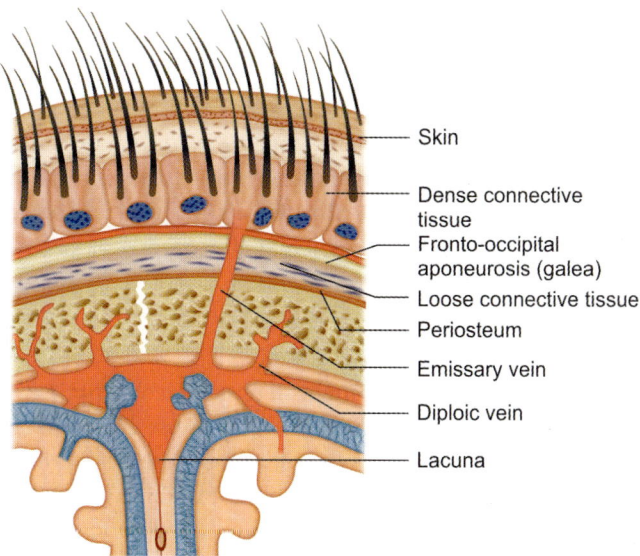

Fig. 3: Layers of the scalp. The dense connective tissue houses the arteries, which tend to evert following an injury. The galea aponeurotica should be included in the sutural bite, as it is the toughest layer and prevents spread of infection to the underlying loose connective tissue housing the emissary veins draining into the cranial venous sinuses.

Scalp Suturing

Injuries to the scalp constitute a major share of a houseman's work in surgical emergency room (ER). Because of its rich vascularity and the tendency for arteries in the dense connective tissue layer to evert once injured **(Fig. 3)**, scalp injuries can bleed a patient to death, if left unattended. Therefore, even in a patient with severe TBI, after resuscitation, top priority has to be given for hemostasis of a bleeding scalp wound. Before wound closure, thorough irrigation with saline and microbicidal solution should be given and underlying depressed fractures or brain injury should be carefully sought for. The wound edges are generously infiltrated with local anesthetic adrenaline combination. Ideally, the contaminated wound edges have to be minimally excised and wound closed with interrupted sutures in two layers. If done in a single layer, it is always necessary to include the galea aponeurotica while taking the bite, which should be 5–10 mm from the wound edge. This is to protect the underlying loose areolar tissue rich in emissary vein that is vulnerable to infection. In the frontal region, galeal suturing is required to prevent a cosmetic deformity. Torrential bleeding can, sometimes, pose problems to the beginner. In such a case, tight compression head bandage with elastocrepe after sufficient padding can temporarily control bleeding in almost all cases. Staples, although easy to apply, are less hemostatic and are useful when there are no significant bleeders. After repair, a tight dressing has to be given taking care not to injure the pinna and eyes from pressure effect of the bandage edges.

PATHOPHYSIOLOGY AND IMAGING OF TBI

Skull X-ray

X-ray of the skull is a poor predictor of intracranial pathology and should not be performed to evaluate TBI. Skull films are mainly used for the identification of skull fractures in cases of suspected child abuse, and not for the evaluation of intracranial pathology in children or adults.

Computed Tomography

Skull fractures can be classified as linear, depressed, comminuted, compound (open), or diastatic. The linear fracture is the most common type of skull fracture. Isolated linear fractures without associated intracranial pathology are usually clinically insignificant. Depressed fractures are often associated with an underlying cortical contusion. When a fracture involves the skull base, communicates with the overlying scalp, or involves the paranasal sinus, it is called a compound fracture. An external compound fracture is typically caused by a penetrating injury and is commonly associated with a depressed, comminuted skull fracture **(Figs. 4A and B)**. An internal compound fracture is usually caused by blunt injury and includes those that extend from the mastoid, middle ear, and paranasal sinuses into the cranium. Compound fractures frequently result in pneumocephalus (intracranial air), and they have an increased risk of infectious complications. In a compound depressed fracture, the underlying dura is exposed under the fracture site. Diastatic fractures occur from separation of the cranial sutures and are more frequent in children than in adults. Temporal bone fractures can cause facial palsy and/or disturbances in hearing and equilibrium.

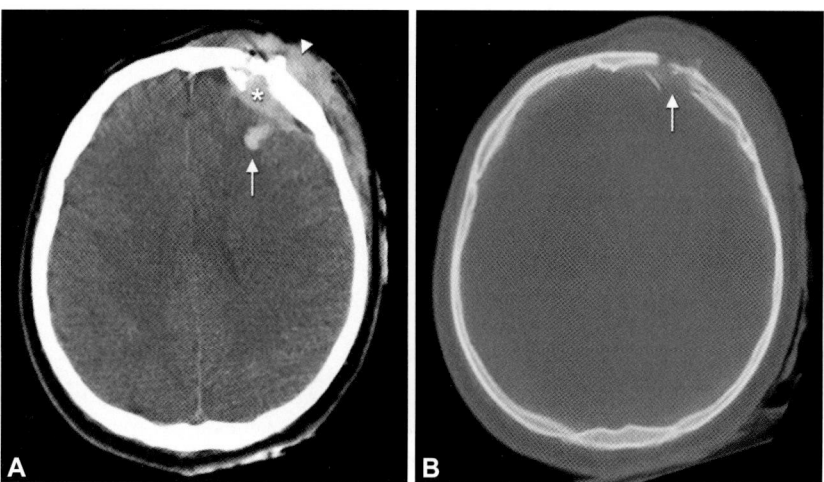

Figs. 4A and B: (A) CT scan showing left frontal scalp laceration (arrowhead), underlying extradural hematoma (*), and a parenchymal contusion (arrow); (B) Corresponding bone window image showing a depressed and comminuted left frontal bone fracture.

Extradural hematomas are usually arterial bleeds associated with a skull fracture and commonly occur in the squamous temporal region due to tearing of meningeal arteries, which are partially embedded in the bone. Being subperiosteal, the hematoma between the dura and inner table of the skull forms an ovoid collection that rarely crosses the cranial sutures, as the outer periosteal layer of the dura is firmly attached at sutural lines.

On CT, an acute EDH appears as a well-defined biconvex hyperdense collection within the epidural space that causes focal brain compression **(Fig. 5)**. Imaging findings associated with a worse prognosis are:

- *Swirl sign*: Presence of low-density areas within the hyperdense hematoma, which represents active arterial bleeding and the chance of expansion.
- Midline shift more than 1 cm and brainstem compression in CT scan point toward raised ICP and need for emergent surgical intervention.

Subdural hematomas (SDHs) are usually venous bleeds that usually occur due to tear of a bridging cortical vein during sudden head deceleration. It is common in the elderly with cerebral atrophy, as the enlarged extra-axial space allows for increased movement between the brain parenchyma and the skull. As it is located between the loosely attached dura and the arachnoid, the blood layers along the entire cerebral convexity in contrast to an EDH.

On CT, an acute SDH is crescent shaped, hyperdense, and located over the convexity **(Fig. 6)**. Unlike EDH, they occur at the contrecoup site (opposite to the side of impact) and are often associated with parenchymal injury and hence a poorer prognosis. The density of SDH decreases with time due to protein degradation. Thus, subacute SDH (around 1–3 weeks old) can have

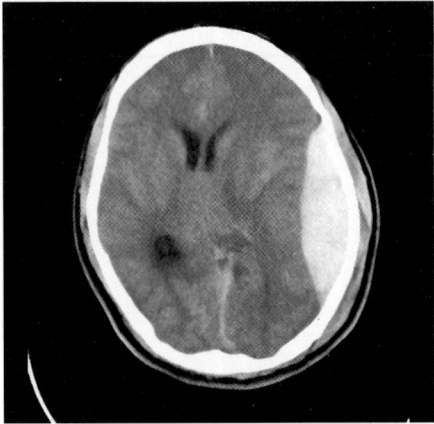

Fig. 5: Large left parietal extradural hematoma with shift of midline to right. Note the biconvex nature of the hematoma, which is compressing the brain and displacing the frontal horns to the right side of the midline.

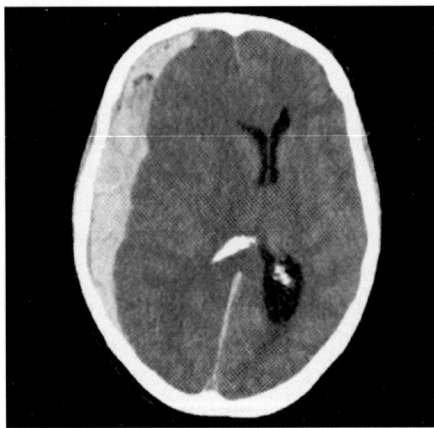

Fig. 6: Acute subdural hematoma over right cerebral convexity. Note the crescent shape of the hematoma that tends to layer along the entire cerebral convexity in contrast to epidural hematoma. There is significant midline shift to left as evidenced by the displacement of the frontal horns.

a density similar to brain parenchyma making it difficult to distinguish in plain CT scan **(Fig. 7)**. In such cases, indirect imaging findings like sulcal effacement, displacement of the gray-white junction away from the inner calvarium (white matter buckling), distortion of ventricles, and midline shift can point toward an isodense SDH. After 3 weeks, a chronic SDH with density similar to CSF forms, which is one of the common curable causes of dementia in the elderly.

Traumatic subarachnoid hemorrhage (SAH) occurs as a result of rupture of small pial vessels or contiguous extension from a contusion or hematoma. On CT, sulcal SAH appears as linear or serpentine areas of hyperdensity

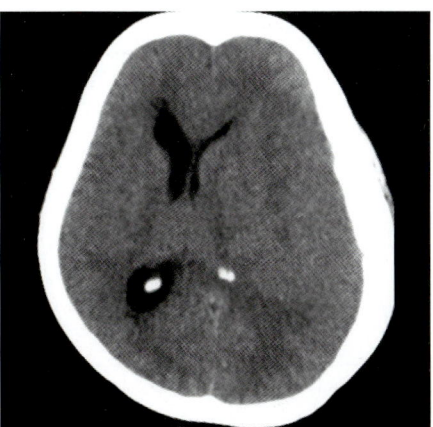

Fig. 7: Subacute subdural hematoma (SDH) can be easily missed in CT scan. Carefully observe the isodense SDH on the left side causing midline shift to right.

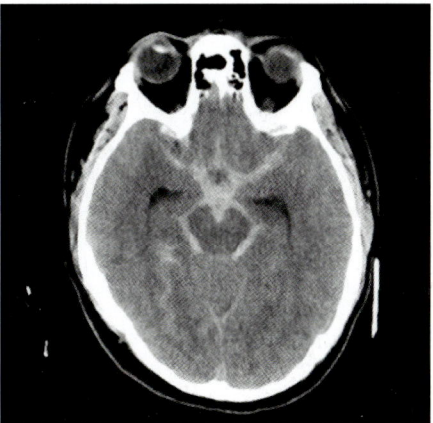

Fig. 8: Subarachnoid hemorrhage in the cisterns around the brainstem. It is always advisable to perform cerebral vascular imaging in such cases to rule out a ruptured aneurysm.

conforming to the cerebral sulci or cisterns. SAH can also be seen in the cisterns surrounding the brainstem **(Fig. 8)**.

Traumatic *intraventricular hemorrhage* (IVH) results from tearing of subependymal veins or as a direct extension of parenchymal hematoma. On CT, acute IVH appears as hyperdensity within the ventricular system **(Fig. 9)**. One should always look for hydrocephalus (enlargement of ventricles) in such cases, as blood, especially in the fourth ventricle, can obstruct the flow of CSF.

The *cortical contusion* is a hemorrhagic parenchymal brain "bruise" involving the superficial gray matter occasionally extending into the underlying white matter. Brain parenchyma in close contact with the rough inner surfaces of the skull is typically affected. On CT, contusions appear as hypodense areas and are often difficult to notice in the early stages.

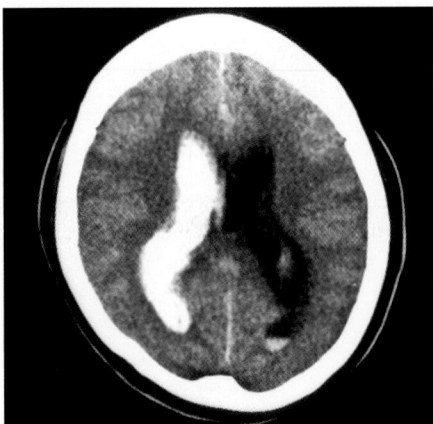

Fig. 9: Intraventricular hemorrhage predominantly in the right lateral ventricle. Note the small amount of blood layered in the left occipital horn.

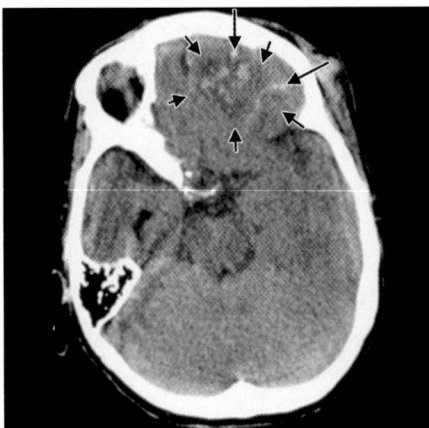

Fig. 10: Right frontal hemorrhagic contusion (arrows). Note the relatively superficial nature and mottled appearance due to hemorrhagic areas (hyperdense) within the contusion (hypodense). In contrast, a parenchymal hematoma is uniformly hyperdense (as shown in Fig. 11).

Hemorrhagic contusions appear as mottled areas of high density within the superficial gray matter. They may be surrounded by larger areas of low density from associated vasogenic edema. As the contusion evolves, the characteristic "salt and pepper" pattern of mixed areas of hypodensity and hyperdensity becomes more apparent **(Fig. 10)**.

Intracerebral hematoma (ICH) results from shear-induced hemorrhage of small intra-parenchymal blood vessels or expansion and joining of adjacent cortical contusions. They are located deeper than contusions. On CT, the acute ICH is a rounded hyperdense mass lesion **(Fig. 11)**. As the hematoma evolves, a low-density rim, due to edema and pressure necrosis, can be observed. Appearance of delayed intraparenchymal hematomas few days after the initial injury is associated with a poor prognosis.

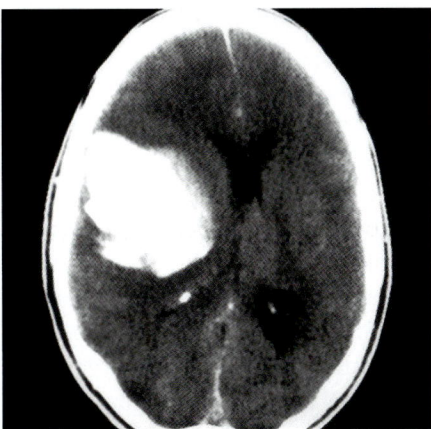

Fig. 11: Right frontoparietal intracerebral hematoma. Note the deeper extent of the hematoma compared to a contusion as shown in Figure 10.

Cerebral edema in TBI is usually of the cytotoxic type. On CT, effacement of the cerebral sulci and compression of the ventricles are the common findings. There is loss of gray-white differentiation and obliteration of cisterns around the brainstem. Increasing mass effect leads to a variety of brain herniation syndromes of which tonsillar herniation into the foramen magnum can be catastrophic. The various types of brain herniation are shown in **Figure 1**.

Magnetic resonance imaging (MRI) of the brain is rarely indicated in acute head trauma.

Severe TBI

In general, TBI is divided into two discrete periods—primary and secondary brain injuries. The primary brain injury is the physical damage to parenchyma (tissue and vessels) that occurs during a traumatic event, resulting in shearing and compression of the surrounding brain tissue. Numerous secondary brain insults, both intracranial and extracranial or systemic, may complicate the primarily injured brain and result in secondary brain injury. Secondary intracranial brain insults include cerebral edema, hematomas, hydrocephalus, intracranial hypertension, vasospasm, metabolic derangement, excitotoxicity, calcium ions toxicity, infection, and seizures. Secondary systemic brain insults are mainly ischemic in nature, such as:
- Hypotension [systolic blood pressure (SBP) < 90 mm Hg]
- Hypoxemia (PaO_2 < 60 mm Hg; O_2 saturation < 90%)
- Hypocapnia ($PaCO_2$ < 35 mm Hg)
- Hypercapnia ($PaCO_2$ > 45 mm Hg)
- Hypertension [SBP > 160 mm Hg, or mean arterial pressure (MAP) > 110 mm Hg]
- Anemia (hemoglobin < 10 g/dL, or hematocrit < 0.30)
- Hyponatremia (serum sodium < 130 mEq/L)

- Hyperglycemia (blood sugar > 180 mg/dL)
- Hypoglycemia (blood sugar < 80 mg/dL)
- Hypoosmolality (plasma osmolality < 290 mOsm/kg H_2O)
- Acid–base disorders (acidemia: pH < 7.35; alkalemia: pH > 7.45)
- Fever (temperature > 36.5°C)
- Hypothermia (temperature < 35.5°C).

The idea of early neurosurgical referral is to prevent or limit the secondary insults so that the morbidity and mortality due to severe head injury can be drastically reduced. The various techniques for intensive neuromonitoring including ICP monitoring, recent advances like cerebral microdialysis, jugular venous oxygen saturation, brain tissue oxygen tension, etc. are beyond the scope of this textbook. Basic cerebrovascular physiology is purposefully omitted from this discussion to keep it simple.

CRITICAL CARE MANAGEMENT

Analgesia, Sedation, and Paralysis

Adequate pain relief is absolutely essential in a patient with head injury. Endotracheal intubation, mechanical ventilation, trauma, ICU procedures, etc. are all potential causes of pain, which contribute to raised ICP and poor outcome. Especially in mechanically ventilated patients, narcotics like morphine or fentanyl should be used as they provide analgesia, mild sedation, and depression of airway reflexes.

Adequate sedation limits agitation, prevents harmful movements, decreases cerebral oxygen consumption, and facilitates nursing care and mechanical ventilation. Benzodiazepines like midazolam and lorazepam can be given as continuous infusion or intermittent boluses. They are short acting and do not interfere with periodic neurologic assessment. Moreover, they provide amnesia and anticonvulsive effect. Another alternative is propofol which reduces ICP, but should be used with caution in hypotensive patients; high dose propofol is associated with significant morbidity. Routine use of neuromuscular-blocking agents to paralyze patients with TBI is not recommended.

Mechanical Ventilation

Patients with severe TBI are usually intubated and mechanically ventilated. Hypoxia, defined as O_2 saturation < 90% or PaO_2 < 60 mm Hg, is an independent predictor of poor outcome following TBI. The ventilatory settings should be adjusted to maintain oxygen saturation (SpO_2) of 95% or greater and/or PaO_2 of 80 mm Hg or greater and to achieve normoventilation (eucapnia) with $PaCO_2$ of 35–40 mm Hg. Prior to suctioning, the patient through the endotracheal tube (ETT), preoxygenation with a fraction of inspired oxygen (FiO_2) = 1.0, and administration of additional sedation are recommended to avoid desaturation and sudden increase in the ICP. Suctioning ETT must be brief and atraumatic.

Hemodynamic Support

Hypotension, defined as SBP < 90 mm Hg or MAP < 65 mm Hg, is a major determinant and an independent predictor of poor outcome of severe TBI. Among predictors of outcome of TBI, hypotension is the most amenable to prevention, and should be avoided and aggressively managed.

Aggressive fluid administration to achieve adequate intravascular volume so as to maintain central venous pressure (CVP) around 8–10 mm Hg is the first step in resuscitating a patient with hypotension following severe TBI. Isotonic crystalloids, specifically normal saline solution, are the fluid of choice for fluid resuscitation and volume replacement. Blood and blood products may be used as appropriate. Anemia and coagulopathies should be corrected appropriately.

Excessive and inappropriate fluid administration is associated with fluid overload and acute respiratory distress syndrome (ARDS), and should be avoided. Even with target CVP, if hypotension persists, vasopressors should be used. Norepinephrine, titrated through a central venous line, is recommended. Dopamine can be given via a peripheral intravenous cannula until a central venous access is established. Dopamine can cause cerebral vasodilation and increase ICP and is not the preferred agent. Phenylephrine, a pure α-agonist vasoactive agent, is recommended in TBI patients with tachycardia.

Hypertension, defined as SBP > 160 mm Hg or MAP > 110 mm Hg, is also a secondary systemic brain insult that can aggravate vasogenic brain edema and intracranial hypertension. This is a compensatory mechanism in response to raised ICP and hence aggressive BP lowering should not be done, as it can impair cerebral perfusion. The target MAP should ideally be guided by the cerebral perfusion pressure (CPP) value obtained after ICP monitoring.

Fluid and Electrolytes

Isotonic crystalloids, preferably normal saline, are recommended solution for fluid management. A target CVP of 8–10 mm Hg so as to maintain euvolemia or moderate hypervolemia is the goal. Negative fluid balance is associated with an adverse outcome and should be avoided. Likewise, aggressive use of normal saline is associated with hyperchloremic metabolic acidosis. Hypotonic solutions [1/2 NS, 1/4 NS, dextrose 5% in water (D5%W), D5% 1/2 NS, D5% 1/4 NS, RL] can decrease serum osmolarity leading to raised ICP and should be avoided. Also, glucose-containing solutions can increase ICP and should be avoided, especially in the first 48 hours, except in cases of hypoglycemia.

Serum electrolyte disturbances are common complications after TBI. The most common causes for hypernatremia (Na^+ > 150 mmol/L) in patients with TBI are central or neurogenic diabetes insipidus, osmotic diuresis (mannitol), and the use of hypertonic saline solution (HSS). Correction of severe hypernatremia (Na^+ > 160 mmol/L) should be gradual, as abrupt changes in serum osmolarity and rapid fall of serum sodium concentration would worsen cerebral edema. Fluid resuscitation of hypovolemic hypernatremic TBI patients should be initially only with NS. Hyponatremia is detrimental and a major secondary systemic brain insult in patients with severe TBI, as it leads to exacerbation of brain edema and an increase in ICP. It is usually secondary to cerebral salt wasting syndrome, or to the syndrome of inappropriate antidiuretic hormone secretion (SIADH). Hypophosphatemia and hypomagnesemia are common complications in head-injured patients and they lower the seizure threshold.

Hyperosmolar Therapy

Mannitol is an osmotic diuretic that reduces ICP by creating a temporary osmotic gradient by increasing the serum osmolarity to 310–320 mOsm/kg H_2O. Twenty percent mannitol is given in a dose of 0.25–1 g/kg intravenously over 15–20 minutes. Mannitol should be given only in patients with symptoms of raised ICP (severe headache, vomiting, etc.), signs of transtentorial herniation (bradycardia, reduced pupillary reactivity, asymmetrical dilatation of pupil, focal neurologic deficits, etc.), progressive neurologic deterioration, or documented raised ICP by formal monitoring. Prophylactic administration of mannitol is not recommended. Mannitol should not be used in patients with hypotension. Once administered, adequate fluid replacement has to be done to maintain euvolemia. Mannitol should not ideally be administered, if serum osmolarity is >320 mOsm/kg H_2O. Due to risk of pulmonary edema and heart failure, it is contraindicated in patients with renal failure. It should be used with caution in patients with extradural hematoma and pneumocephalus, as it can potentiate these by reducing the cerebral swelling. Prolonged administration of mannitol leads to intravascular dehydration, hypotension, hyperkalemia, and prerenal azotemia. It can also lead to rebound increase in ICP by passing the blood–brain barrier, accumulating in the brain, leading to reverse osmotic shift and increased brain osmolarity. The diuretic action and thereby reduction in ICP by mannitol is potentiated by the administration of intravenous furosemide (10–20 mg) given few minutes later.

Recent studies have highlighted the benefits and role of hypertonic saline (3% and above) as an alternative to mannitol. HSS causes faster expansion of intravascular volume (with small volumes), increased cardiac output and pulmonary gas exchange, reversal of immunomodulation caused by hypotension, and decreased CSF production. It produces osmotic dehydration and viscosity-related cerebral vasoconstriction. When compared to mannitol, it does not cause renal failure or pulmonary edema. Hypertonic saline is also associated with potential side effects including sudden hypertension, hypernatremia, altered consciousness, and seizures. Mannitol still remains the current standard of care for reducing ICP.

Seizure Prophylaxis

Post-traumatic seizures can be early (occurring within 7 days of injury) or late (occurring after 7 days following injury). Prophylactic therapy is not recommended for preventing late post-traumatic seizures. It may be given in patients with TBI who are at high risk for seizures. The risk factors include—GCS score < 10, cortical contusion, depressed skull fracture, subdural hematoma, EDH, intracerebral hematoma, and penetrating TBI. Phenytoin is the recommended drug for the prophylaxis of early post-traumatic seizures. A loading dose of 15–20 mg/kg administered intravenously over 30 minutes followed by 100 mg, intravenously or per oral every 8 hours, for 7 days is recommended.

Deep Vein Thrombosis Prophylaxis

Mechanical thromboprophylaxis, including graduated compression stockings and sequential compression devices, is recommended and should be continued until patients are ambulatory. In the absence of a contraindication, low-molecular weight heparin or low-dose unfractionated heparin should be used in combination with mechanical prophylaxis. However, the use of pharmacological prophylaxis is associated with an increased risk for expansion of intracranial hemorrhage.

Stress Ulcer Prophylaxis

Severe TBI is a well-known risk factor for stress ulcers (Cushing's ulcer) in the ICU. Prophylaxis includes early enteral feeding and pharmacological prophylaxis such as H_2-blockers, proton-pump inhibitors, and sucralfate.

Nutritional Support

There is evidence to suggest that malnutrition increases mortality rate in TBI patients. Early enteral feeding is recommended in patients with severe TBI, as it is safe, cheap, cost-effective, and physiologic. Transgastric jejunal feeding is recommended to reduce the incidence of ventilator-associated pneumonia.

Glycemic Control

Hyperglycemia has repeatedly been associated with poor neurological outcome after TBI. But, maintaining low-blood glucose levels within tight limits is controversial in patients with severe TBI, because hypoglycemia, a common complication of tight glucose control, can induce and aggravate underlying brain injury. Hence, most studies do not support tight glucose control (maintenance of blood glucose levels below 110–120 mg/dL) during the acute care of patients with severe TBI.

Steroids

There is level I evidence to refute the use of steroids in head injury. Moreover, steroid can be detrimental in trauma patients, as it leads to increase in infection rates.

Barbiturate Coma

Barbiturates reduce cerebral metabolism and cerebral blood flow (CBF) and lower ICP. High-dose barbiturate administration is recommended to control elevated ICP refractory to maximum standard medical and surgical treatment. Hemodynamic stability is essential before and during barbiturate therapy. Administration of barbiturates to induce burst suppression measured by EEG as prophylaxis against the development of intracranial hypertension is not recommended.

General Measures for Reducing ICP

- *Raising head of bed to 30–45°*—reduces ICP and improves CPP and lowers the risk of ventilator-associated pneumonia.
- *Keeping the head and neck of the patient in a neutral position*: This would improve cerebral venous drainage and reduce ICP.
- Avoiding compression of internal or external jugular veins with tight cervical collar or tight tape fixation of the ETT that would impede cerebral venous drainage and result in an increase in the ICP.
- Turning the patient regularly and frequently with careful observation of the ICP.
- Administering a bowel regimen to avoid constipation and increase of intra-abdominal pressure and ICP.

Special Situations

Diffuse Axonal Injury

Diffuse axonal injury (DAI) is a frequent result of traumatic acceleration/deceleration or rotational injuries and a common cause of persistent vegetative state in patients with TBI. DAI is suggested in any patient who demonstrates clinical symptoms disproportionate to CT scan findings. Among patients eventually proven to have DAI, 50–80% demonstrate a normal CT scan upon presentation, and MRI is usually indicated in such patients. The prognosis of DAI depends on the severity and extent of the injury, those with involvement of the brainstem having the worst prognosis.

Cerebrospinal Fluid Rhinorrhea

Cerebrospinal fluid rhinorrhea is seen in 2% of all head traumas, and up to 30% of all basilar skull fractures. The most common presentation is unilateral watery rhinorrhea and CSF β-2 transferrin is the preferred method of confirming a fluid as CSF. In an acute setting, there should be a high index of suspicion, as it may be missed due to presence of blood. Available guidelines are against administration of prophylactic antibiotics, as they have not been shown to reduce the risk of meningitis. But most centers use a combination of parenteral third-generation cephalosporin with aminoglycoside for a period of up to 1 week. It usually subsides with

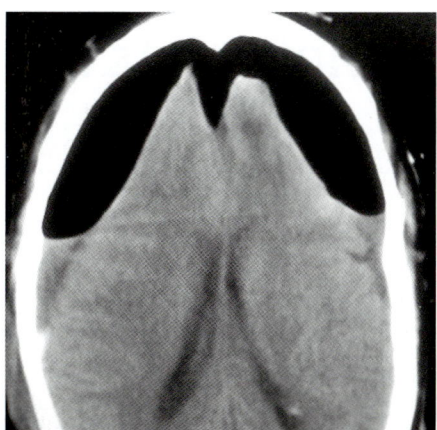

Fig. 12: Mount Fuji sign due to large pneumocephalus. Tension pneumocephalus is a neurosurgical emergency and requires drainage of intracranial air.

conservative treatment including strict bed rest, head end elevation, and avoidance of ICP raising maneuvers, over a period of 1 week. Refractory cases are dealt by CSF diversion or endoscopic/open surgical repair. CSF otorrhea is also managed more or less similarly.

Depressed Fractures

Open depressed skull fractures with contamination require urgent neurosurgical intervention. Also in cases of associated dural tear with pneumocephalus or an underlying intracranial hematoma requiring evacuation, neurosurgical referral is required for a depressed calvarial fracture. Otherwise, most surgeons prefer to elevate a fracture, if the depressed segment is below the inner table of the adjacent normal bone or is producing a neurological deficit. Depressed fractures with cortical injury or compression are likely to cause seizures. All open depressed fractures following trauma shall be deemed contaminated and need parenteral antibiotic therapy.

Pneumocephalus

Pneumocephalus is the presence of gas within the cranial cavity, commonly occurring after trauma or a surgical procedure and indicates damage to the dura or air sinus. Mild-to-moderate pneumocephalus can be managed with analgesics, intermittent oxygen inhalation, and close clinical/radiological follow-up.

If there is a valve mechanism, which allows air to enter the skull but prevents it from escaping, a tension pneumocephalus can occur, which is a neurosurgical emergency. CT scan of patients with tension pneumocephalus typically shows air that compresses the frontal lobes of the brain, which results in a tented appearance of the brain in the skull known as the Mount Fuji sign **(Fig. 12)**.

Use of Antiseptics and Ointments for Wound Management

R Dayananda Babu

CARE OF THE WOUND

Skin is responsible for primary defense against wide range of bacterial invaders. When the integrity of skin is compromised accidentally or intentionally, the natural defense weakens. Once a wound is there, it has to be protected either by covering with plain dressing or by some antimicrobial or antiseptic dressing. Different types of wound care products are available in the market.

Wound care products can be classified as:
- Gauze
- Alginates
- Antiseptics
- Enzymatic products
- Antimicrobial or biocides
- Hydrogels
- Hydrocolloids
- Foams.

Antiseptics

Chemical agents are primarily used to decrease the risk of infection for intact skin or minor wounds. Most antiseptics are not suitable for open wounds, as they impede wound healing by direct cytotoxic effects on keratinocytes and fibroblasts. The commonly used antiseptics are:
- *Alcohols and iodophores (povidone iodine)*: They have rapid action but the action is not persistent.
- *Chlorhexidine*: The action is slow but it has got persistent action.

Generally, the above substances are used to clean the intact skin surrounding the wound and not inside the wound.

Substances used for the Management of Infected Wounds

- Povidone iodine
- Hydrogen peroxide (100% toxic to the cell)
- 1% acetic acid (for *Pseudomonas* infection)
- Dakin solution

- *Edinburgh university solution (Eusol)*: Hypochlorite
- Silver nitrate
- Silver sulfadiazine.

All these agents will impair wound healing.

Eusol and Dakin Solution

These solutions are of historical significance. They were widely used during World War-II because of their broad-spectrum activity against gram-positive and negative organisms. Because of their high potential for cytotoxicity, they are abandoned now.

Hypochlorite is now used for cleaning the floor of HIV patient's room.

Hydrogen Peroxide

This is a very commonly used agent, which is used for chemical debridement of necrotic tissue by irrigation. The reactive hydroxyl radicals produced by it will damage the DNA and it is 100% cytotoxic to the cell. They also inactivate the bacterial housekeeping enzymes.

Note: The best form of debridement is mechanical.

Precautions to be taken while using hydrogen peroxide:
- Use only in wounds with necrotic tissue as irrigation
- Use only half strength
- Always rinse with normal saline after irrigation.

Disadvantage of hydrogen peroxide: If it is instilled into wound cavities under pressure, it will result in air embolism.

Povidone Iodine

Food and Drug Administration (FDA) has not approved this agent for use in wounds.

Mode of action: It destroys the microbial protein and DNA. It has broad antibacterial and antifungal spectrum.

Disadvantages:
- It is cytotoxic to fibroblasts (unless diluted to 1:1,000)
- Acidosis in burns patients
- It impairs the ability of the wound to fight infection, therefore, increases the chance for infection
- Neuropathy
- Cardiovascular, renal, and hepatotoxicity.

Normal Saline (0.9%)

This is the best noncytotoxic solution for wound care. This is very useful for partial and full-thickness wounds. It is used for wet to dry dressing.

Dressing changes are required 2–3 times a day. If the dressing is saturated and changing is not done, maceration of the skin surrounding the wound will occur.

Silver Nitrate

They are used in burns because of the broad antibacterial spectrum. However, it will slow the epithelialization and cause electrolyte abnormality in large burns. Most important disadvantage is that it stains the cloth.

Silver Sulfadiazine

This is the ointment which is commonly used in burns. It accelerates epithelialization, promotes neovascularization, and has broad-spectrum activity.

Disadvantages:
- Transient neutropenia (bone marrow suppression)
- Poor penetration into the eschar
- Poor Gram-negative and anaerobic coverage.

Note: It should be avoided in glucose-6-phosphate dehydrogenase (G6PD)-deficient patients. There is no FDA approval for its use in wounds.

Mafenide Acetate

It is used in burns because of the better eschar penetration and better Gram-negative and anaerobic coverage.

Adverse effects:
- It prevents epithelialization
- It can cause acidosis.

Antibacterial Ointments

Conventionally, they are used to treat infected wounds. The antibacterial activity will last for 12 hours. They are soothing to apply and lubricate the wound.

The antibacterial ointments available are:
- Neomycin (for Gram-negative)
- Neosporin (polymyxin + bacitracin + neomycin)
- Bacitracin (for Gram-positive cocci and bacilli)
- Polymyxin B (for Gram-negative)
- Polysporin (polymyxin + bacitracin).

Neosporin

Neosporin increased re-epithelialization in experimental wounds by 25% when compared to no dressing.

Newer Agents

Platelet-derived growth factor: This will promote wound healing once the wound is granulating. It is used only in following situations:
- The wound should be free of infection
- Free of necrotic tissue
- Free of osteomyelitis
- The wound must have adequate blood supply.

Collagen-based Products

Collagenase is an enzymatic debriding agent derived from *Clostridium histolyticum* belonging to the metallopeptidase family. Collagenase will specifically hydrolyze the peptide bonds and digest all triple helical collagen. It will not degrade any other protein lacking the triple helix. It is a unique feature of collagenase.

Uses of Collagen-based Dressing

- Useful in chronic dermal ulcers and severe burns
- Liquefies necrotic tissue
- Promotes granulation tissue and epithelialization of wounds.

NB: The activity is impaired in pH higher or lower than 6–8 range.

Papain-based Products

Papain is a nonspecific proteolytic enzyme, which is derived from the fruit of papaya (*Carica papaya*). The papain breaks down the fibrinous material in necrotic tissue. The presence of sulfhydryl group such as cysteine is required for its activity. It will not digest collagen.

SUMMARY

- Povidone iodine and silver sulfadiazine are not approved by FDA for use in wounds.
- Povidone iodine has no role in wound care. It impairs wound healing and has systemic toxicity.
- Hydrogen peroxide should be avoided in large cavities and it should not be instilled under pressure. Always rinse the wound with 0.9% saline after using hydrogen peroxide.
- Normal saline is the ideal agent in partial and full-thickness wounds.
- The best form of debridement is mechanical and not chemical.
- Neosporin is the ideal antibiotic ointment in wounds.
- Platelet-derived growth factor is useful only in clean uninfected wound with adequate vascularity without any necrotic tissue.

43 Bandaging Techniques

John S Kurien

INTRODUCTION

Bandaging is an art, evolving since the days of Achilles' heel injury, and it has still not gone out of style. Bandaging is more about practice than theory and a well-applied, neat-looking bandage is well appreciated by most patients.

A bandage may be applied for one of many reasons—to immobilize and support a body part or joint to allow it to heal, to provide compression in an area of the body which is bleeding, and to hold sterile dressings in place covering infected body parts. Whatever be the reason to apply a bandage, there are some general bandaging principles which the surgeon has to follow and may also have to improvise depending on the resources at hand.

GENERAL PRINCIPLES

The most commonly and widely used bandages are made of gauze, although many specialized bandages made up of nylon, polyester, and viscose are now available. Elastic crepe bandages are also available, made of cotton, that can stretch to many times its length, but recoils to its original length.

The width of the roller bandage should always depend on the size of the area being bandaged. Any discrepancies as such will give rise to an ugly looking bandage.

Always position the patient before starting to apply the bandage and, if necessary, have an assistant nearby, as they may have to support the part of the patient's body that you are bandaging.

A rolled bandage should always be rolled over the body part by keeping the outer surface of the roller bandage in contact with the skin throughout the procedure. It offers much easier maneuverability than to start by keeping the inner surface of the bandage in contact with the skin.

The initial two turns should completely overlap each other. This offers stability at one end of the bandage. Thereafter, every turn of bandage should leave one-third of the previous turn of bandage uncovered. Always give a complete turn of bandage at the end and, if necessary, fix it with a micropore plaster or tie it.

It is advisable to keep open wounds and bony prominences well padded before bandaging and to keep the tension same throughout the area bandaged.

A wet bandage will shrink after it has dried which is dangerous, as too tight bandage may cause vascular compromise to the bandaged area. If bandaged for too long, this may lead to tissue death. At the same time, a bandage that is too loose will easily give away and may not serve its purpose.

THE BASIC TURNS

Circular Bandage

When a bandage is rolled out over an area with each turn completely overlapping the previous one, it is simply called a circular bandage. It is usually used for small wound dressings.

Spiral Bandage (Fig. 1)

When we have to bandage a large area of uniform dimension throughout (e.g., upper arm), we use this technique. Each turn overlaps one-third of the previous turn, preferably going from inferior aspect of the area, upwards or from proximal to distal in limbs.

Reverse Spiral Bandage (Fig. 2)

When we are to apply bandage over an area not uniform in its circumference throughout (e.g., forearm), we use a reverse spiral bandaging technique. After the first two turns to secure the bandage, the next turn onwards the procedure

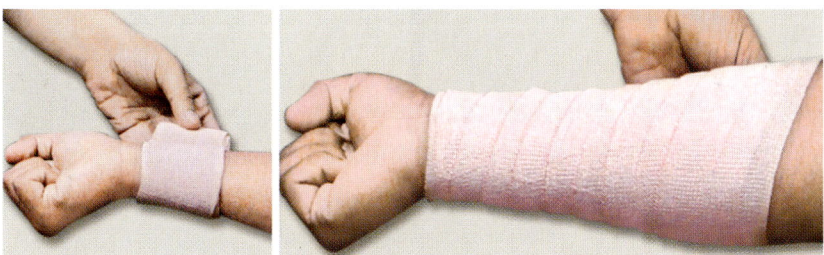

Fig. 1: Spiral bandage.

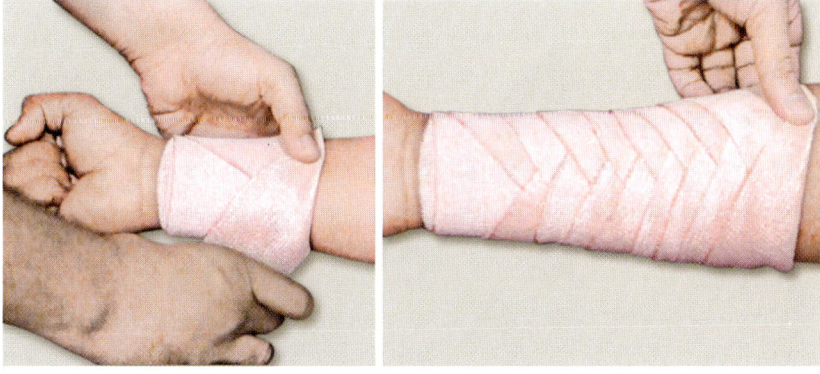

Fig. 2: Reverse spiral bandage.

is same as the spiral bandage, except that each surface of the bandage should alternately touch the part being bandaged. This can be achieved if after every turn, the bandage is neatly folded over itself so that for the next turn, the surface of the bandage in contact with the skin now comes to face outwards.

Figure of Eight Bandage (Fig. 3)

It is usually used over ankle, knee, and elbow joints. It is called so because each complete turn of this technique follows the shape of the number 8.

Recurrent Bandage (Fig. 4)

It is usually used to cover a large area like a head or amputation stumps, especially large uneven surfaces like the thigh. After a couple of turns around the head to secure the bandage, it is taken from the glabella anteriorly to the occiput posteriorly. Thereafter, a series of alternating turns to and fro, from glabella to occiput, are taken anteroposteriorly, spreading laterally from the sagittal plane and partly covering the previous turn, but always being folded

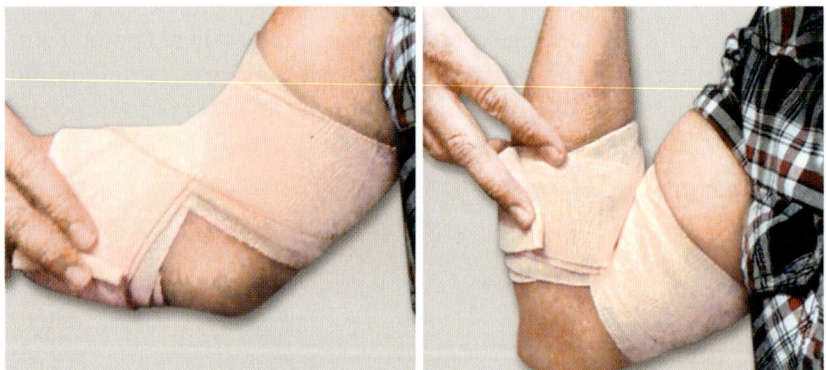

Fig. 3: Figure of eight bandage.

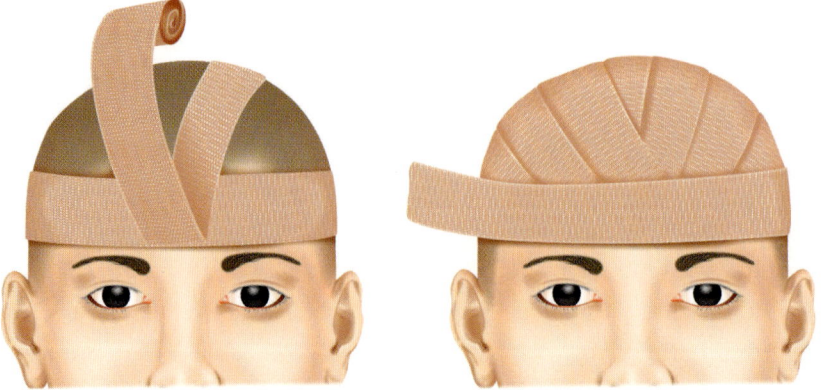

Fig. 4: Recurrent bandage for head.

at the same 2 points. An assistant may be needed to place his finger over these points so that the folded portions do not give away and your hands are free to do the bandaging. When the entire area is covered, circular turns are made around the head, making sure they cover the folded areas that the assistant was previously keeping in place, thereby securing them. Alternatively, this bandaging can be directed in the coronal plane, placing the folded points on two points above the ears.

HEAD BANDAGE

- *Recurrent bandaging*: As explained above, head bandaging can be done using the recurrent technique using a single roller bandage.
- *Barton's bandage*: This method is simple and is used to maintain compression on the chin in fractures of the lower jaw.
- *Four-tailed bandage* **(Fig. 5)**: This method is good for any protruding part of the body like chin or nose.
- *Capeline bandage* **(Fig. 6)**: There is another method to bandage the head using two roller bandages, the free ends of which are tied together. Each roller bandage held in one hand, the surgeon keeps the tied ends centered

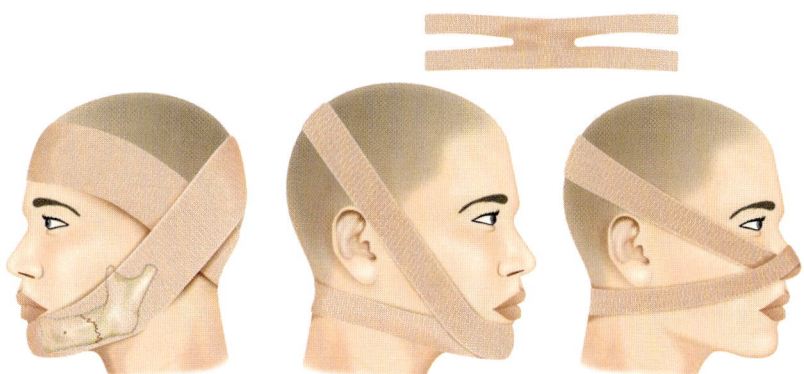

Fig. 5: Four-tailed bandage.

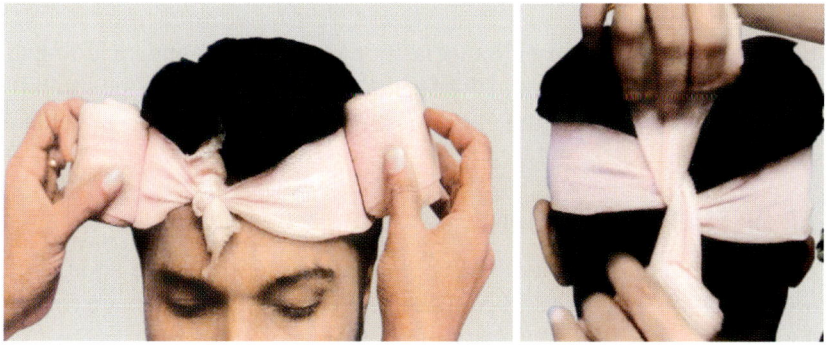

Fig. 6: Capeline bandage.

in the midline on the forehead and applies two turns with each bandage, one going clockwise and the other anticlockwise, always meeting in the center ventrally and dorsally. This secures the bandage and marks the starting point.

Then the left bandage is taken over the right in the center of the forehead. The right one is folded on it and directed from left frontal to temporal to the parieto-occipital region. Now, the left bandage is continued in a circular fashion till the occiput over the right one. Again, the right bandage is folded above the left one and directed to a similar path to reach the starting point. The left bandage is brought to the starting point in a circular fashion. Both bandages are now again at the starting point.

In this case, the right bandage gives traction to the left one while it is folded back and forth to cover the whole head. Finally, both are turned in a circular fashion once the whole head is covered and tied off **(Fig. 7)**.

- The same method described above can be done with a single roller bandage as well. The same principle is used. Traction is provided by a loop of the bandage lifted off the forehead by the assistants' or patients' thumb. This marks the starting point.

  After taking two circular turns around the head, a loop of the bandage, while taking the third turn, is supported by the patient's thumb. The bandage is looped from under this segment of bandage and pulled to the opposite side (path 1). In **Figure 8**, the roller bandage is looped from right to left, and then directed to cover the right frontotemporoparietal region. Then, it is rolled over from the left occiput, above the left ear to the starting point (path 2), where it is now looped from left to the right, and the process is repeated on the opposite side. After many turns, once the whole head is covered, the end of the bandage is tied with this small U-shaped loop supported by the thumb **(Fig. 9)**.

- *Triangular bandage*: This is done using a triangular piece of cloth, the length of its base being greater than the head circumference. The base is centered on the forehead and the tip is placed near the occiput. This covers the whole skull. The ends of the base are then taken backward and tied over the tip **(Fig. 10)**.

EYE BANDAGE

The bandage is applied in a circular fashion above the ear and including the affected eye. After a few turns in this fashion, the bandage is applied similarly, but this time from below the ear, over the mastoid on the affected side to cover that eye.

EAR OR MASTOID BANDAGE

This technique is same as the eye bandage except that we should not cover the eye this time. Only the affected ear and mastoid region are covered **(Fig. 11)**.

Bandaging Techniques

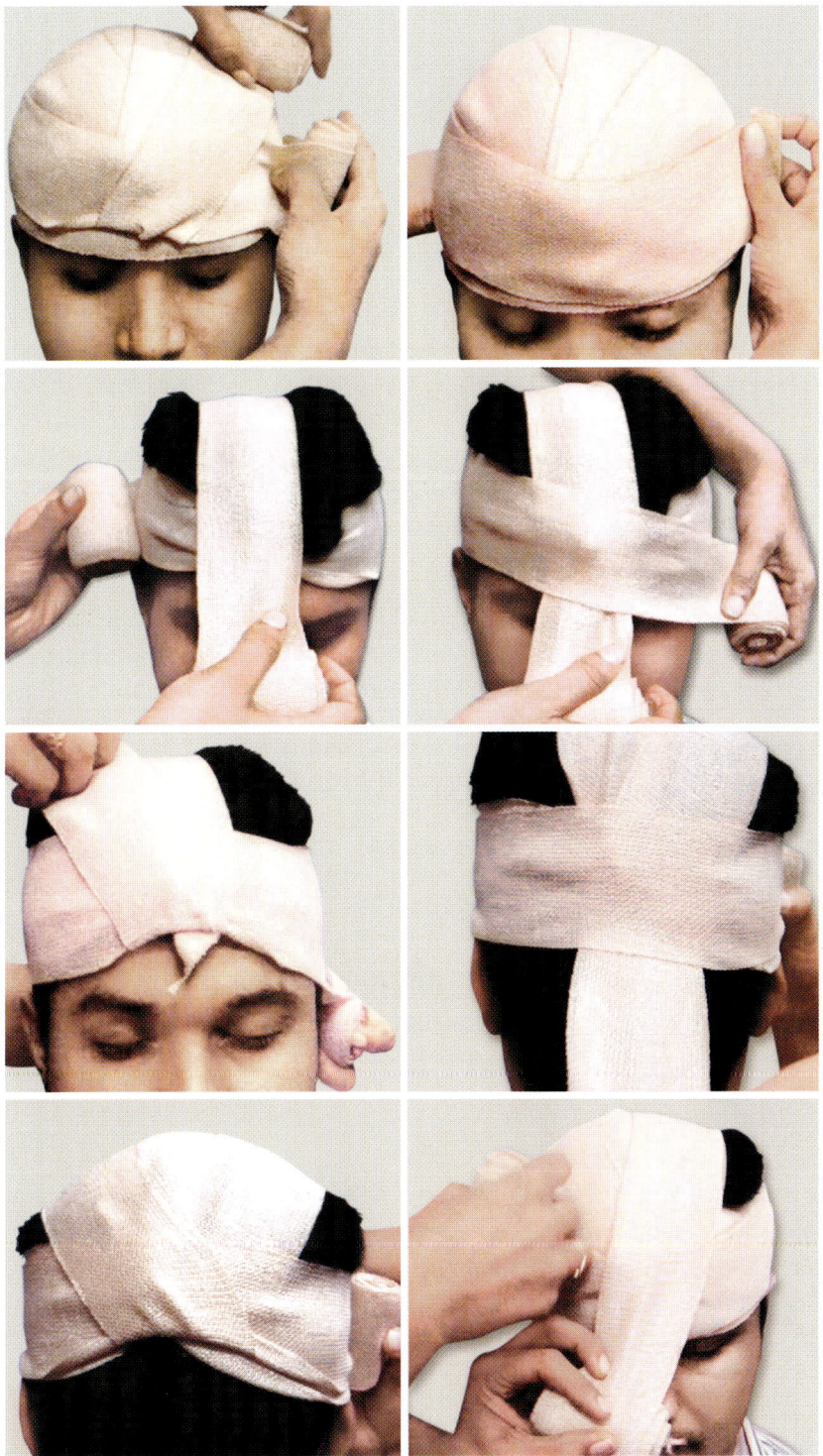

Fig. 7: Different types of head bandage.

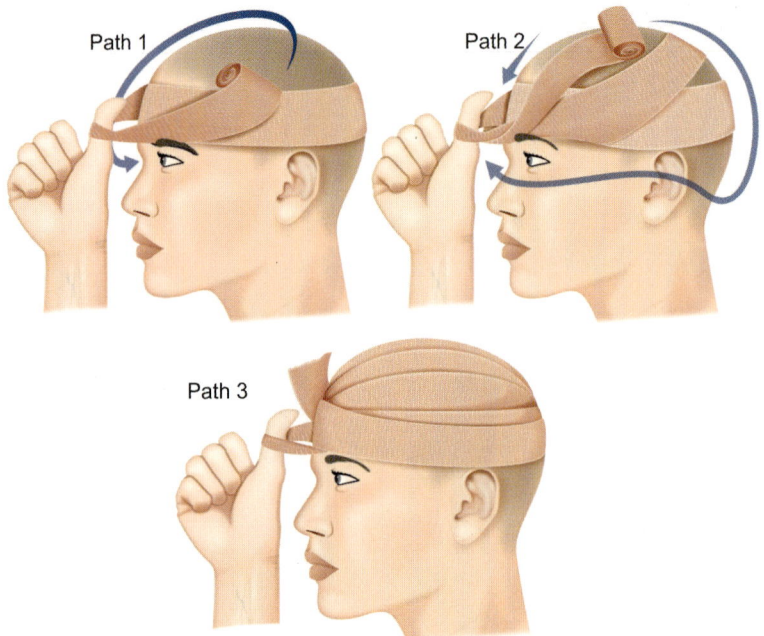

Fig. 8: Schematic representation of bandaging.

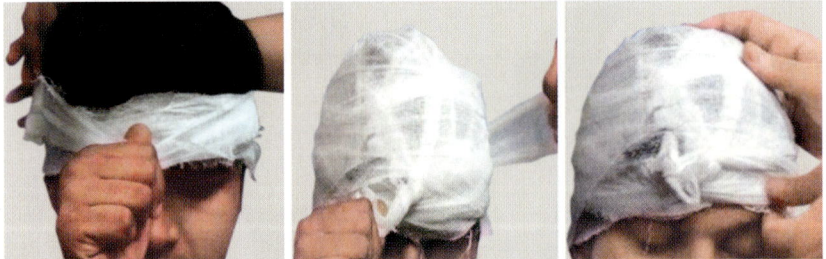

Fig. 9: Bandaging technique.

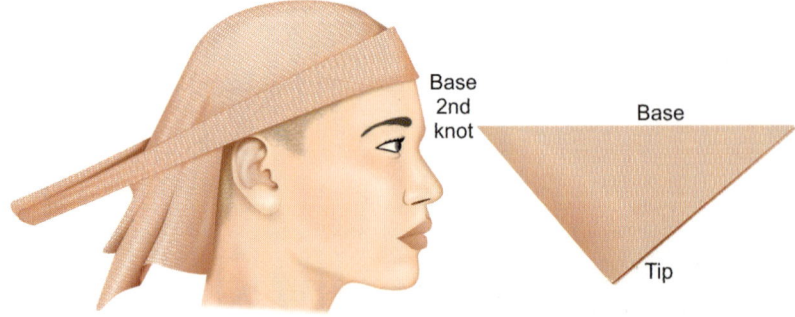

Fig. 10: Triangular bandage.

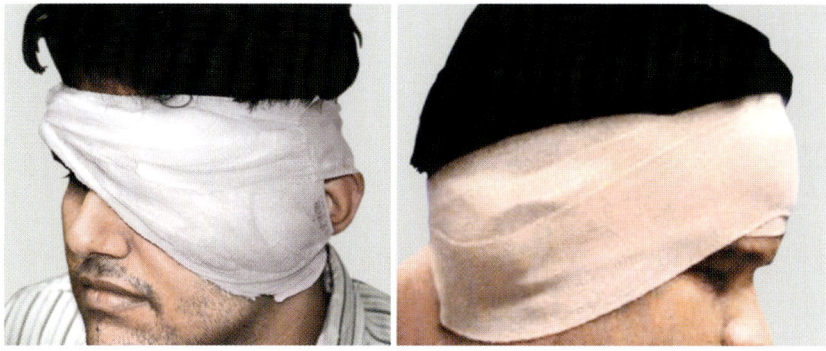

Fig. 11: Ear or mastoid bandage.

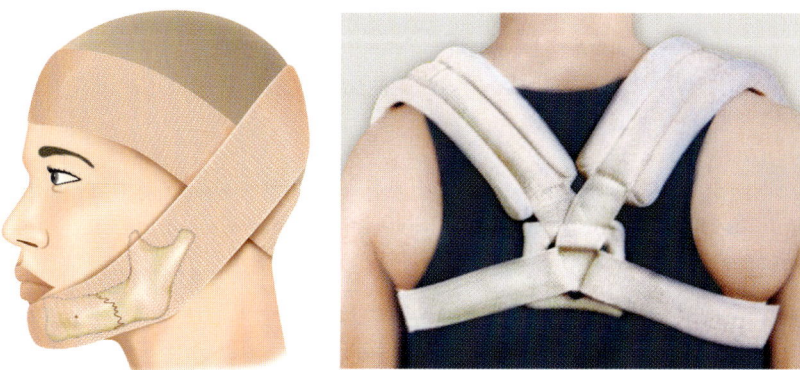

Fig. 12: Barrel bandage and figure of eight.

BARREL BANDAGE

It is used to support the chin in a patient of a fractured jawbone **(Fig. 12)**.

CLAVICULAR FRACTURE

Commercial clavicular braces are available for a fractured clavicle. Nevertheless, a clavicular brace can be made from a roller bandage as well.

After adequate padding under the armpits and on the shoulder, a roller bandage is applied in a figure of eight fashion from under the axilla to opposite shoulder along the back of the patient. In distal acromioclavicular fractures, the joint may be stabilized using adhesive bandages to perform Jones strapping.

BREAST BANDAGE

After a modified radical mastectomy (MRM), an elastocrepe bandage is applied in horizontal circular fashion after adequately padding the surgical site. A compression dressing may help in preventing seroma formation

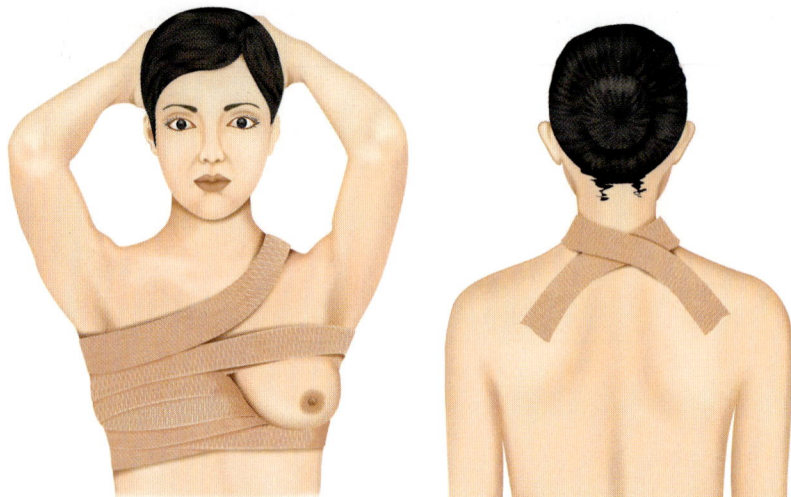

Fig. 13: Breast bandage.

post-MRM. Preferably, do not include the normal breast into the bandage. Applying the elastocrepe from above and under the unaffected breast increases patient comfort **(Fig. 13)**.

NECK BANDAGE

After thyroidectomy and other neck surgeries, application of a circular bandage may give the patient a choking sensation and cause discomfort. For this reason, two separate adhesive bandages are applied in a cross-like fashion extending from the lateral collars of the neck to the anterior chest wall of the opposite side.

AMPUTATION STUMP

An amputation stump can be bandaged in a recurrent or figure of eight pattern. In case of above knee amputations, both patterns can be used together. After giving a compression, bandaging in a recurrent fashion on amputated stump, the whole bandaging can be secured in place by taking the last few turns in a figure of eight pattern from around the waist to the base of the bandage. Compression dressings are very important after an amputation, as they reduce edema, encourage healthy venous return, and tone up the flabby tissue. This results in early rehabilitation using various prostheses. In **Figure 14**, the dotted lines represent the bandage outline behind the patient.

T-Bandages

After hemorrhoidectomy, anal fistulectomy, abdominoperineal resection, and other perineal procedures require the use of a T-bandage in the

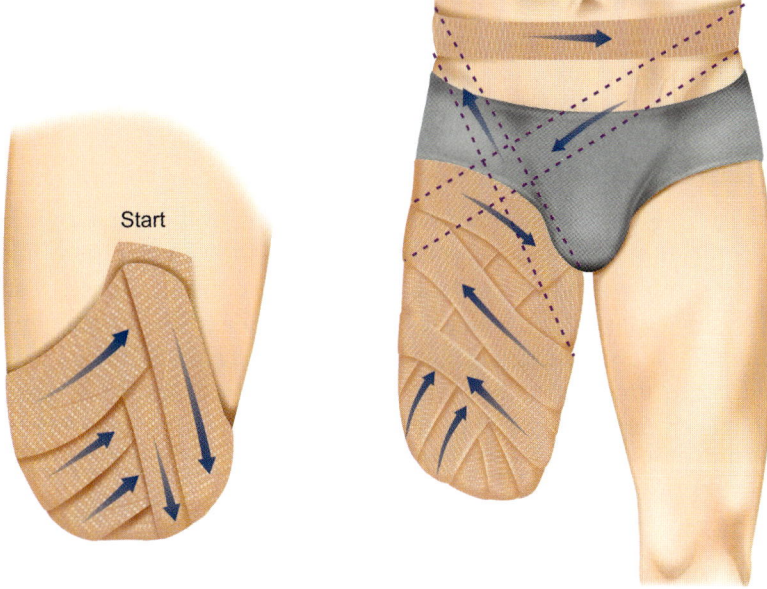

Fig. 14: Amputation stump bandage.

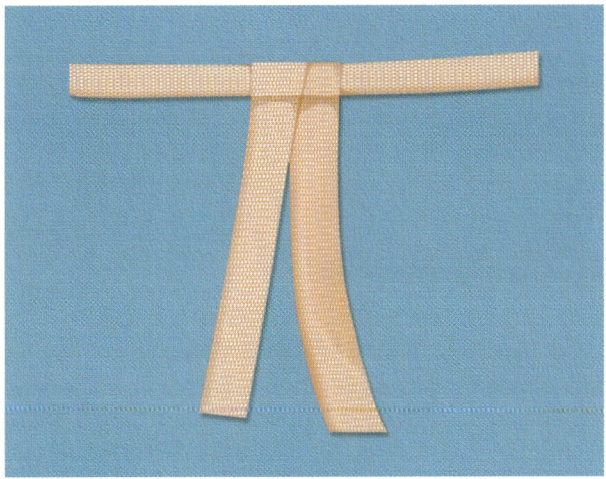

Fig. 15: T-bandage.

postoperative period. The horizontal part of a T-bandage is tied across the abdomen, while the vertical portion is taken from under the genitals and perineal region and tied to the abdominal part. This provides support to the perineal dressing **(Fig. 15)**.

ABDOMINAL BINDERS

Postlaparotomy patients, especially the elderly and obese, may benefit from an abdominal binder, in view of avoiding wound dehiscence. Some believe that abdominal binders are often soaked with wound discharge, and wearing the same belt day after day could lead to wound infections. Cloth-made abdominal binders are available or may be stitched, which can be washed daily to avoid such complications **(Fig. 16)**.

BUTTERFLY STRAPPING

When an abdominal surgical wound gets infected, debridement is done after removing skin sutures and the wound is left open for secondary suturing. In such cases, the wound edges can be brought closer using a butterfly strap with adhesive elastocrepe bandage to improve healing. The central portion of a butterfly strap is narrow and nonadhesive since it is folded on itself, while the edges are broad and adhesive. Hence, multiple dressings can be changed without even removing the strap, using an artery forceps to introduce fresh gauze. But if the strap gets soiled, it may be a focus for infection and must be changed **(Figs. 17A to C)**.

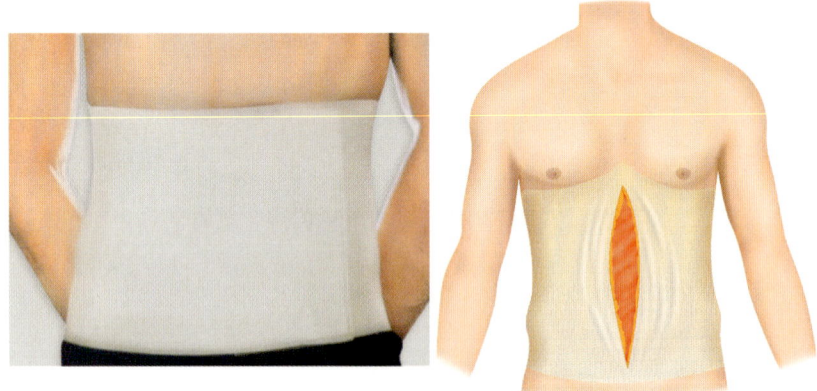

Fig. 16: Abdominal binder.

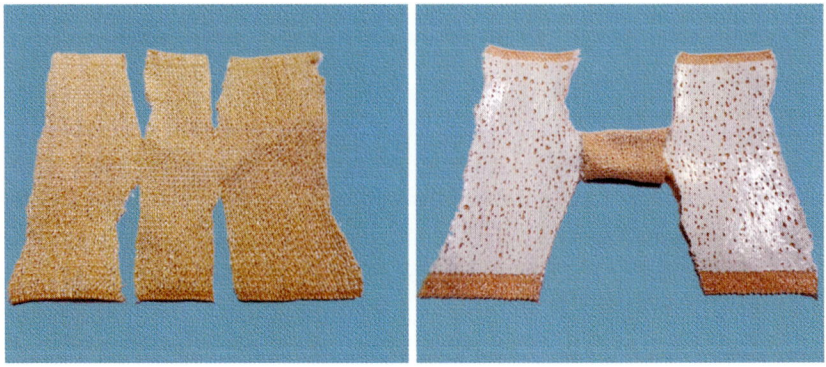

Fig. 17A

Bandaging Techniques

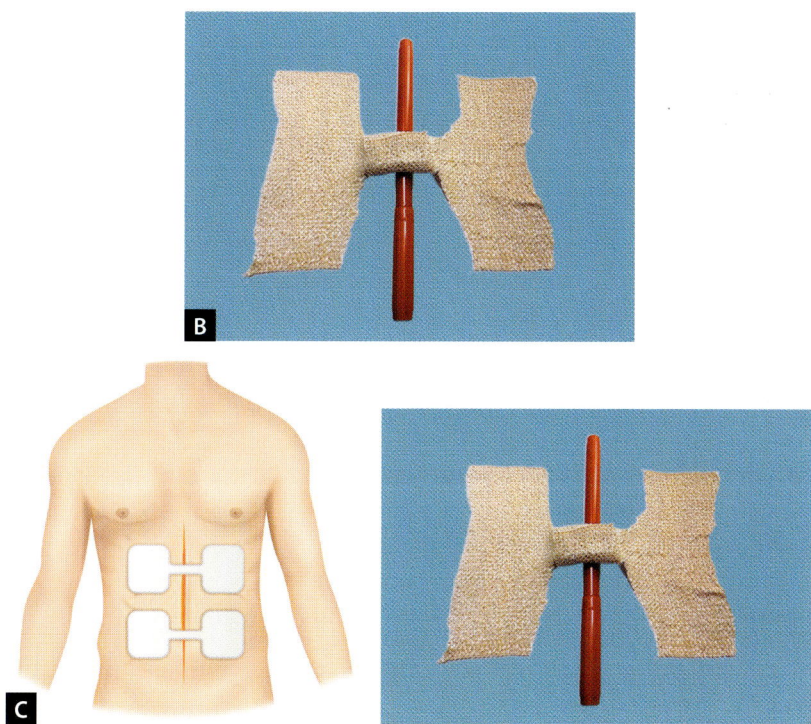

Figs. 17B and C

Figs. 17A to C: Butterfly strapping of the abdomen.

First cut an elastocrepe adhesive bandage of the following shape.

Note the shape of the elastocrepe cut out. Hence, it is called butterfly strapping. The pen can easily pass under the central portion since it is nonadhesive. In the same way, daily dressings can be changed in the central portion without removing the butterfly strap. Also, note how the laparotomy wound edges come closer after butterfly strapping.

Medical Negligence (Professional Negligence/Malpractice)

R Dayananda Babu

What is medical negligence?
It is the failure to execute *reasonable degree of skill and care* or *willful* negligence of a medical practitioner which causes some harm or bodily injury or death. It may be an *act of omission* (not doing something a reasonable man would do) or *act of commission* (doing something a reasonable man would not do).

ELEMENTS OF NEGLIGENCE

The liability for negligence arises if the following conditions are satisfied (*four D's*):
1. Duty—the skill in deciding what is his/her illness and what is the treatment needed. The care in administration of proper treatment also comes under duty.
2. Dereliction of duty—the failure to maintain applicable standard of care and skill.
3. Direct causation—there should be causal connection between the negligent act and injury.
4. Damage.

Burden of proof—the patient should prove all four elements of negligence.

REASONABLE SKILL AND CARE AND TIMELY REFERENCE

The medical practitioner should execute skill and care expected from a man of his caliber at that time. High caliber of an expert or specialist cannot be expected from an ordinary practitioner. The doctor should keep abreast of recent developments in medical science and should refer the patient in time not to make his condition complicated. *Timely reference* of the patient is also the duty of medical practitioner otherwise, it may amount to negligence. If a general practitioner treats a case as a specialist which clearly lies within a specialized medical field, he will be held liable for failure to use skill equal to that of a specialist.

DOCTRINE OF RES IPSA LOQUITUR (THE THING SPEAKS FOR ITSELF)

Examples are:
- Failure to remove swabs or instruments after operation **(Fig. 1)**
- Operation on wrong patient/wrong part of the patient
- Loss of hand due to prolonged splinting
- Too tight plaster cast causing gangrene
- Failure to give antitetanus serum resulting in tetanus.

In all these situations, the burden of proving the innocence lies upon the doctor. The doctrine of res ipsa loquitur is related to the doctrine of common knowledge and is applied in both *civil* and *criminal* negligence.

NOVUS ACTUS INTERVENIENS

In the case of an assault or an accident, the normal sequence of events may change during treatment due to the carelessness of doctor. The responsibility for subsequent disability or death may pass from the original incident to negligent action of the doctor. This plea is not generally accepted by the court. Sometimes, the patient may take treatment from another doctor without the knowledge of the first doctor. The first doctor cannot be held responsible by applying this rule.

CIVIL AND CRIMINAL NEGLIGENCE

As per Indian law, there is no definition for civil negligence. Section 304A Indian Penal Code (IPC) deals with criminal negligence—"whoever causes death of any person by doing a *rash* or *negligent* act *not amounting to culpable homicide* shall be punished with imprisonment up to *2 years* or with fine or with both". In such cases, a gross negligence from the part of the doctor which

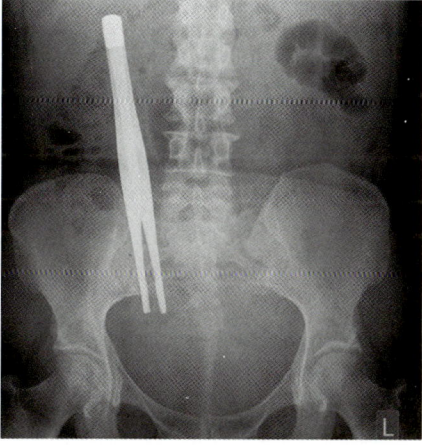

Fig. 1: Plain X-ray showing instrument inside abdomen.

causes the death has to be proved. In *civil negligence*, the onus of proof lies with the patient.

In *criminal negligence*, the doctor has to prove innocence.

PROCEDURES TO BE FOLLOWED BEFORE GIVING CHARGE TO THE DOCTOR FOR NEGLIGENCE

The cases have to be referred to an expert panel constituted by the district medical officer, in which a medicolegal expert is a member. The medical board will examine the case and will give a report. If the board finds that the doctor is negligent, then a charge of negligence is given against the doctor. For criminal negligence, the guilt should be proved beyond reasonable doubt.

EXAMPLES OF CRIMINAL NEGLIGENCE

- Amputation of wrong limb/wrong patient
- Removing healthy eye instead of diseased eye
- Leaving instruments, tubes, sponges, or swabs in the abdomen
- Performing criminal abortion and patient dies
- Gross mismanagement of delivery and subsequent death
- Gross incompetent anesthesia and death of the patient
- Doing surgery under the influence of alcohol/drugs causing gross damage
- Removal of wrong organ
- Mismatch transfusion and complications
- Ligation of ureter, bile duct, etc.
- Paralysis and gangrene after splints and plaster.

If there is no criminal negligence, the case can be referred to *Consumer Redressal Forum* for compensation of damages. In all hospitals, deaths with alleged criminal negligence, the police will charge a case under Section 304A IPC. There is no other section in IPC to deal with it. The death from road traffic accident as a result of rash or negligent driving and death of a patient while the doctor is trying to save life, acting in good intention comes under the same category in IPC. Therefore, an amendment of law is required in this matter and should be taken up legally in the Supreme Court.

DEFENSE AGAINST MEDICAL NEGLIGENCE

- *Calculated risk doctrine*: There is a calculated risk of 5–10% death in cardiac surgery and it becomes *professional accident*.
- *Contributory negligence*: This is only a partial defense where there is unreasonable conduct of the patient and medical negligence. Examples are:
  - Refusing to take the suggested treatment
  - Leaving the hospital against medical advice
  - Failure to give accurate medical history
  - Failure to cooperate and carry out the instructions.

- *Vicarious liability (respondent superior) (let the master answer)*: For the negligent action of a subordinate doctor, the responsibility always lies on the superior; both may be sued by the patient. For example:
  - The negligent action of house surgeon or postgraduate doctor in training, the unit chief will be responsible.
  - If one qualified doctor assists another doctor in the operating room, the assistant is considered an employ of the principal surgeon and both are liable.
  - A surgeon is not responsible for the negligence of anesthesiologist and vice versa.
  - The responsibility lies with the doctor for a negligence on the part of the nurse.
  - The physician/surgeon is responsible for the acts of interns/residents working under his/her direct supervision.
  - The superintendent of the hospital is not responsible for the action of any doctor or staff if he/she is appointing qualified persons.
  - Nursing superintendent is responsible for mistakes of trainee nurses.
  - Hospital authorities cannot be held responsible for the negligence on the part of doctors—"Captain in the ship doctrine".
- *Corporate negligence*: The hospital administration should provide standard equipment and competent employees, otherwise they will be held responsible.
- *Products liability*: Defective or negligently designed medical or surgical instrument or drug, the manufacturing company is responsible.
- *Medical maloccurrence*: In spite of good medical attention and reasonable skill and care, inevitable accidents may happen. Doctors cannot be blamed for the death of a patient if he/she had executed care and skill, e.g., recurrent laryngeal nerve injury in thyroidectomy, idiosyncratic response to drugs.
- *Therapeutic misadventure (similar to medical maloccurrence)*: Examples are:
  - Diagnostic procedures using dyes, catheters, etc.
  - Adverse reactions to drugs.
- *Error in judgment*: A doctor cannot be held negligent if he/she has executed reasonable skill and care. Each case is considered on its own merit and analyzed.
- *Res iudicata*: Negligent case against a doctor should be filed within 2 years from the date of alleged negligence. After the stipulated time, a case of negligence cannot be filed.
- *Res judicata (things have been decided)*: Once a case is completed between two parties, it cannot be tried again.
- *Composite negligence*: In a case of negligence of two or more doctors, the compensation should be split between the defendants.

- *Good Samaritan doctrine*: If one doctor is encountering a serious problem during performing a surgery and takes the help of another surgeon, the helping surgeon cannot be charged with contributory negligence. *Informed consent is not a defense in negligence cases.*

PRECAUTIONS TO AVOID NEGLIGENCE CHARGE

- Always take informed consent
- Establish rapport with the patient
- Keep full and accurate medical records
- Employ reasonable skill and care
- Do necessary investigations to arrive at a diagnosis
- Immunization should be given against tetanus
- Sensitivity tests should be given before injections
- Get the opinion from another doctor in cases of doubts (second opinion)
- Do all necessary tests for early detection of malignancy
- Inform the relatives in critical situation (proper communication)
- Do not give too much promise to the patient
- Do not guarantee a cure
- Convey each step of your treatment to the patient and relatives
- If facilities are inadequate, refer the patient to a higher center
- In multistage treatment, specific separate consent should be taken
- Keep the operation sterilized and infection free
- Every medical act must be in accordance with the prevailing practice
- Record meticulously the changing clinical profile of the patient
- Always join in one of the medical indemnity insurance schemes (professional protection scheme).

45 Breaking the Bad News

R Dayananda Babu

INTRODUCTION

The desired outcome of consultation while breaking bad news would be "to convey threatening information in a way which promotes understanding, recall, and support for the patient's emotional response and a sense of ongoing support". However, well-communicated bad news is still bad. It is important to understand how the patient may respond to the bad news. The aim to minimize the impact, to remove needless fears, to instill realistic hope, and to reassure the patient that he/she will not be abandoned. When the news is really bad (disclosure of cancer), the five steps described by Elisabeth Kübler-Ross in her book titled "On Death and Dying" becomes very relevant. The possible reactions from the patient are:

1. Denial
2. Anger
3. Bargaining
4. Depression
5. Acceptance.

Not everyone goes through the same stages and not in the same sequence as mentioned by Elisabeth Kübler-Ross herself. The physician's job is to find out the persons feelings, react appropriately, and help the person to come to the state of acceptance.

DENIAL

The usual initial response of the patient will be "this cannot be true, this cannot be happening to me". This is usually a passing phase, but once in a while a patient may continue in denial. For sometime, it is a good coping strategy. When the person is unable to deny anymore, there may be a higher emotional impact to the bad news.

ANGER

The anger at the situation may get redirected in the form of "shooting the messenger"—anger at the doctor or nurse or often anger may be directed at whatever is close to the patient such as the spouse, close friends, close family members, or threatening usually the security staff, reception staff, junior doctors, etc. Anger is a response to feeling of helplessness, distress, and fear. It may also be a negative result of an ineffective communication.

BARGAINING

Bargaining may be with God and may accompany offers to "go straight" hereafter. It may also take the form of "doctor shopping" or "system hopping"—trying different systems of medicine one after another.

DEPRESSION

It is normal to grieve when there is bad situation and grieving people may need help and support. Sometimes, the patient may go into clinical depression, which needs to be identified and treated.

ACCEPTANCE

This is the state when the patient says to himself/herself—"well, this has happened, I cannot undo it, let us see what we can do about it" is the healthiest of all.

How to manage denial?
Denial is a defense mechanism and it varies in its severity, leading onto poor compliance to treatment. The main problem of denial by the patient is that it will cause delay in diagnosis and further management, which will lead onto more severe disease. By denial, the patient is avoiding the eventual painful situations, which are likely to happen in the course of the disease. Continued efforts are required to make the patient realize the problem, so that one can proceed with the treatment. The patient may sometimes completely refuse the treatment. The patient has to be counseled by conveying that the treating physician will give care to him and the patient is not alone. Ask the patient about the illness and the seriousness of it. Estimate how much the patient has understood about the illness and what are his/her future plans. Rule out psychiatric problems objectively.

Active listening is required by proper body language and eye contact. Make sure that the denial is not due to the lack of understanding. If the patient is frightened, provide emotional support. Always a nonconfrontational approach is adopted in such situations. Give the feeling that the patient will not be abandoned at any cost by comforting words.

How to manage anger?
The anger is a feeling of helplessness and is often unleashed on very close people like spouse, close family members, friends, doctors, nursing staff, and paramedical staff. Try to calm down the patient and make the patient sit down for a dialog. One should be empathetic and positive during the conversation. Let the patient express feelings and emotion. Give them an opportunity for participatory decision-making after explaining the details of

the disease process. Use positive nonverbal communications, which may be useful. Assure all support for the patient.

How to manage patient's family?
There are situations where the family members will conspire among themselves and with professionals to withhold the information from the patient under the pretext that it will cause emotional harm to the patient. Explain to them that the patient has the right to information. The consequences of withholding the diagnosis from the patient can affect the patient's future plans, if any. Assess whether the family is having correct understanding of the diagnosis and treatment options including the palliative care. The patient may be sometimes in the bargaining phase. The treating physician can facilitate a conversation between patient and family, if they find it difficult to handle.

Talk to the patient and assess the wishes of the patient. Inform the family members regarding the patient's wishes and what has been discussed with the patient. Sometimes, the patient may request the physician to withhold information from the family. It is a very difficult and sensitive situation because the patient has to give permission for disclosure to the family.

STEPS FOR EFFECTIVE COMMUNICATION

- *Relationship building*: Time and privacy—sitting down at eye level of the patient, not too close to invade private space, but close enough to lean forward and touch the patient if the need arises. Convey empathy without expression—"I see that you are very worried". The important thing is to convey that you care.
- *Open the discussion*: "It looks like life is a burden for you right now". Acknowledgment of suffering makes the patient feel that he/she is understood:
    - *Listen actively*—active listening involves eye contact
    - *Body language*—ideally should be leaning forward
    - *Verbal responses* like—"Yes", "I see", "and?", "hmm", "oh", etc.
    - *Appropriate facial expression* on the part of the listener is also important.
- *Information gathering*: Explore and find the patient's level of knowledge, what does he/she know?, use open questions or statements—"what do you think might be the problem?", "what worries you the most?", and "that must have come as a shock to you".
- *Assess the patient's perspective*: How does the patient feel about it? An emotional reaction should be expected and the doctor can be prepared for it. It may be an extreme emotional reaction or can be a mild one depending on the patient's current mental status. The physician could ask the patient to share his/her feelings or thoughts which may give the patient some form of relief.

- *Share information*: The patient has a right to know everything. Confirm what the patient really wants to know. Use common conversational language. Check understanding at every stage.
- *Come to an agreement regarding the course of action which is acceptable to the patient*: Summarize the problem and suggest a course of action acceptable to the patient. Tell the patient that the plans are negotiable. Answer any questions and doubts from the patient.
- *Leave the door open for further talk*: Review and summarize discussion before finishing. Always leave the door open to talk again.

Orthopedics

Tigy Thomas Jacob

FRACTURES AND DISLOCATIONS

Fracture is a break in the normal trabecular pattern of bone. There are two types of bones—(1) cortical bone and (2) cancellous bone. In cortical bone, the basic units called osteons or Haversian systems are tightly packed. In the cancellous bones, which are commonly found in the metaphysis, the bones have a lattice pattern with thin medullary interspaces separating.

Definitions

Dislocation is a total loss of contact between the two articulation surfaces of a joint **(Fig. 1)**. Subluxation is the partial loss of contact between the articulating surfaces of a joint. Sprain is usually used to describe tear of the ligaments. Strain is used to describe a tear of the muscle.

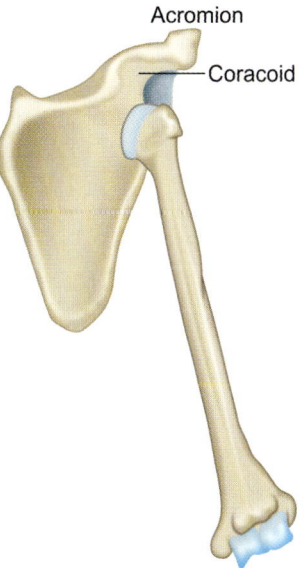

Fig. 1: A dislocated shoulder.

TYPES OF FRACTURES

Simple Fracture

A fracture, which has two fragments and has not broken the skin (not open). A simple fracture is divided into three types **(Fig. 2)**:
1. *Transverse fracture*: It is usually caused by a direct blow or impact at the site of fracture. This essentially points to a three-point force system.
2. *Oblique fracture*: Fracture is at an angle to the bone. One bone may be trapped.
3. *Spiral fracture*: It is caused by rotational stress, often due to weight of the body rotating about a fixed point such as the foot in contact with the ground.

Open or Compound Fracture

Here, the fracture hematoma communicates with the exterior. The compounding may be inside out (where the bone fragment pierces the skin and comes out) or outside in (external object penetrating) **(Fig. 3)**.

Comminuted Fracture

There are three or more fragments **(Fig. 4)**.

Segmental Fracture

There are three or more fragments, but it involves the circumference of the bone. Since most of the present injuries are high-velocity injuries, the segmental fractures are much more common now **(Fig. 5)**.

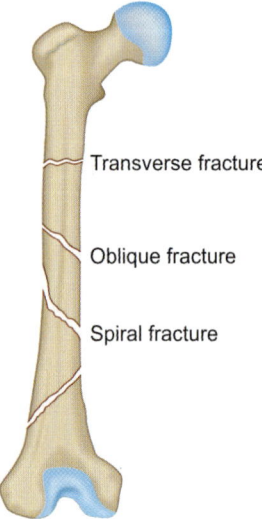

Fig. 2: Simple fractures.

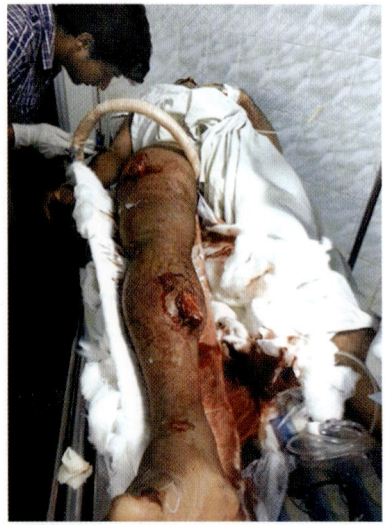

Fig. 3: An open fracture on Thomas splint.

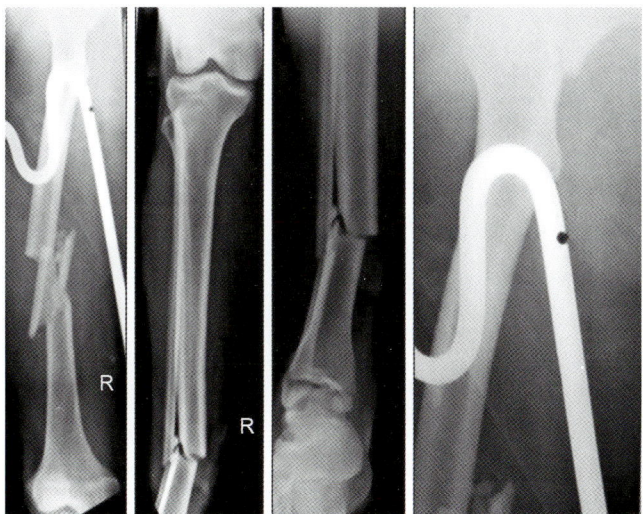

Fig. 4: Comminuted fracture.

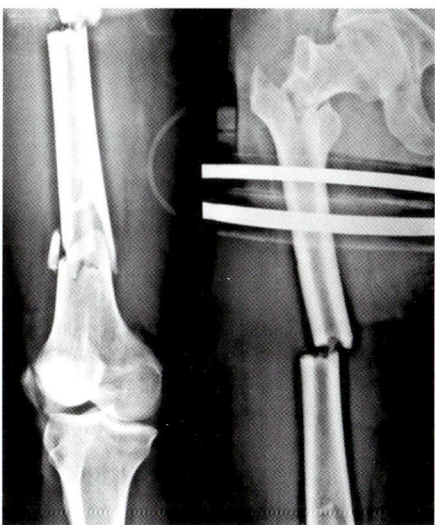

Fig. 5: Segmental fracture.

Avulsion Fracture

Where the musculotendinous junction is avulsed. Surgical correction will be a necessity in such conditions **(Fig. 6)**.

Compression Fracture

These fractures are primarily seen in the metaphysis of bones. Since vertebra is a very common site of metaphysis, vertebral compression fractures belong to this fracture type. These fractures can also be seen in the metaphysis of long bones such as the tibial plateau and the lower radius.

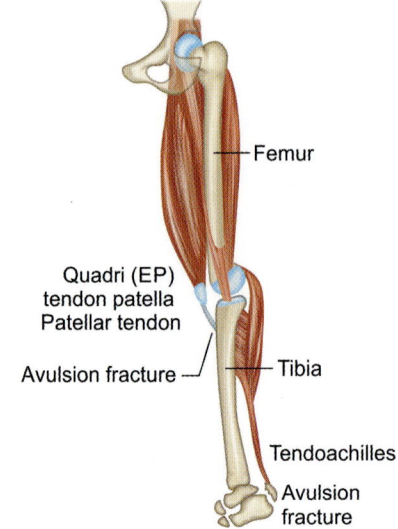

Fig. 6: Quadriceps mechanism.

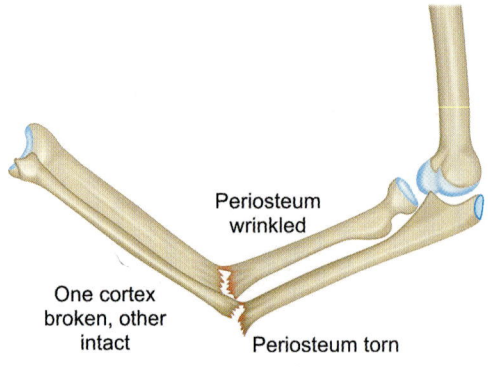

Fig. 7: Greenstick fracture.

Greenstick Fracture

These types of fractures are seen in children. These plastic-like bones deform or they fracture in such a way that one cortex fractures and the periosteum ruptures. The other cortex only compresses and the periosteum will fold. When these fractures are reduced, it is important to note that the cortex on the concave side should be broken and the fracture overcorrected and a plaster should be put according to three-point concept so that the bent plaster may produce straight bones **(Fig. 7)**.

1. *Depressed fracture*: This is predominantly seen in the skull **(Fig. 8)**.
2. *Stellate fracture*: They are seen in patella and denote the shape of the fracture.
3. *Pathological fracture*: These are fractures seen in a bone already weakened by a pathological process. The weakening may be due to malignancies, infections, or metabolic causes **(Figs. 9 and 10)**.

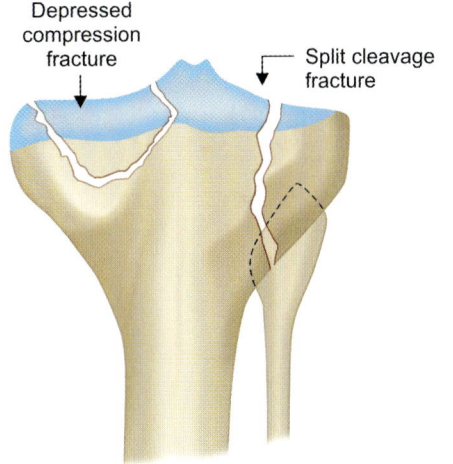

Fig. 8: Depressed fracture and split fracture of tibial condyle.

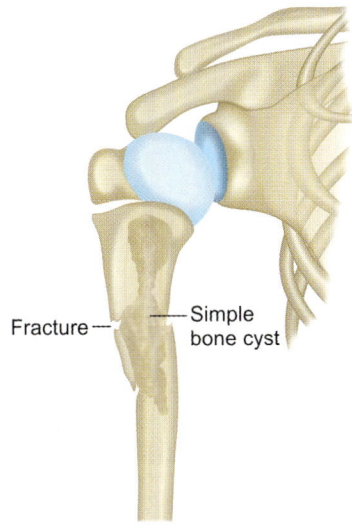

Fig. 9: Pathological fracture (unicameral bone cyst).

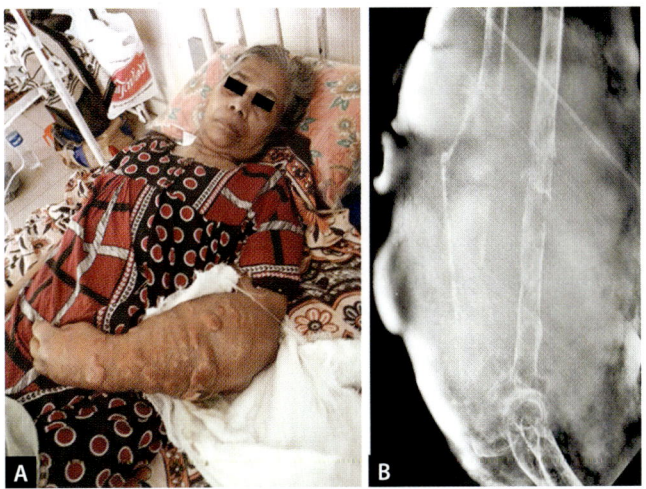

Figs. 10A and B: Pathological fracture (lymphoma).

Pseudofracture

These are not true fractures but the Looser's zones or Milkman's zones are seen due to vessel pulsations on bone weakened by osteomalacia (**Figs. 11 to 14**).

FRACTURE UNION

Stages [Brighton, Carl T, and Robert M Hunt (1991)]: There are three major phases of fracture healing, two of which can be further subdivided to make a total of five phases:

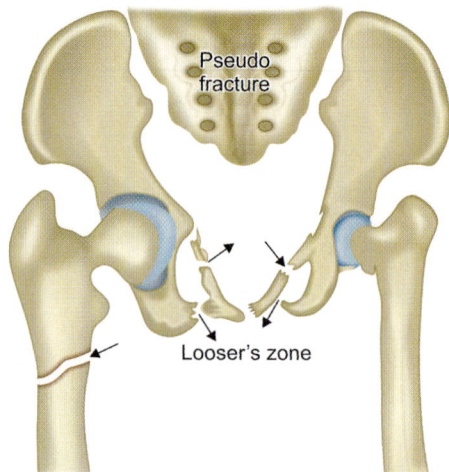

Fig. 11: Osteomalacia and Looser's zone.

1. *Reactive phase*:
    - Fracture and inflammatory phase
    - Granulation tissue formation.
2. *Reparative phase*:
    - Cartilage callus formation
    - Lamellar bone deposition consolidation.
3. *Remodeling phase*: Remodeling to original bone contour.

DIAGNOSIS

As in several conditions, the importance of clinical examination is the most relevant and absolutely irreplaceable. Conventional radiography comes next supplemented by other special investigations like CT scan, MRI scan, bone scan, etc.

HISTORY

A proper history of the accident can have a great bearing on the subsequent course and outcome and should modify treatment. If the patient is not conscious or is under the influence of alcohol, the proper history may not be elicited. If there was a severe crush initially, the patient may have pain but the internal degloving and subsequent avascularity and gangrene and sloughing of the overlying skin may not be appreciated. Alcohol and head injury can also mask a compartment syndrome and can have catastrophic outcome.

Another quite underdiagnosed condition in out setup is the battered baby or other abuses. Special vigilance has to be kept in mind when several injuries in different stage of healing and fracture shaft of femurs in very young age are encountered **(Figs. 15 and 16)**.

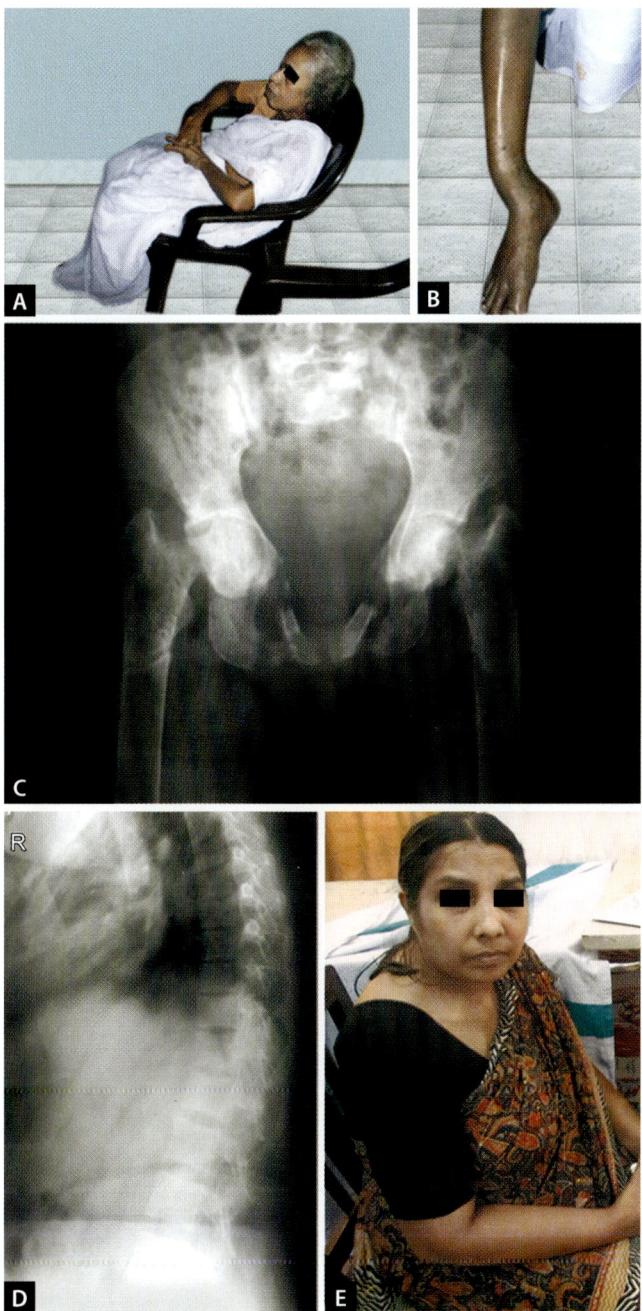

Figs. 12A to E: Osteomalacia.

Pain

Pain is the most common symptom. But pain will vary with the site and mobility of the fracture. Severe pain at one site may distract our attention from other fractures. We may diagnose a fracture of the metacarpal or phalanx

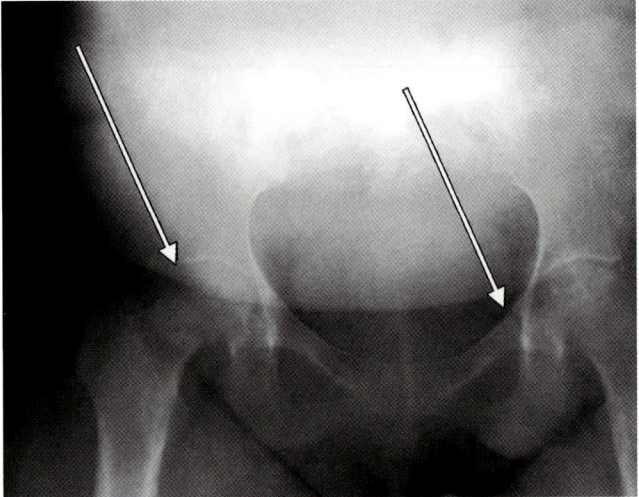

Fig. 13: Looser's zone.

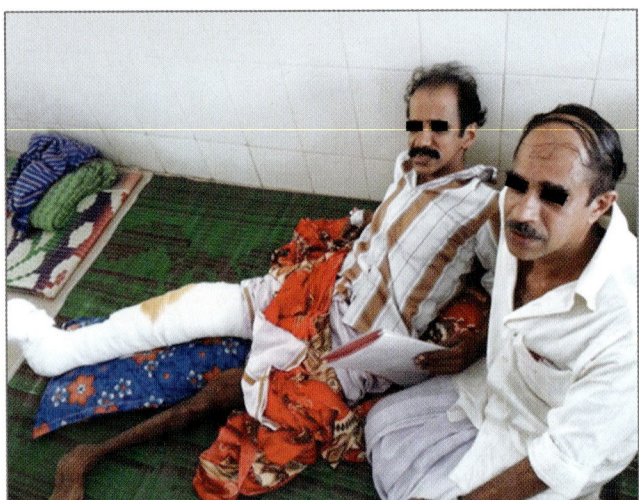

Fig. 14: Brothers with dentinogenesis imperfecta.

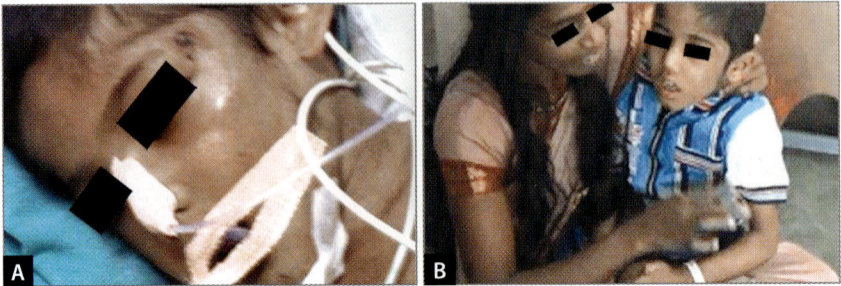

Figs. 15A and B: Battered baby.

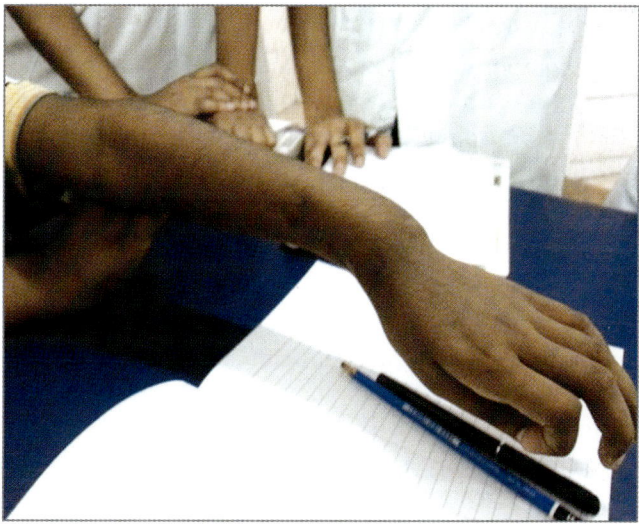

Fig. 16: Garden spade deformity.

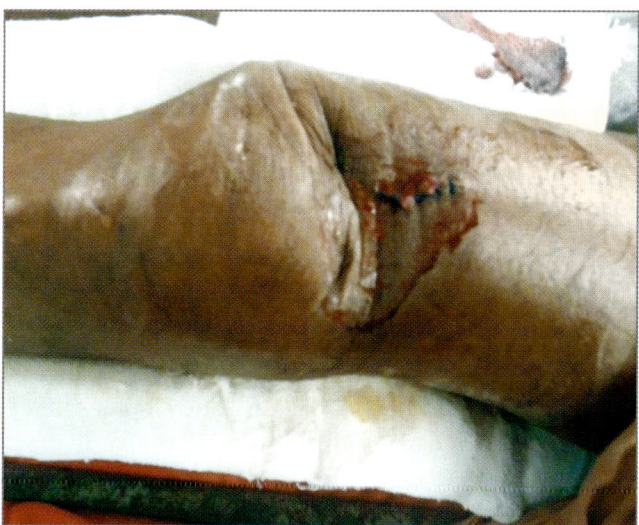

Fig. 17: Puckering due to impending compounding.

only later unless we practice sufficient care and do a meticulous examination **(Fig. 17)**.

Loss of Function

It is almost always present to some degree in the affected area or limb. The limb may be splinted, and the patient may be reluctant to move it. The surgeon should also elicit sufficient care and must be gentle and should always have the trust and confidence of the patient.

Loss of Motor Power or Sensation

Neurovascular complication of a musculoskeletal injury must be promptly diagnosed. It should be elicited whether the limb or extremity was numb or feeling dead or if the patient is unable to move the joints. Most patients in spite of the pain will be able to make the difference. This will also be relevant on a medicolegal point of view.

PHYSICAL SIGNS

External Appearance

Attitude and deformity may vary and classical appearances are seen in different fractures. The following are some of the classical deformities seen:
- Colles' fracture dinner fork/silver fork deformity
- Smith fracture garden spade deformity
- The "S" deformity in supracondylar fractures of humerus in children
- The external rotation deformity of the lower limb is seen in both intracapsular and extracapsular (trochanteric) fractures of the neck of the femur.

Tenderness

This is one of the most important, valuable, and constant physical signs. It is very important to actually do a proper clinical examination including gentle palpation. Even though tenderness in superficial fractures can be palpated easily, deeper injuries may not be that amenable to examination.

Swelling

It is seen in all fractures. In certain fractures like Colles' fracture, this will be the predominant feature along with the deformity. In Colles' fracture, the classical abnormal mobility and loss of transmitted mobility may not be seen.

Initially the swelling may be minimal but it can rapidly increase. A very rapid increase should arouse the suspicion of a vascular injury. In certain fractures like the upper tibial, lower tibial, ankle and calcaneal fractures, severe swelling and probably blebs may contraindicate an internal fixation.

Swelling near a joint may be due to bleeding into the joint.

In some injuries such as the fracture acetabulum and probably proximal femur, the so-called Morel-Lavallée lesion may be an evidence of severe trauma including internal degloving. Such injuries may have a bad result complicated by sloughing and infection when an internal fixation is embarked upon.

Local temperature rise is also seen in fractures.

Abnormal Mobility

This is a classical feature of fractures. A conscious effort to elicit it should not be attempted.

Loss of function is always present whenever there is a fracture and the patient will resist all attempts to use the limb.

However, many a times, the doctor fails to identify a neurovascular injury. Missing a vascular injury can have catastrophic complications like losing the limb or chronic disability following a compartment syndrome. Missing a nerve injury can have profound disability and has litigation potential.

RECORDS

Documentation and proper records are crucially important. However, this is an aspect which is always not up to the required standards. Immediate and prompt detailed recording should be done after the initial assessment. The neurovascular status has to be clearly depicted. This can have very severe legal implications when a previously nonmentioned injury is later detected.

RADIOLOGICAL EXAMINATION

There is no orthopedics without proper radiographs. AP and lateral views must be taken. Special views are sometimes needed:
- Two views of the whole bone
- Two limbs—to rule out an epiphyseal injury in a child
- Two sites—like the spine and the calcaneum when falling from height
- Two joints in Monteggia, Galeazzi, and also to rule out an ipsilateral fracture shaft and neck of femur
- Two occasions must be taken to rule out fractures. This is necessary in certain fractures such as the fracture scaphoid where the fracture line is visible only after 2 weeks.

MANAGEMENT

X-rays provide the following information:
- Localized fractures or dislocation
- Degree and direction of displacement
- Pre-existing pathology
- Foreign body
- An additional injury
- Air suggesting penetrating injury.

First Aid

The ABCDEF of orthopedics is:

*A*irway, *B*reathing, *C*irculation, *D*igestive system, *E*xcretory system, *F*ractures.

The immediate goal is to prevent any further injury to the patient. Control of bleeding can be done by application of external pressure. Any clean cloth can be used for bandaging or keeping firmly over the bleeding site. When the patient is moved, a manual pressure can be given.

Tourniquet

It is not routinely employed since it may actually increase bleeding by impairing venous return and may be left too long inadvertently.

Splint

Splinting should be done by whatever method available. Lower limb can be splinted with the other limb (bandaging both legs together) or can be splinted using wood or umbrella, etc.

Plastic splints, Cramer's wire splints, and inflatable splints may also be available.

An injured leg may be splinted in reasonable anatomical positions but undue force must not be used to attain this position. So, the limb may be splinted as it lies, if necessary.

Injury to the spine should be cared for and the head should be moved carefully to avoid neck injury and the movement of the fractured spine may need several helpers.

DEFINITIVE MANAGEMENT

- *Reduction*: Reduce
- *Retention*: Hold
- *Rehabilitation*: Move.

Is there any immediate complication? Wound closure?

Getting a satisfactory wound closure is a major step to get a good result. Skin is considered as the best dressing. But, great care and judgment must be applied before wound closure. Premature closure may be needed to both ischemia and infection. 6 hours is the "golden period", after that the bacteria will multiply and wound infection may occur.

External fixator is the preferred method of skeletal stabilization for open fractures. Since the orthopedic fraternity is definitely moving toward a closed interlocking nail, more and more wounds are closed after debridement. A clean incised wound may be closed even if it is several hours late. But a badly contaminated wound with much necrotic tissue may be left unclosed.

A proper debridement of all necrotic tissue should be done. But, all viable tissue should be preserved. Fasciotomy may be done, if there is suspected compartment syndrome. Bony fragment with soft tissue attachment should be preserved.

Wound may be closed by skin apposition or split skin grafting. All exposed tendons and articular cartilage should be covered. If primary closure is not obtained, delayed secondary closure should be done.

Ischemia of the Limb

If there is an ischemia or suspected ischemia, urgent intervention is needed. If the fracture is not reduced, gentle reduction by manipulation or open reduction may improve vascularity.

Will reduction be necessary?
As far as possible, all fractures should be reduced. Reduction may be needed to avoid:
- Malunion
- Cosmetic impairment
- Nonunion and delayed union
- Soft tissue interposition.

Malunion in the plane of movement of the joint may be accepted. This is seen in the acceptance of extension component of supracondylar fracture humerus in children, but not accepted in the medial tilt, which may lead to gunstock deformity.

In femur, shaft fracture in children bayonet of apposition is accepted but angulation may not be acceptable. Even though in humerus, a little malposition is accepted; in the present state of knowledge, no malposition at all is accepted in fracture of BBs forearm.

How will reduction be achieved?
Closed reduction
Manipulation: Even though for Colles' fracture, anesthesia is not sought in every case, as a rule manipulation, may be always ideal under anesthesia. Even though surgery is the rule now, a malposition like a dislocated ankle has to be reduced initially since a displaced portion can lead to severe soft tissue compromise and may contraindicate an open-reduction later.

Traction: The traction method of definitive management of fractures is becoming obsolete. But even now before a closed interlocking nail is carried out for a fracture shaft of femur, a preliminary skeletal traction either upper tibial or lower tibial (if it is a intercondylar supracondylar fracture femur) traction is given. A traction given routinely may be a fixed femoral traction in young children, even though internal fixation using elastic nails and other implants is more resorted to even in these fractures.

Open reduction internal fixation (ORIF): Operative intervention is the most preferred and used method for attaining reduction at present. The risks such as further soft tissue damage, periosteal stripping, and the ever present danger of infection are there, precaution and care has considerably reduced these risks and surgery is embarked upon almost in all cases. Indications are:
- Close manipulative reduction has not achieved the desired position.
- When there is a fracture of necessity (a fracture which needs open reduction such as Galeazzi, Monteggia, intra-articular fractures such as talus, patella, etc.).
- A close manipulative reduction and fixation (e.g., in the case of fracture of neck of femur) does not involve opening the fracture site.
- Sometimes, an open reduction may not involve fixation like in radiocapitellar dislocation.

How will position be maintained?
If the reduced fracture is inherently unstable to hold the fracture, some form of splintage is necessary. Splintage can be an external or internal.

External fixation
- *Splintage*: The most commonly used external splintage is plaster of Paris. Other newer splintage such as the scotch casts are also in use. Plaster of Paris [Gypsum plaster] is produced by heating gypsum to about 300°F (150°C). $CaSO_4 \cdot 2H_2O + heat \rightarrow CaSO_4 \cdot 0.5H_2O + 1.5H_2O$ (released as steam) is cheap, easily available, fairly strong, versatile, and easy to apply. It absorbs secretions to certain extent. But they are rather heavy, warm, unyielding, and may lead to pressure effects. Ischemia and septicemia are catastrophic complications. But the advantages outweigh the disadvantages. The newer Scotchcast synthetic casting materials are composed of knitted fiberglass fabric impregnated with a water-activated polyurethane resin. In its unhardened state, the resin contains a very low volatility form of diisocyanate, commonly known as MDI.
- *Traction*: It may be used to achieve and maintain reduction of fracture.

This can be either skeletal traction or skin traction. This can also be a fixed traction or balanced traction.

Skin traction is given in synovitis of the hip of the knee. The disadvantages of skin traction are seen when the skin condition is not good. They may also lead to nerve involvement rarely.

Skeletal traction is routinely used and they can be upper tibial, lower femoral, lower tibial, or skull tractions. Skin tract infection is a complication.

A fixed traction is given in association with a Thomas splint occasion.

A balanced traction is when the weight attached is balanced by the weight of the patient. Since the present goal of the orthopedic management is rehabilitation by movement, any treatment option confining the patient to his bed is not acceptable.

Internal fixation
Almost all fractures are reduced by open reduction and internal fixation nowadays.

The advantages are:
- Accurate reduction
- Maintenance of position
- Rehabilitation
- Early union
- Diminished hospital time.

The disadvantages are:
- Infection
- Inadequate fixation
- Subsequent surgery to remove the implant
- Delayed mobilization in nonoptimum surgery.

Indications of internal fixation:
- External fixation inadequate
- Long period of immobilization is not desirable
- Early mobilization
- Polytrauma.

Hybrid fixation: In certain fraction, a combination of internal and external fixation may be used. These types of fixations are called hybrid fixation.

Internal fixation devices:
- *Plates*:
  - Dynamic compression plates
  - Locking compression plates
  - Reconstruction plates.
- *Screws*:
  - Cortical screws
  - Cancellous screws
  - Nails.
- *Rush nails*:
  - Küntscher nails
  - Interlocking nails
  - Wires.
- Kirschner wires.

How long should the fracture be held?
- A long bone may need at least 12 weeks to unite. An easy way to remember is 100 days ± 20 days.
- Cancellous bone may need about 6–8 weeks.
- In children < 12 years, this can be halved.
- In children < 2 years, this can again be halved.
- In a neonate, a femur may unite in 1–2 weeks.

Rehabilitation
- Life is movement and movement is life.
- Mobilizing the patient is the ultimate goal of orthopedic management. If the rehabilitation part is not looked upon, the end result may not be satisfactory.

COMPLICATIONS

Immediate Complications

Hemorrhage

In an era of high-velocity injuries, multiple fractures are the dictum now. A thorough examination may reveal undetected fractures. Polytrauma can produce hemorrhage from several sites. Scalp and face bleeding has to be addressed immediately in the triage or during primary assessment itself. A fracture of femur may have about 500 mL of blood loss. This may not be the only reason for a state of shock.

Injury to Important Organs

In any case of polytrauma, unexplained shock should alert as to an associated soft tissue injury and organ trauma. The important organs injured in association with fractures are the bladder and digestive system in a pelvis fracture and the spleen and the liver in association with the spine and rib fracture. Missing such injuries can lead to unsalvageable clinical situations.

Neurovascular Injury

The term complicated fracture is used to describe damage to important structures in association with the fractures. Time and time again, a lapse in proper and thorough clinical examination of the circulation and neurology is repeated. Even though compartment syndrome can coexist with the presence of distal pulsations, an absent distal pulsation is always a loud and ominous sign. In certain areas like the upper third leg and the notorious elbow fractures, the compartment syndrome should always be ruled out.

Anatomical knowledge will help us to identify the nerves injured in individual fractures and dislocations. Axillary nerve in shoulder dislocation and neck of humerus fractures, radial nerve in distal third humerus fractures, anterior interosseous nerve in supracondylar fractures humerus, posterior interosseous nerve in Monteggia, ulnar nerve in Galeazzi, medial nerve in Colles', sciatic nerve in hip dislocations, and peroneal nerve in neck of fibula are some of the classical associations. If there was activity in the muscles supplied by the nerve and then later neurological involvement is seen, a neurapraxia is suspected and recovery is expected. Usually, only open injury leads to neurotmesis and in such situations, an exploration is warranted.

Skin Loss or Damage

In degloving injuries, a distally based skin flap will result in loss of the protective cover. In the palm of the hand and sole of the feet, the lost cover can never be adequately replaced. Free muscle pedicle graft has been provided as an answer in almost all situations of loss of cover. So, plastic surgery support is imperative in such situation **(Fig. 18)**.

Early Complications

Local Complication

Skin and soft tissue necrosis: As mentioned before, in a distally based flap following a degloving injury, even though the skin will look viable initially,

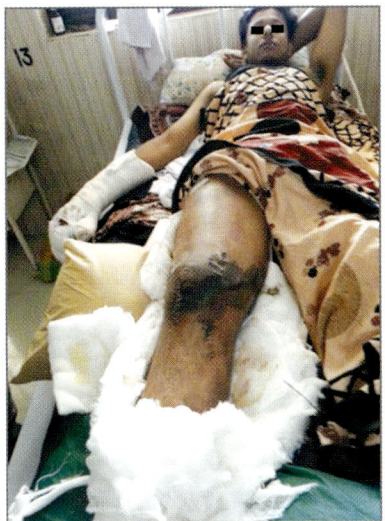

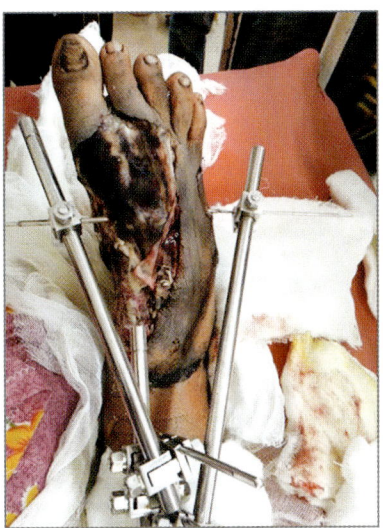

Fig. 18: Skin necrosis.

Fig. 19: Skin and soft tissue necrosis.

ischemia, gangrene, and sloughing may occur. So, a careful guarded approach is very essential in a distally based flap. Thorough debridement and primary grafting or after granulating, the surface formed will provide satisfactory results. Except over cartilage and bare tendon, the split skin graft and flaps are possible **(Fig. 19)**.

Ischemia from vascular damage or external pressure: Loss of distal pulsation, comparative decrease in the temperature, or even cold limb will warn us and a Doppler study will fairly help us to diagnose a vascular injury. The cardiovascular surgeons and the plastic surgeons will help us in revascularization.

Sometimes, a plaster can lead to external constrictions. This is especially true in the case of primary cast applications. All constricting or encircling structures have to be removed. Look for pain, pulselessness, paralysis, pallor, and plum-colored extremities.

Volkmann's ischemic contracture (VIC) is classically seen in the forearm as a result of elbow supracondylar fractures. The peculiar anatomy of the upper limb may also contribute to a compartment syndrome in the upper limb **(Fig. 20)**. Note the anterior interosseous artery is an end artery supplying the deepest muscles, flexor digitorum profundus, and flexor pollicis longus. Stretch pain is ominous. Compartment syndrome leads to ischemia, necrosis, sequestration, fibrosis, and contracture of the muscle leading onto a fixed length phenomenon called VIC **(Figs. 21 to 24)**.

Treatment:
- Remove all external constrictions.
- If the fracture is not reduced, reduce it.

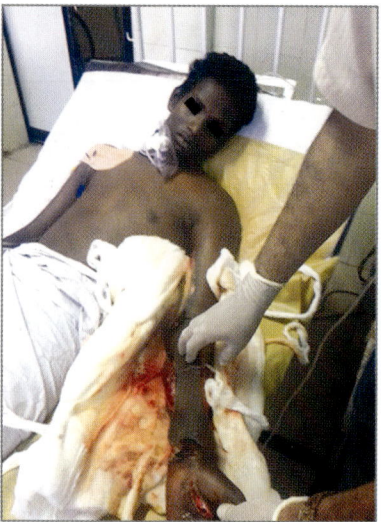

Fig. 20: Gangrene of left upper limb to rule out gas gangrene.

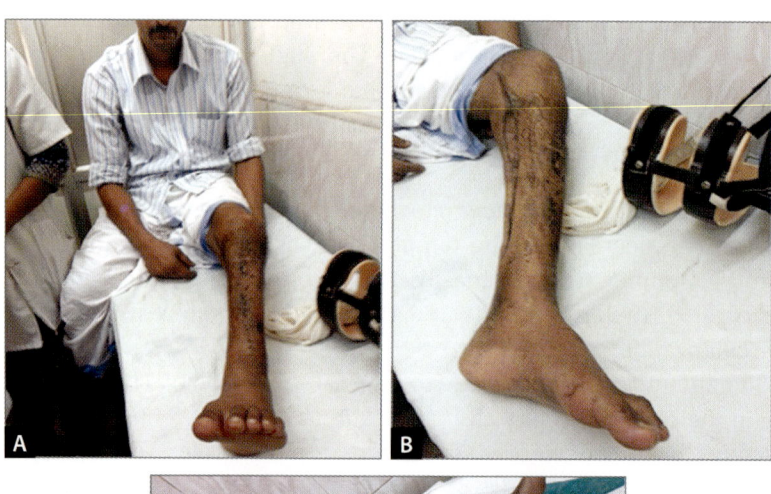

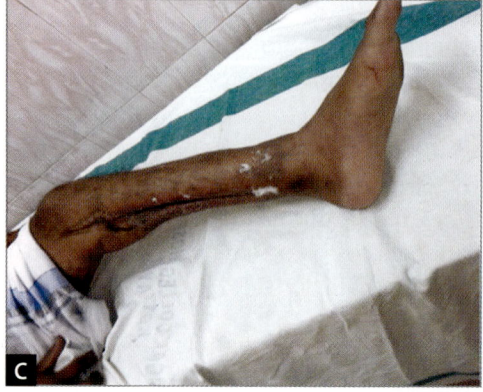

Figs. 21A to C: Postcompartment syndrome sequelae.

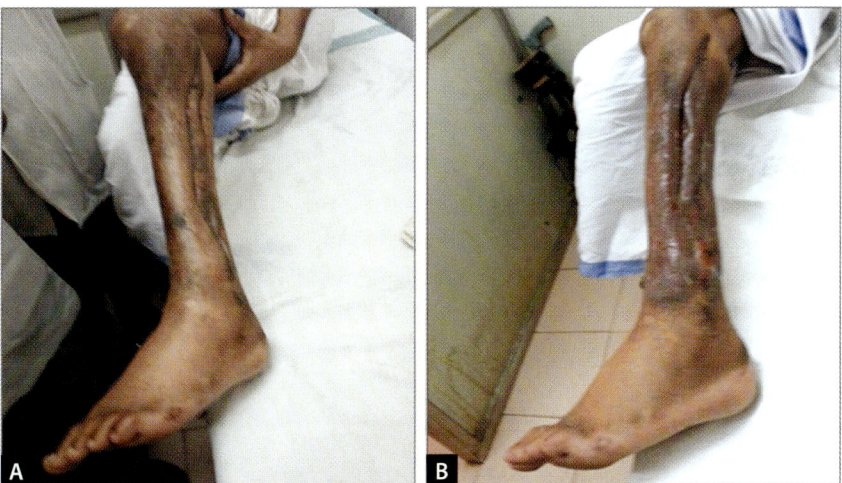

Figs. 22A and B: Compartment syndrome.

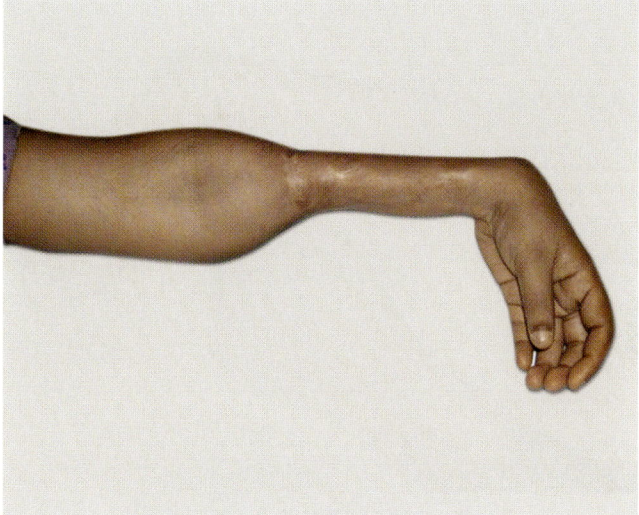

Fig. 23: Volkmann's ischemic contracture.

- If the fracture is reduced, avoid compromising positions such as acute flexion in elbow fractures.
- If the situation does not improve, do a fasciotomy.
- Except in open injuries, vascular damage is a rarity and exploration not routinely done. But if the above methods do not lead to satisfactory results, a vascular exploration itself may be warranted.

Pressure sore: When the plaster is applied, one of the most notorious areas of plaster sore is the heel. So, sufficient padding and care during application is very important to avoid this. The common peroneal nerve, the ulnar nerve, and the radial nerve also have to be protected.

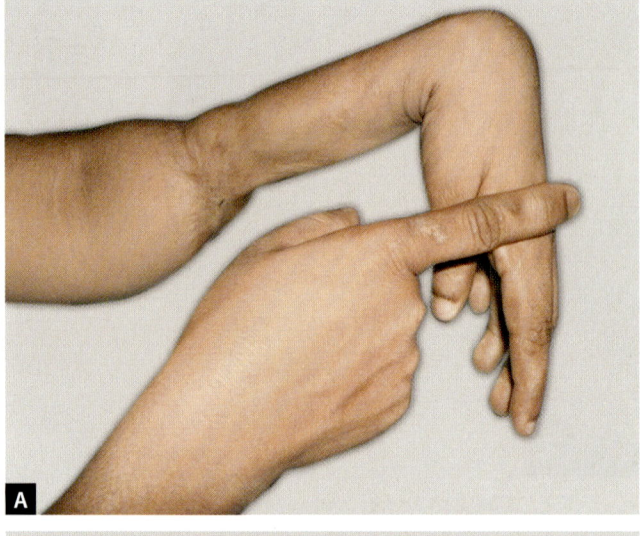
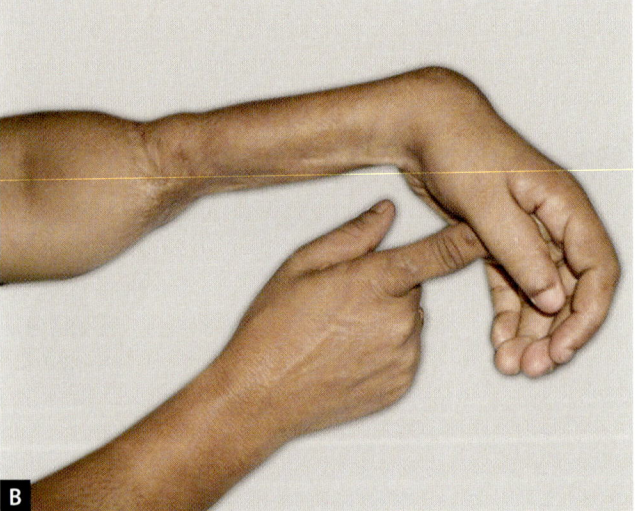

Figs. 24A and B: Volkmann's sign.

Infection and wound breakdown: Of course, the nemesis of the orthopedic surgeon is infection. It is obvious that this is extremely uncommon in closed injuries. But, it is very common in open injuries. The risk is many folds when there is contamination.

Infection inside a plaster is not very easy to detect. Extreme caution should be employed in such situations.

If a surgical wound shows external evidence of inflammation, then watch out for an infection. The antibiotics may need to be started or continued. The sutures may need to be removed. If there is pus, a pus culture and sensitivity may be done. Debridement of the wound can be done. If the implant cannot be left in situ due to persistence of infection, the surgeon may be forced to remove the implant.

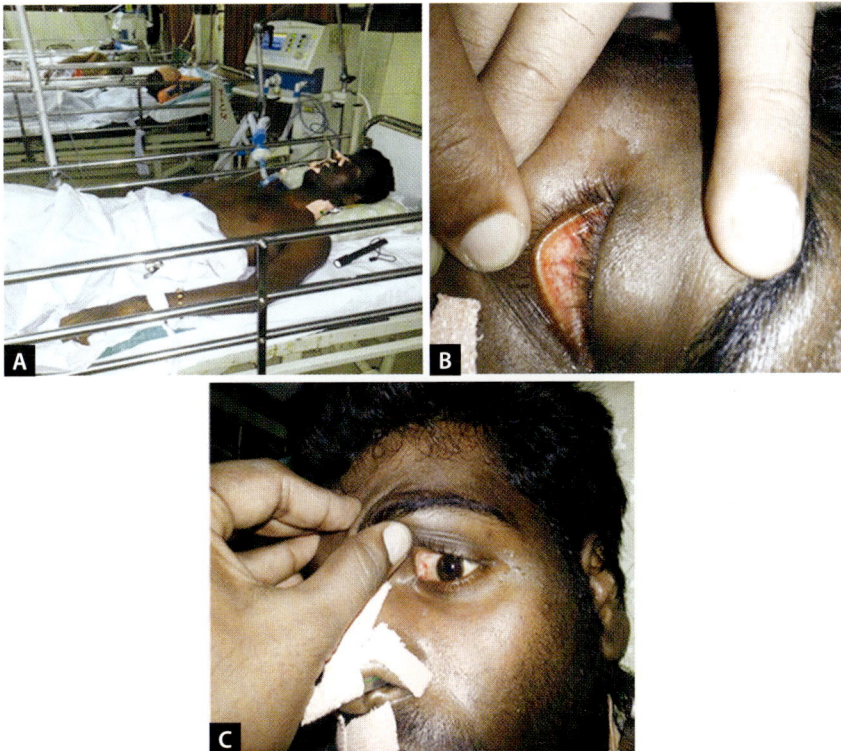

Figs. 25A to C: Fat embolism, *note* the conjunctival petechial hemorrhages.

Loss of position of fracture: When the initial edema subsides, almost all fractures are displaced in plaster. Colles' fracture is the most vulnerable and precarious around day 10. So, an X-ray is warranted at this time to avoid malunion. After 2 weeks, the fracture will be stuck and remanipulation will be difficult.

General Complications
- Fat embolism
- Crush syndrome.

Gurd's Criteria for the Diagnosis of Fat Embolism Syndrome
Major criteria:
- Axillary or subconjunctival petechiae **(Figs. 25A to C)**
- Hypoxemia (PaO$_2$ < 60 mm Hg)
- Central nervous system depression disproportionate to hypoxemia
- Pulmonary edema.

Minor criteria:
- Tachycardia (more than 110 beats per minute)
- Pyrexia (temperature higher than 38.5°C)

- Emboli present in retina on funduscopic examination
- Fat present in urine
- Sudden unexplainable drop in hematocrit or platelet values
- Increasing erythrocyte sedimentation rate
- Fat globules present in the sputum.

Late Complication
- Malunion **(Figs. 26 to 28)**
- Delayed union and nonunion.

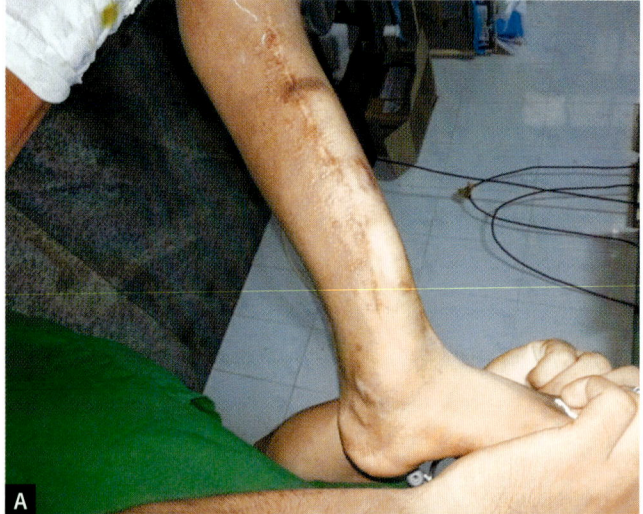

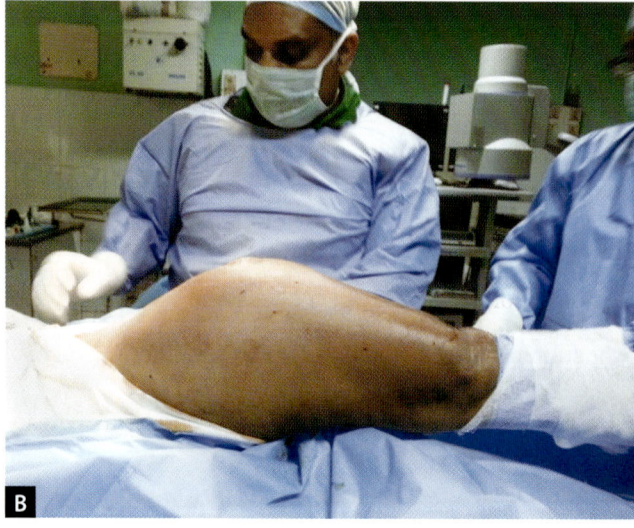

Figs. 26A and B: Malunited fracture.

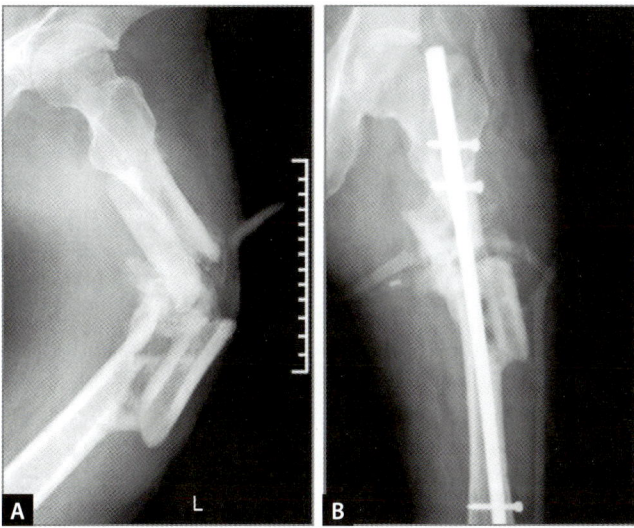

Figs. 27A and B: Malunited fracture: (A) Reduced; (B) Fixed.

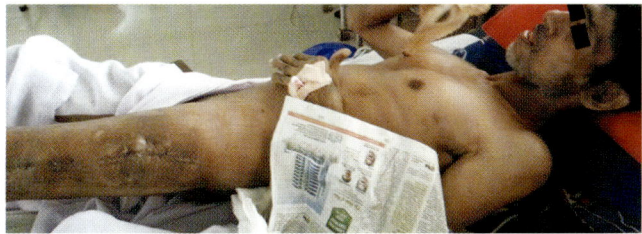

Fig. 28: Patient after reduction of malunited femur fracture.

Nonunion

Nonunion can be defined as a state of the fracture where the biological reparative process has come to a standstill clinically characterized by painless abnormal mobility and radiologically characterized by gap sclerosis of the bone ends and obliteration of medullary cavity.

Causes of nonunion:
- Inadequate hematoma (open)
- Infection
- Insufficient blood supply
- Interposition of soft tissue
- Intact fellow bone
- Insecurely fixed
- Improper immobilization
- Improper contact
- Ill-advised open reduction
- Impatient surgeon
- Impossible patient

- Immunocompromised (AIDS and diabetes)
- Irradiated bone.

Nonunions are classified into two types according to the viability of the ends of the fragments.

In the first type, the nonunion is hypervascular (hypertrophic) or viable and is capable of biological reaction.

The second type of nonunion is classified as avascular (atrophic) or inert and is not capable of uniting without intervention.

Types of nonunions:
Hypervascular **(Figs. 29A to C)**:
- Elephant foot nonunion
- Horse hoof nonunion
- Oligotrophic nonunion.

Hypovascular **(Fig. 30)**:
- Torsion wedge nonunions
- Comminution wedge

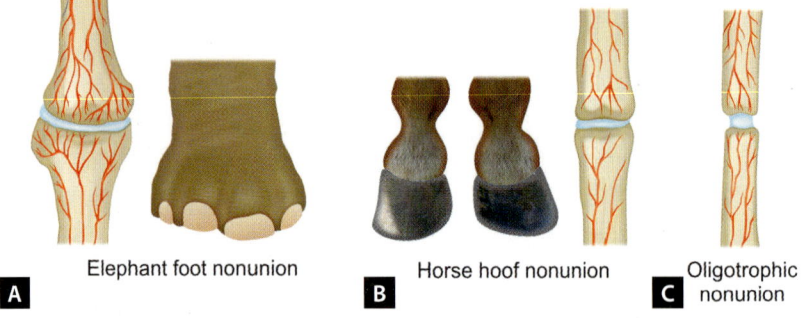

Figs. 29A to C: Types of hypervascular nonunions.

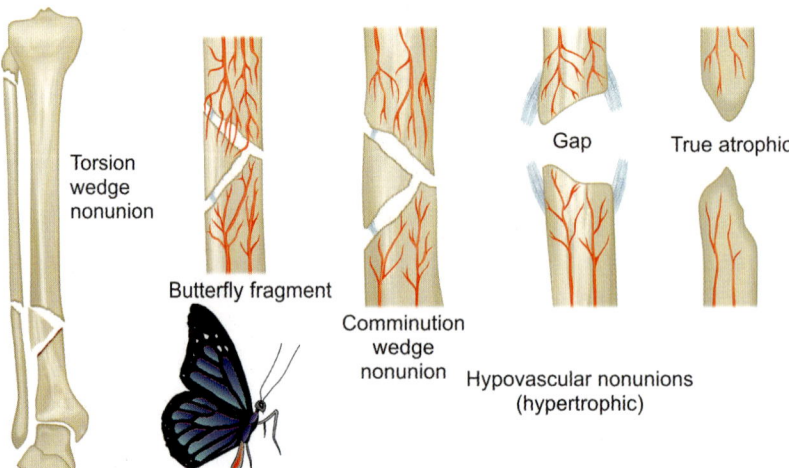

Fig. 30: Types of hypovascular nonunions.

- Gap
- True atrophic.

Treatment of nonunion consists of rigid fixation bone grafting **(Figs. 31 and 32)** and Ilizarov's method of osteosynthesis and bone transport.

Bone grafts can be taken from ilium, greater trochanter, proximal metaphysis tibia, lower radius, olecranon, and excised femoral head.

The grafts can be autogenous/autografts in same person. This can be either cancellous grafts or cortical grafts. Allografts/homografts are taken from the same species, whereas xenografts are taken from another species.

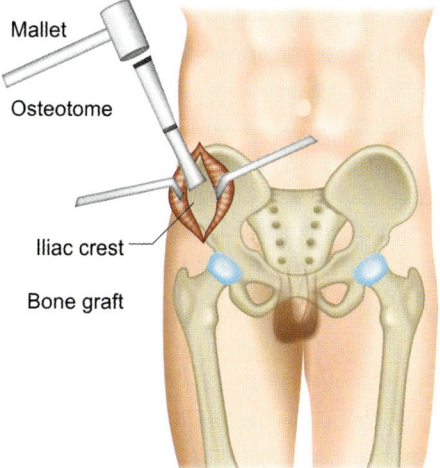

Fig. 31: Iliac crest bone grafting.

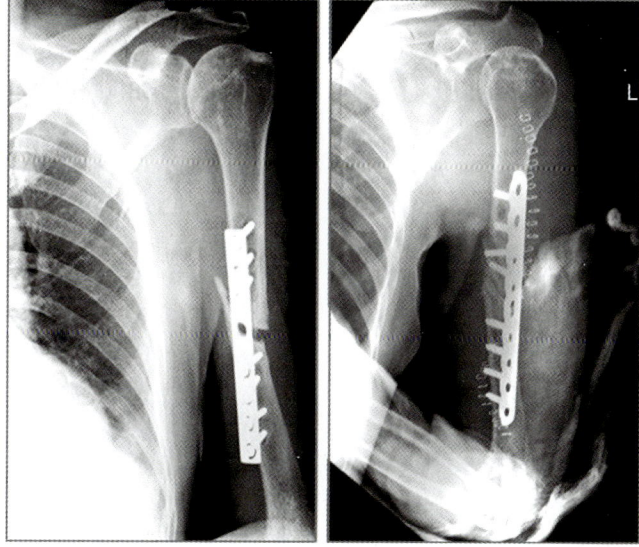

Fig. 32: Failure of internal fixation.

Bone grafts act by osteoinductive (stimulate), osteoconductive (scaffold), stimulation of osteoprogenitor cells in graft bed, partly by cells surviving on host surface, and also by bone morphogenic protein.

Joint Stiffness
Joint stiffness is always associated with fractures and will be considerable when the fracture is very close to the joint. In supracondylar fracture, there will be average 10° of flexion and extension loss of the elbow. Children will have less stiffness, whereas older people have more stiffness. Shoulder is one joint, which is considerably hampered by stiffness. In joints, which are prone to stiffness, early mobilization is a must.

Sudeck's Osteodystrophy
The vicious triad in fractures is diethetic (inherently fearful personality), sympathetic overactivity, and pain due to the fracture. This produces pain and stiffness of the extremity called by several names. Sudeck's osteodystrophy, Leriche post-traumatic dystrophy, and reflex sympathetic dystrophy (Lankford) are synonyms. The recent terminology is complex regional pain syndrome.

Compensation Neurosis
Some people suffer from this.

FRACTURES AND DISLOCATIONS OF SPINE
Fracture Spine
Early management of spine injury:
- *Cervical spine*:
    - Computed tomography (CT)
    - Radiology
    - Treatment.
- *Thoracolumbar injury*:
    - CT
    - Management.
- Lumbar and sacral injury.
- Fracture sacrum coccyx.

Introduction
The spine essentially has an intervertebral disk, which represents a secondary cartilaginous joint and two posterolateral synovial articulations; the whole is connected by multiple ligaments. The cervical, dorsal, lumbar, and sacral vertebrae have different characteristics. Each vertebrae of the above group may also be different.

Three-column Concept of Spine by Francis Denis
The spine is divided into anterior, middle, and posterior columns.

Different Cervical Vertebrae
In the cervical region, the facet joints are arranged in a horizontal plane, which makes it very susceptible to dislocations and fracture dislocations. In the dorsal spine, the facet joint is arranged in a coronal plane, or more specifically, intermediate plane. In the lumbar spine, they lie in the parasagittal plane. The ribs add to the stability of the dorsal spine and the spine here is more stable.

The significance of spinal injury depends upon displacement and stability. The cervical canal is large and can accommodate significant displacement without code injury. Since this spinal cord ends at the level of L1 and the cauda equina occupies distally, fracture of the lumbar vertebrae also accommodates some amount of displacement. However, this is not seen at the level of L1 and above where the spinal cord is most vulnerable. A detailed and careful clinical and radiological examination is essential.

Emergency Management of Suspected Spinal Injury
Any patient with suspected spinal injuries needs to be handled and transported with utmost care and caution to avoid unnecessary cord damage. Patient who is unconscious or having head injury or undergoes influence of alcohol is quite vulnerable. Maximum expertise needs to be sorted for transportation and the patient should be in one piece. The cervical spine should be protected, collar applied, if available, and the other part of spine also should be guarded.

Cervical Spine Injury
Injuries to the cervical spine can be flexion injuries or extension injuries. Usual injuries are flexion injuries. In the "whiplash" injury, there is hyperextension followed by flexion. There is a characteristic nipping of the cervical cord leading onto a central cord syndrome. The telltale evidence in cervical spine injuries are the lacerations or abrasions or injuries on the face or scalp or forehead. In orofaciomaxillary injuries, cervical spine injuries should be ruled out. Teardrop fracture always is an evidence of cervical spine injury. More serious injuries lead to unifacetal or bifacetal dislocations.

Clinical Features
In unconscious patients, those with head injuries and those under the influence of alcohol, red alert should be maintained.

In conscious patient, pain tenderness over the cervical region and neurological deficit must be elicited.

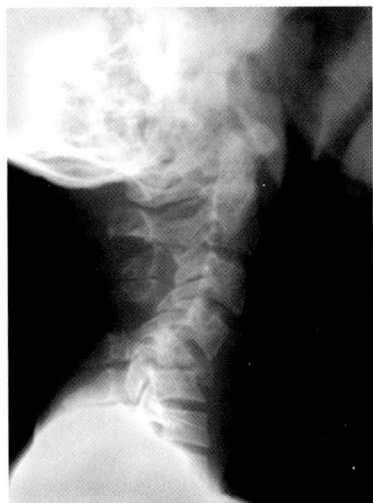

Fig. 33: Fracture dislocation of cervical spine.

Diagnosis

Radiology

X-ray should be taken **(Fig. 33)**. The views are:
- Anteroposterior (AP) view
- Lateral view
- Shoulder pull-down view
- Open mouth view.

A vertebra displaced less than 50% means a unifacetal dislocation and more than 50% means a bifacetal dislocation. Soft tissue anterior to the third cervical vertebrae, if more the 5–7 mm, should alert one to rule out a cervical spine injury.

At last, burst fractures (Jefferson's fractures), odontoid fractures, and lamina fracture of second cervical vertebrae or spondylolisthesis C23 (Hangman's fracture) may all need CT scans for making a proper diagnosis.

Treatment

In stable injuries, hard collar or Philadelphia collar has to be applied for 6 weeks or more. Unstable injuries and burst fractures may need skull traction followed by open reduction and stabilization **(Fig. 34)**.

Traumatic Paraplegia

- Cervical injuries
- Thoracic and thoracolumbar injuries
- Diagnosis of neurological conditions
- Management.

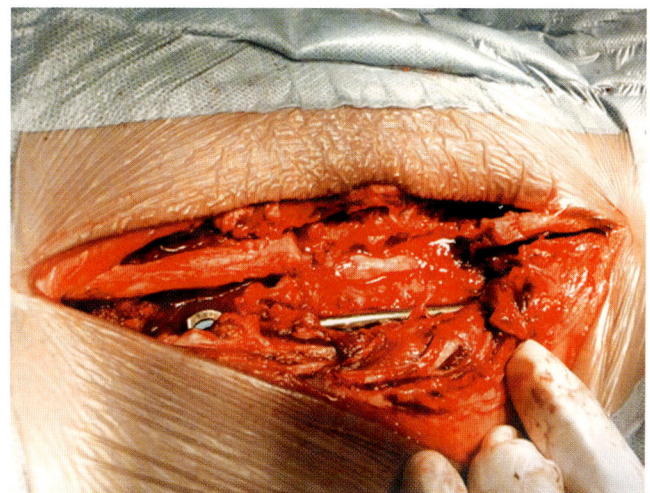

Fig. 34: Moss–Miami posterior stabilization of dorsolumbar spine fracture.

FRACTURES OF PELVIS (FIGS. 35A TO E)
- Stability
- Management
- Complications:
  - Hemorrhage
  - Bladder–urethra injury
  - Rectum–vagina injury
  - Sciatic nerve palsy
  - Diaphragm rupture.

Fracture Dislocation Hip (Figs. 36A to C)

The three types of hip dislocations are:
1. Posterior
2. Anterior
3. Central.

Posterior dislocations outnumber anterior dislocations by approximately three to one.

The typical mechanism for a posterior dislocation is an accident in which the occupant's knee strikes the dashboard with the knee and hip flexed.

Knee injuries including posterior dislocation, cruciate injury, and patellar fractures are most common.

In a posterior dislocation, the leg is flexed, adducted, and internally rotated.

Anterior dislocations present with the extremity externally rotated with varied amounts of flexion and abduction.

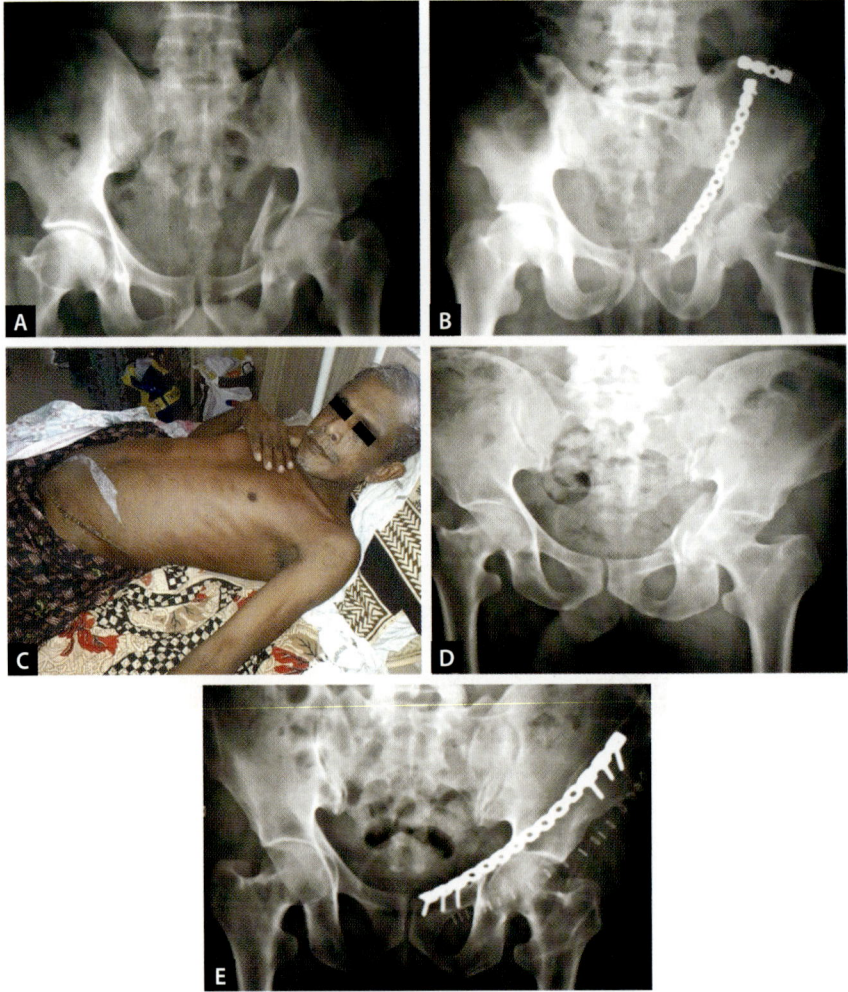

Figs. 35A to E: Central fracture dislocation fixed with plate and screws.

The less common anterior dislocations are the result of hyperabduction and extension. Patients presenting with a hip dislocation or femoral head fracture should be presumed to have multiple injuries **(Figs. 37 and 38)**.

Techniques for reduction of posterior dislocations are:
- Stimson
- Allis maneuver
- East Baltimore lift
- Bigelow's method.

Complications

- *Arthritis*: Osteoarthritis due to cartilage damage, retained fragments, or avascular necrosis (AVN)

Orthopedics

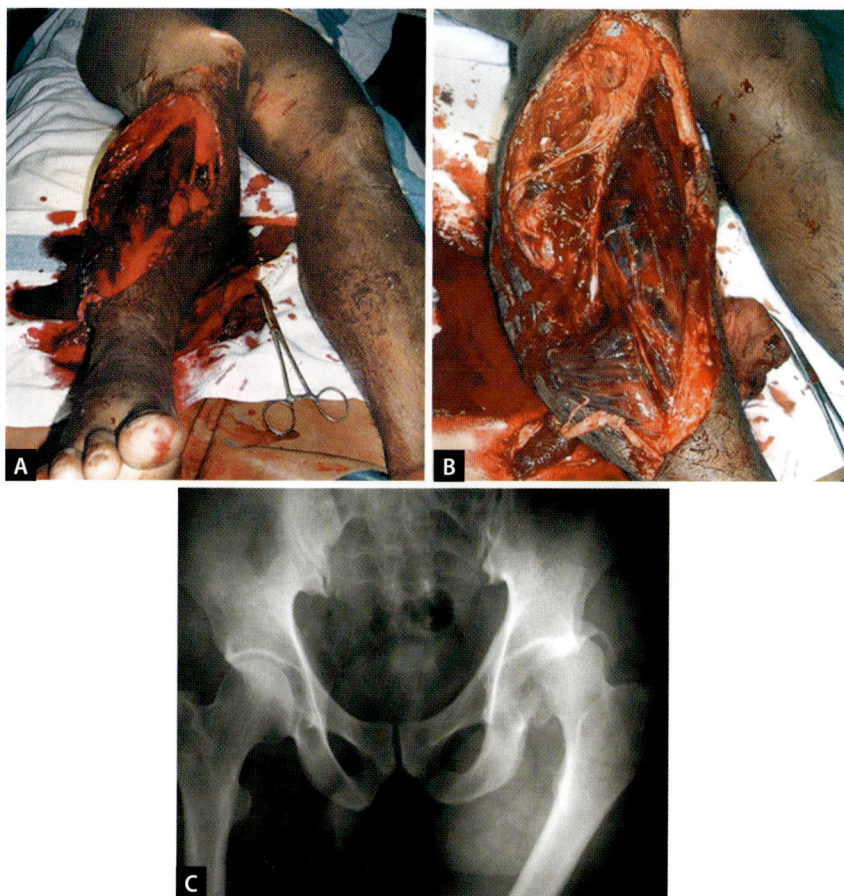

Figs. 36A to C: It is not the very obvious posterior tibial artery, which is important. The fracture dislocation of the hip is also important. *See* the Pipkin fracture of the femoral head.

- Sciatic nerve palsy
- Superior gluteal artery may be torn
- AVN 10% in PDH
- If treatment delayed by few hours, the AVN is 40%
- Myositis is uncommon complication.

Fracture Neck of Femur

Regarding fracture neck of the femur, the crucial aspect is the precarious blood supply, which causes complications. The blood supply is essentially a distally based one, the retinacular vessels from the ascending cervical and the lateral epiphyseal being the predominant supply. The proximally based foveal blood supply is insignificant. There are two arterial rings—(1) the subsynovial and (2) the extracapsular rings **(Fig. 39)**.

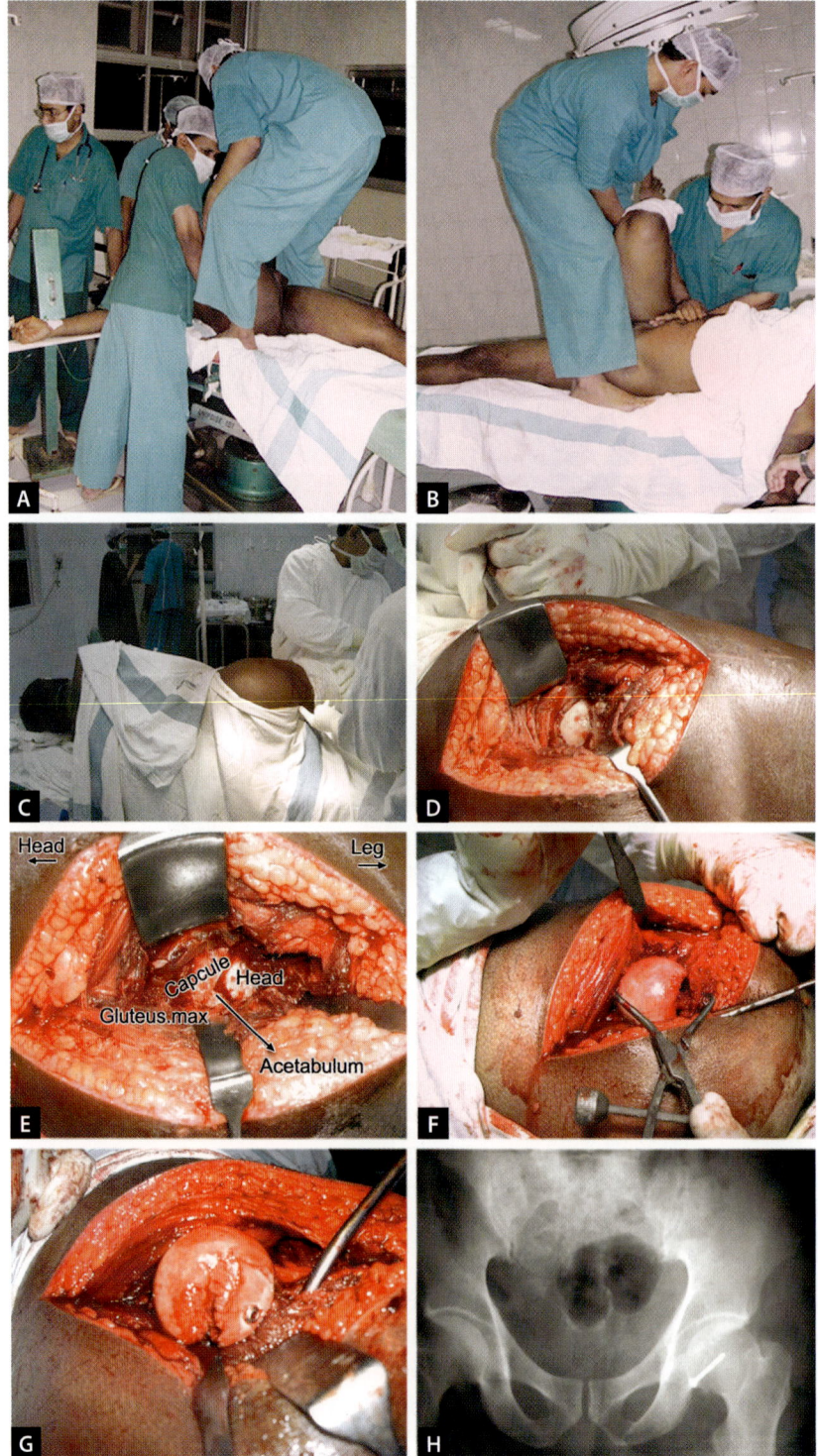

Figs. 37A to H: Close manipulatory reduction of a hip dislocation.

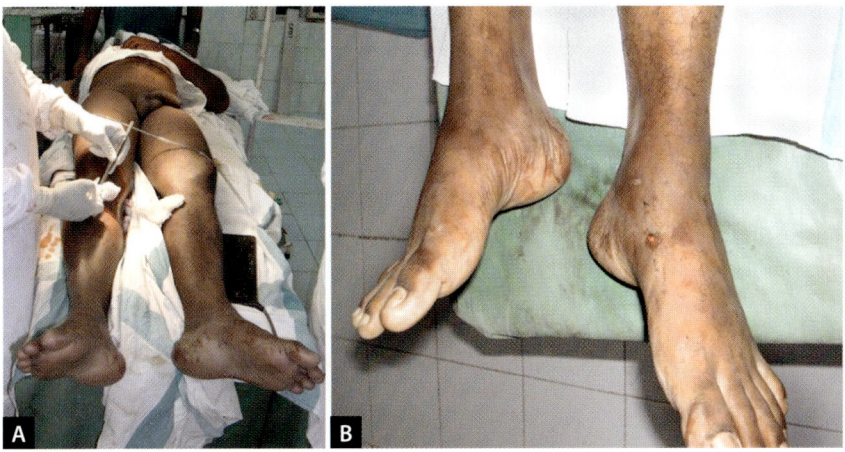

Figs. 38A and B: Postoperative pictures of reduction of the fracture dislocation of the hip.

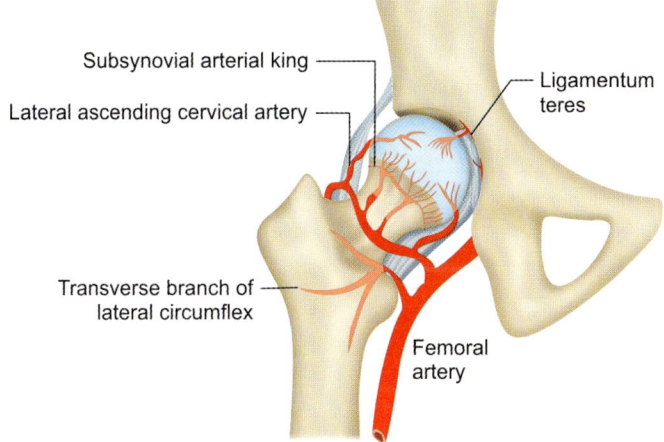

Fig. 39: Distally based blood supply of the femoral head.

The old classification of Pauwel's depends upon the angle which the fracture line makes with the horizontal—30°, 50°, and 70° **(Fig. 40)**.

The Trabecular Pattern of the Proximal Femur (Figs. 41 and 42)

- Primary tension
- Primary compression
- Secondary tension
- Secondary compression
- Trochanteric.

The classical Garden's staging depends upon the displacement of the fracture **(Figs. 43A to D)**:

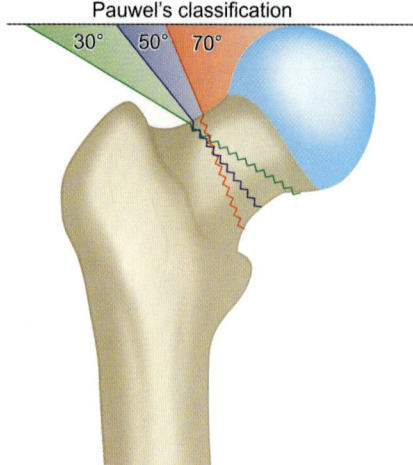

Fig. 40: Pauwels' classification of fracture neck of femur depending on the fracture line.

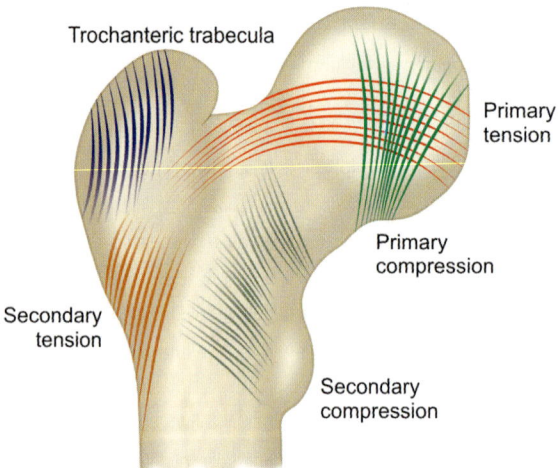

Fig. 41: Trabecular pattern of the proximal femur.

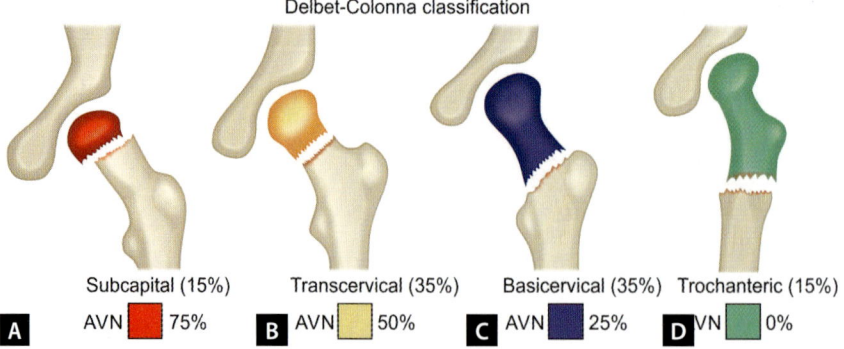

Figs. 42A to D: Different types of fractures of the proximal femur and the avascular necrosis associated.
(AVN: avascular necrosis)

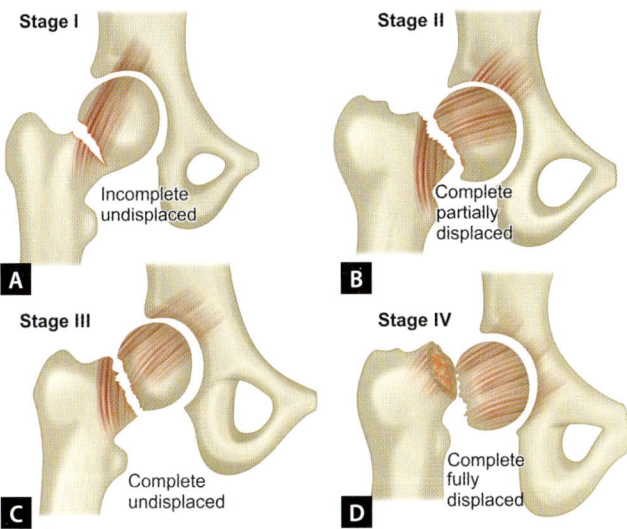

Figs. 43A to D: Garden's staging of fracture neck of femur.

- *Stage 1*: Incomplete (the trabeculae of the neck, the head, and the acetabulum are in alignment).
- *Stage 2*: Complete undisplaced (the neck and the head are not in alignment but the head and the acetabulum are in alignment).
- *Stage 3*: Complete partially displaced (the neck, head, and the acetabulum are not in alignment).
- *Stage 4*: Complete fully displaced (the neck and the head are not in alignment but the head is aligned with the acetabulum).

Causes of Nonunion (Fig. 44)

The distally based blood supply is a major factor for nonunion. The more displaced the fracture is, the higher will be the chance of nonunion. Pauwels' has already stated that in higher fracture angle, the shear stress will be more and so the nonunion will be more. In young adults, comminution will further complicate the issue. Older people with poor bone quality have lesser union. Hip tamponade due to hematoma will impede vascularity. Absence cambium layer of periosteum, chondrogenic factors in synovial fluid which inhibit callus formation, lack of hematoma formation by synovial fluid, washing away, and dilution of osteogenic factors will all lead to nonunion.

In children, a hip spica may suffice but osteosynthesis is the goal in all fracture neck of femur. After 65 years and now, since physiological age is considered 75 years, the head may be sacrificed and prosthetic replacement is done. If there is preexisting arthritis, total hip replacement may be opted.

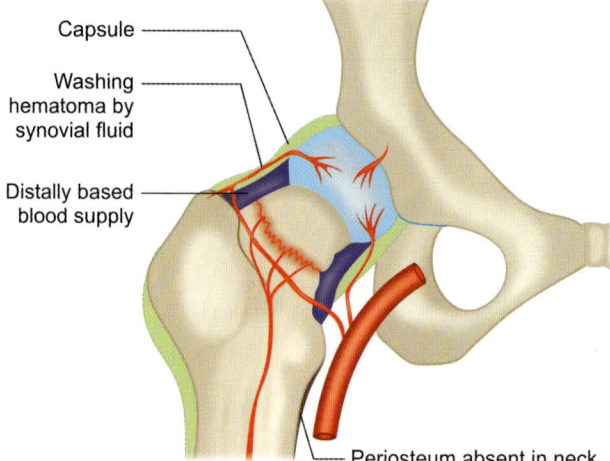

Fig. 44: Causes of nonunion of fracture neck of femur.

Extracapsular FNOF

These fractures occur in slightly younger patients when compared with fracture neck of femur. In trochanteric fractures, the rule is union and malunion to be precise. This is due to the cancellous bone of the metaphysis and good blood supply. But since there is malunion, there will be shortening and limping. Another problem in old age is the metabolic syndrome and encephalopathy, which follows dehydration and uremia. This may further be complicated by sacral source and other decubitus ulcers. So, a simple fall in a bathroom can lead to mortality. So, early stabilization using some internal fixation devices, such as the dynamic hip screws or the proximal femoral nail, has to be done **(Figs. 45 and 46)**.

Fracture Shaft of Femur

This is one of the most common types of fracture where considerable violence may be involved. Fractures can be subtrochanteric, upper third, middle third, or lower third. Neurovascular injury is uncommon. More than 500 mL blood loss is unlikely. If there is shock, think of other causes such as the blunt abdominal trauma **(Figs. 47A to C)**.

Management

In newborns to 6 months of age, a primary hip spica can be applied. Bryant's or Gallows traction or even a Pavlik harness can be considered.

From 6 months to 6 years, immediate or early spica may be applied. If the displacement is more than 2 cm, a skin or skeletal traction may be initially given. External fixators are reserved for open fractures.

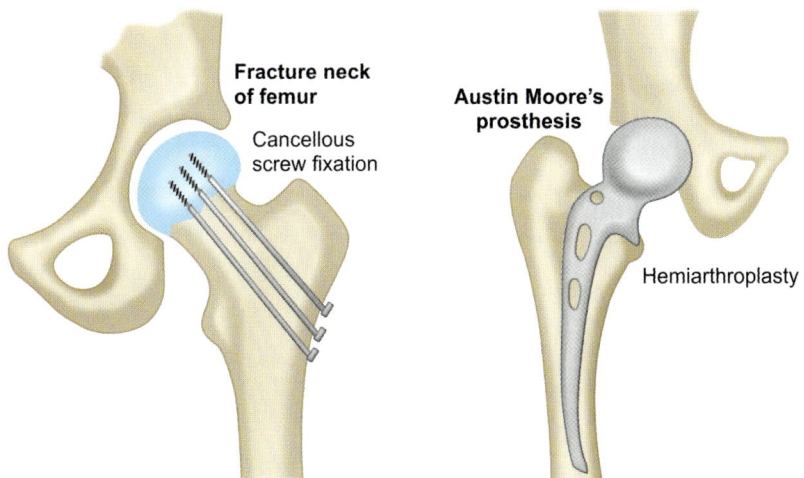

Fig. 45: Screw fixation (osteosynthesis) of fracture neck of femur and Austin Moore's prosthetic replacement.

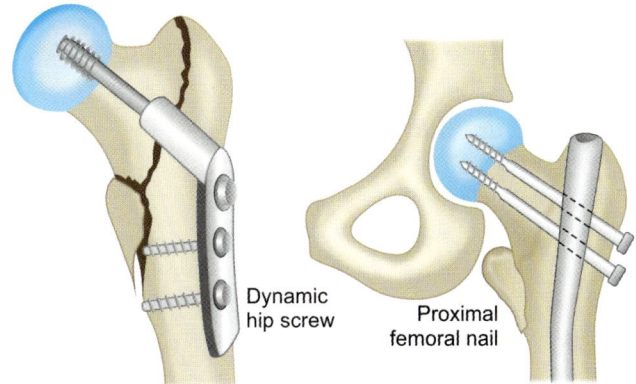

Fig. 46: Dynamic hip screw and proximal femoral nail fixation for trochanteric fractures.

From 6 to 11 years of age, treatment of fracture shaft of femur is highly controversial. There is a shift from conservative to surgical management. Intramedullary flexible rodding is getting popular. Locking plates also may be applied.

Patients with 12 years of age and above, the management is mainly surgical. If the epiphysis is closed, the ideal management is changed from open retrograde intramedullary clover-leaf Kuntscher nailing to closed antegrade intramedullary interlocking nails **(Fig. 48)**.

In supracondylar fractures of the femur the treatment options are a tip-locking interlocking nail **(Fig. 49)**, dynamic condylar screws, distal femoral locking plates, and intramedullary supracondylar nails. A Thomas splint is used for initial stabilization of fractures of the shaft of the femur.

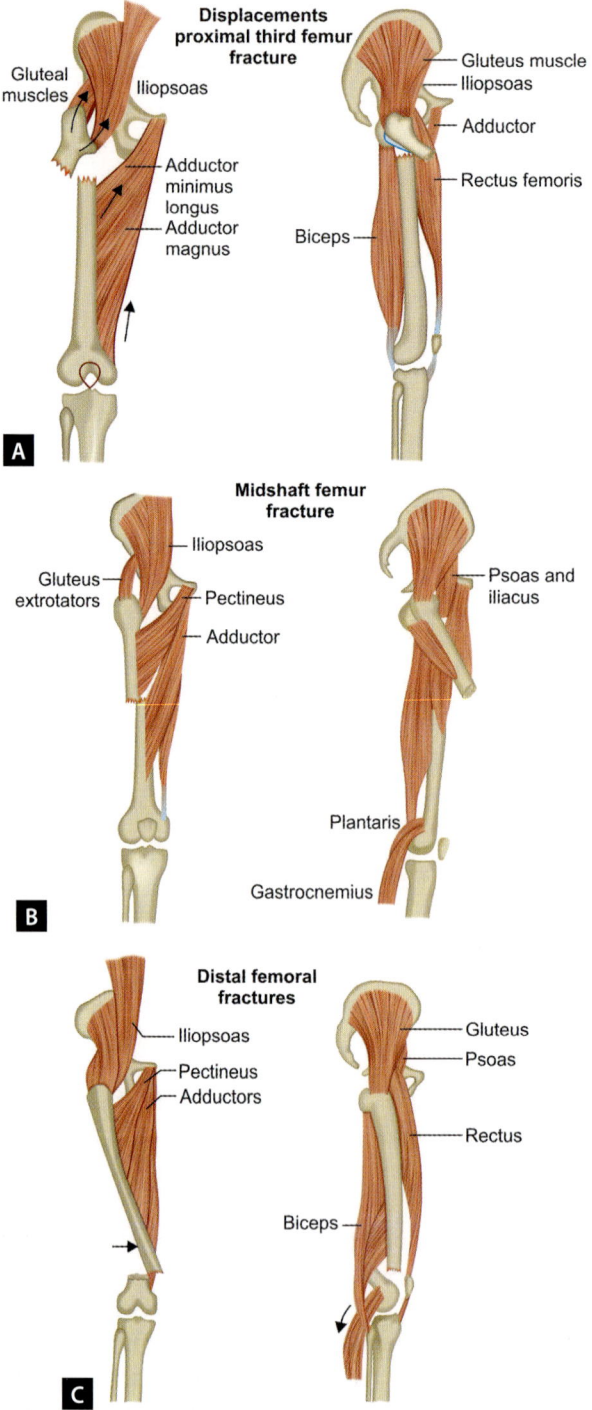

Figs. 47A to C: Displacements in different shaft of femoral fractures.

Orthopedics

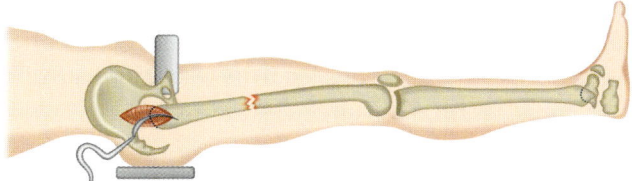

Fig. 48: Method of closed antegrade intramedullary interlocking nail.

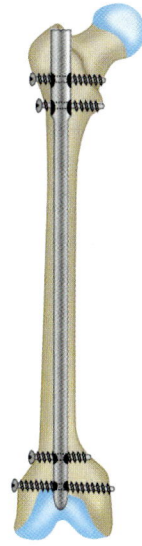

Fig. 49: Interlocking nail of femur.

PATELLA DISLOCATION

An acute dislocation of the patella is usually lateral and may be easily reduced. Sometimes, the knee may be flexed and the patella irreducible. Reduction is by manipulation. If not properly immobilized (3 weeks) initially, a recurrent dislocation of the patella may be a sequella.

Q Mechanism

It consists of the quadriceps muscle, quadriceps tendon, patella, patella tendon, and tibial tuberosity. Any disruption of this mechanism has to be repaired surgically.

Patella

Patella fractures may be the undisplaced fractures, displaced transverse fracture, lower pole patella fractures, upper pole patella fracture, comminuted patella fracture, and vertical fracture of patella. The tense hemarthrosis may be aspirated under sterile conditions and definitive management may be continued. The management options include conservative management for intact quadriceps mechanism, total patellectomy for comminuted fractures, superior or inferior patellectomy, tension band wiring for transverse fracture, and screw fixation for vertical fractures.

Ligaments and Menisci of the Knee

Knee is a Pandora's box with the collateral ligaments, cruciate ligament, and the menisci enclosed. The road traffic accidents and the sporting accidents frequently cause injury to these structures. They may cause significant disability due to the poor healing because of the poor vascularity. The tests employed in the diagnosis of the knee injuries are valgus and varus stress tests, anterior and posterior drawer, Lachman's test, McMurray test, Apley's grinding test, and various pivot shift and jerk tests **(Figs. 50 and 51)**.

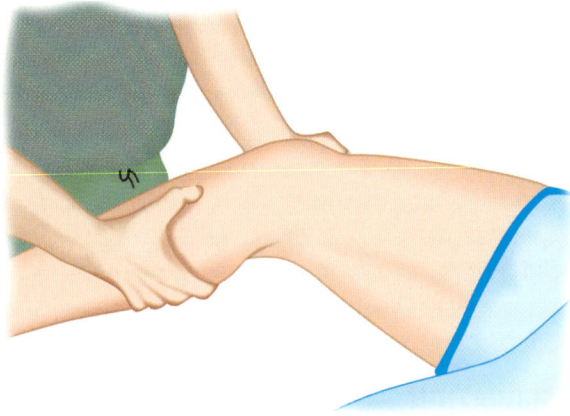

Fig. 50: Lachman's test.

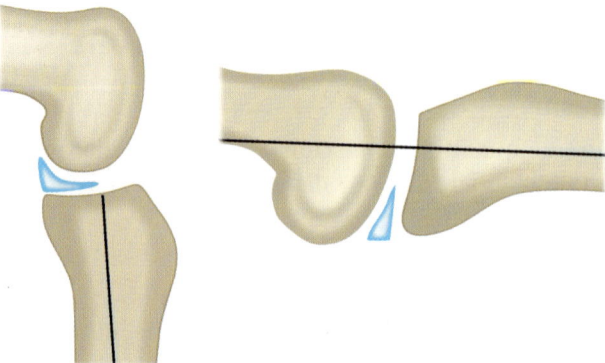

Fig. 51: The door-stop effect in Drawer's test makes Lachman the ideal test in cruciate injuries.

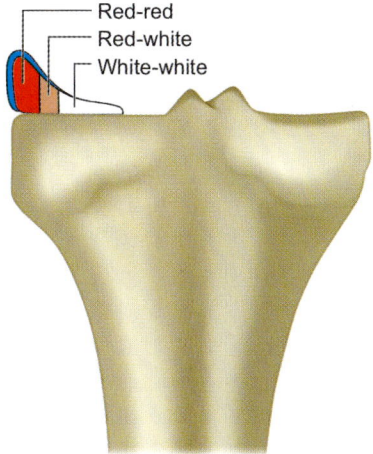

Fig. 52: The various zones of the meniscus.

Management

The collateral ligament mild injuries may be managed by plaster immobilization, but moderated severe injuries require surgical repairs. The cruciate ligaments usually need reconstruction either open or closed and may be done by using either bone-tendon-bone (BTB) graft or Hamstring graft. The BTB graft is taken from patella, patella tendon, and tibial tuberosity. The semitendinosus and gracilis tendons are taken for Hamstring graft. The arthroscopic method uses the medial and lateral portals and the large incisions are avoided.

Meniscal Injuries

The lateral meniscus forms a larger part of a small circle and medial meniscus forms the smaller part of a large circle. Miller, Warner, and Harner have divided the meniscus into three zones—(1) the red, (2) the red-white, and (3) the white-white zones depending upon the vascularity **(Fig. 52)**.

The major meniscal injuries are longitudinal, radial, oblique, peripheral, substance or horizontal, and flap tears **(Fig. 53)**. The longitudinal tear is otherwise called the bucket handle tear **(Fig. 54)**. The oblique tear is also called the parrot beak tear. The longitudinal tear has the worst prognosis and peripheral tear is the best prognosis.

Locking and giving way of the knee should warn us toward the possibility of a meniscal injury.

KNEE DISLOCATION

It can be anterior or posterior. Immediate reduction and reassessment of neurovascular status should be done. The preferred management is to

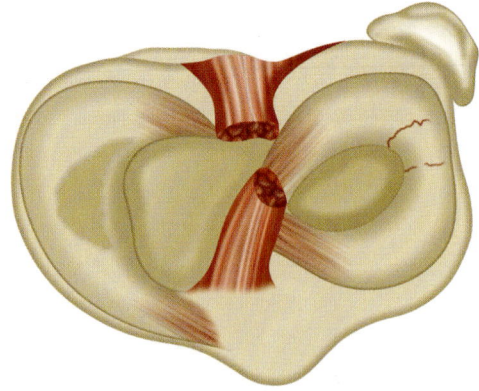

Fig. 53: Different meniscal injuries.

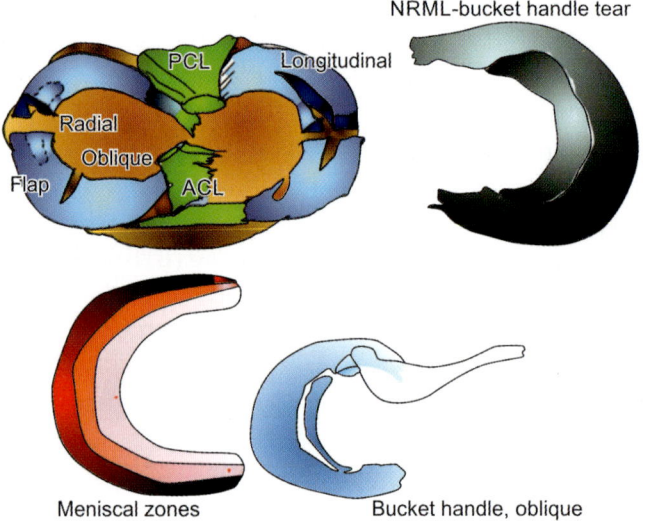

Fig. 54: Various meniscal injuries.

reduce the dislocation and opt for a conservative management. If there is internal derangement at 2 months, arthroscopic/open repair may be done.

TIBIA FRACTURE UPPER

Fractures Knee Tibia

The proximal tibial fractures are intra-articular fractures and surgery is an absolute necessity. Different types of tibial buttress plates and tibial-locking plates are available. Compartment syndrome should be ruled out in proximal tibial fractures. The injury may be a depressed fracture or a cleavage fracture. Physiotherapy and mobilization are absolutely necessary.

Fracture of Both Bones of Leg

One of the most common orthopedic injuries can be due to road traffic accidents, sports, or any trauma. The subcutaneous location makes this, especially vulnerable to compounding.

Management of Closed Injuries

Almost all both bone (BB) fractures are managed surgically now. Intramedullary closed interlocking nailing is the rule now. Plating of the tibia is becoming obsolete due to the preponderance for infection. Conservative managements such as closed manipulative reductions (CMRs) and slab followed by cast immobilizations are infrequent now.

Management of Open Injuries

All type I, type II, and even type IIIa/b are attempted interlocking nailing, if the soft tissue allows. The preferred skeletal stabilization of open fractures, i.e., the external fixators are reserved for extremely comminuted and type IIIc injuries. The wounds are managed preferably in cooperation and consultation with plastic surgeon. In certain situations, flap cover may be needed and in other situations, the orthopedic surgeon may be able to get away with a split skin grafting. In a mangled extremity, experience is important in judging—which limb can be salvaged and which requires amputation.

Early weight bearing will help in fracture healing. If you are using a single crutch for walking, it should be used on the side of the strong leg.

In an open fracture with multiple sinuses or gaps, the preferred method of management is distraction osteosynthesis using an Ilizarov ring external fixation.

ANKLE FOOT

Ligament Strains

The lateral ligament complex includes the anterior talofibular ligament, posterior talofibular ligament, calcaneofibular ligament, and lateral talocalcaneal ligament. The anterior talofibular ligament is most commonly injured. The cause is usually an inversion strain.

The ankle may be swollen. In severe injury, the ligament may be ruptured and surgical repair may be needed.

It is better to fracture than to sprain. Careful management of ligament injuries will prevent disability.

Simple strains are protected by strapping. Moderate injury needs a plaster immobilization and severe injuries need surgical repair.

Deltoid ligament injuries are rare.

RICE—Rest, Ice, Compression, Elevation is a management protocol.

Ankle Fractures

The ankle is formed by the lower end of the tibia, fibula, and the talus. The anterior tibiofibular ligament, the posterior tibiofibular ligament, the deltoid ligament, and the lateral ligament complex may be involved. The anterior tibial lip is called chaput tubercle and the posterior tibial lip is called Volkmann's triangle.

Figures 55A to C show the surgeons who contributed to the ankle fracture findings.

Lauge–Hansen's Classification (Fig. 56)

- Supination adduction injury **(Fig. 57)**
- Pronation abduction injury
- Supination external rotation injury **(Fig. 58)**
- Pronation external rotation injury **(Fig. 59)**
- Vertical compression injury.

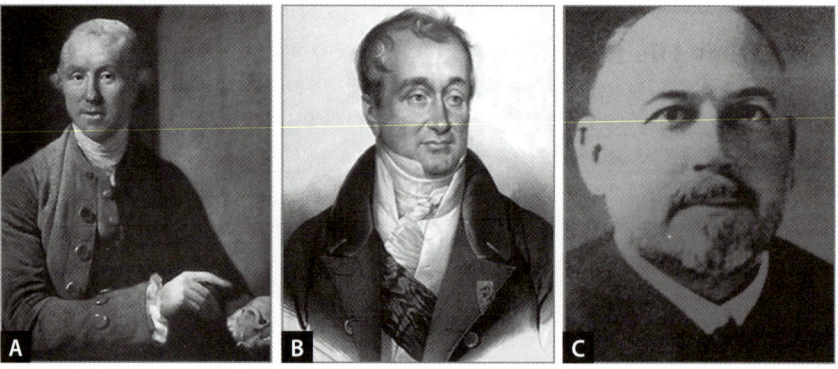

Figs. 55A to C: (A) Percivall Pott; (B) Baron Guillaume Dupuytren; (C) JF Cotton.

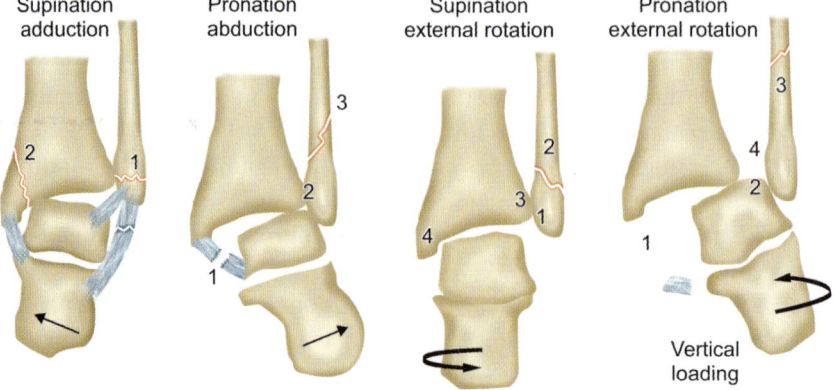

Fig. 56: Lauge–Hansen's classification.

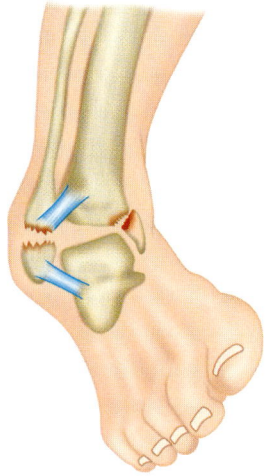

Fig. 57: Supination adduction injury.

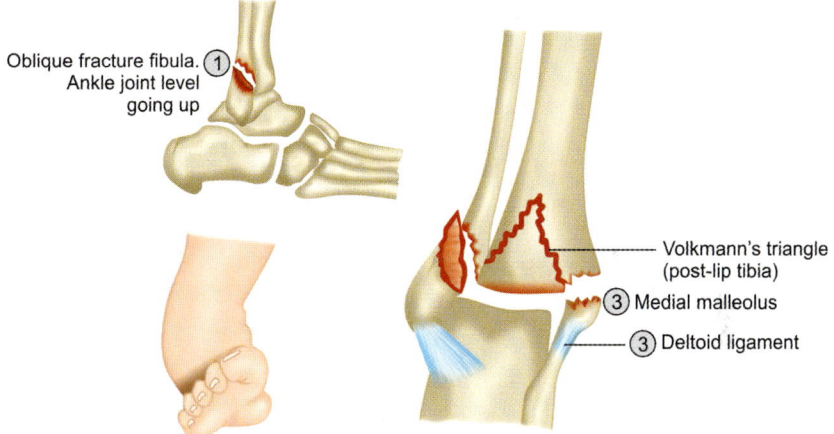

Fig. 58: Supination external rotation injury.

Danis–Weber Classification (Fig. 60)
- Infrasyndesmotic fibula fracture
- Trans-syndesmotic fibula fracture (supination external rotation injury)
- Suprasyndesmotic fibula fracture (pronation external rotation injury).

Synonyms
- Potts's fractures—bimalleolar fracture
- Dupuytren's fracture—bimalleolar fracture
- Cotton's fractures—trimalleolar fracture
- Tillaux-Chaput fractures—avulsion of the tibial part of anterior tibiofibular syndesmotic ligament

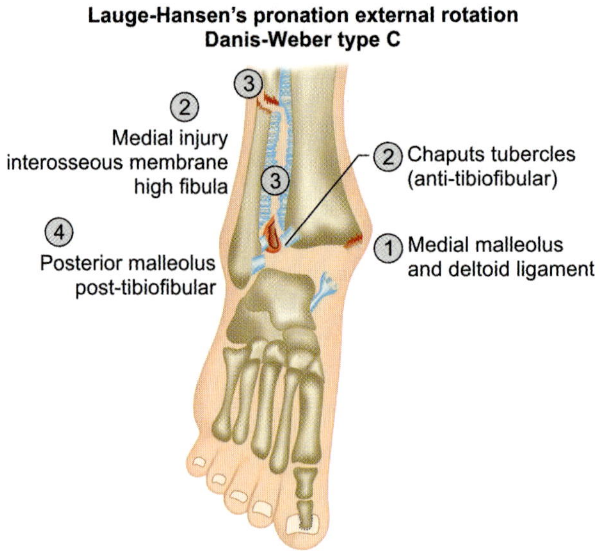

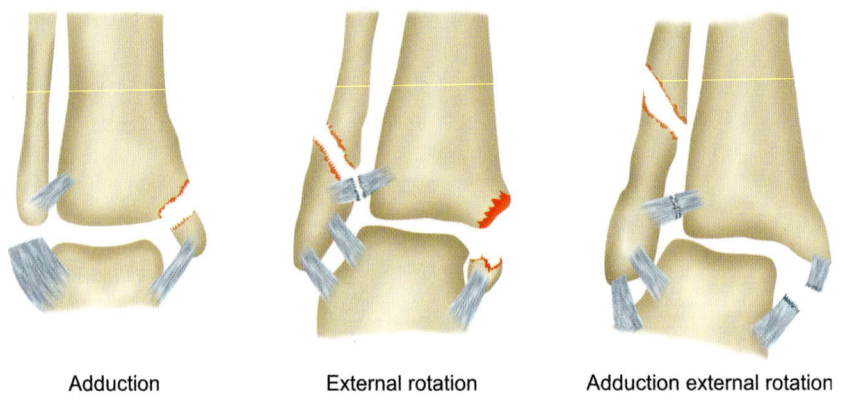

Fig. 59: Pronation external rotation injury.

Fig. 60: Danis–Weber classification based on level of fibular fracture.

- LeFort–Wagstaffe fracture—avulsion of the fibular part of anterior tibiofibular syndesmotic ligament.

TALUS (FIG. 61)

Talar fractures are not very common. This is one of the few areas in the body with a distally based blood supply along with the head of the femur and the proximal pole of scaphoid. The fractures can be a body fracture, neck of talus fracture, or posterior tuberosity fracture. The Hawkins classified talar neck fractures into four types **(Fig. 62)**. Management is anatomical reduction and fixation with screws.

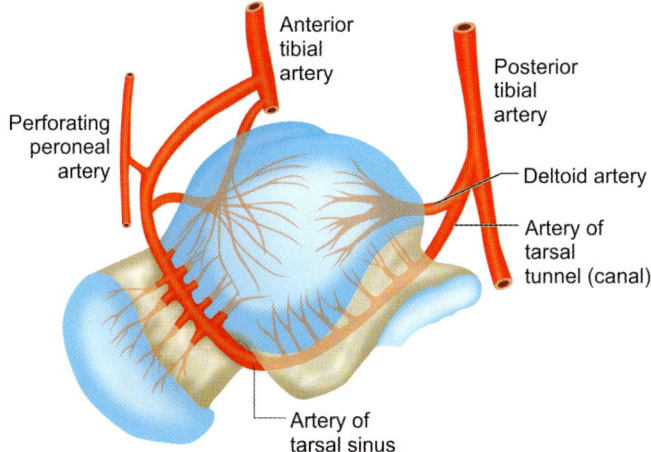

Fig. 61: The distally based blood supply of talus makes the neck of talus fractures prone for nonunion and avascular necrosis of the body.

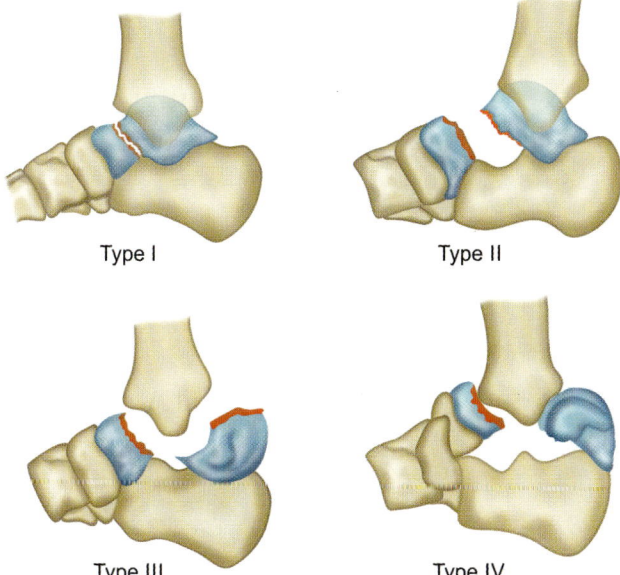

Fig. 62: Hawkins classifications of talar neck fractures.

Treatment

Anatomical reduction of the fracture is the goal. The medial malleolus is usually fixed with malleolar screws or 4 mm cancellous screws. The fibula is usually fixed with plates. The tibiofibular syndesmosis, if unstable, is fixed with a screw. If the posterior malleolar fracture is more than 30%, it should also be fixed.

CALCANEUM

This is one of the bones injured in fall from height. Spine fractures should always be ruled out in such situations. The fractures may be tongue fracture **(Fig. 63)** or a depressed fracture **(Fig. 64)**. In depressed fracture, the thalamus or the area between the subtalar articular surfaces may be driven into the substances of the bone.

Management

Previously, the management was a plaster immobilization for undisplaced fractures or the Essex–Lopresti procedure of Steinman pin manipulation of the subtalar joint. This is replaced by the open reduction and internal fixation using plates. Initially a medial incision was used and now it is largely replaced by a lateral "L" shaped incision. Protection of the sural nerve and the peroneal tendon has to be done.

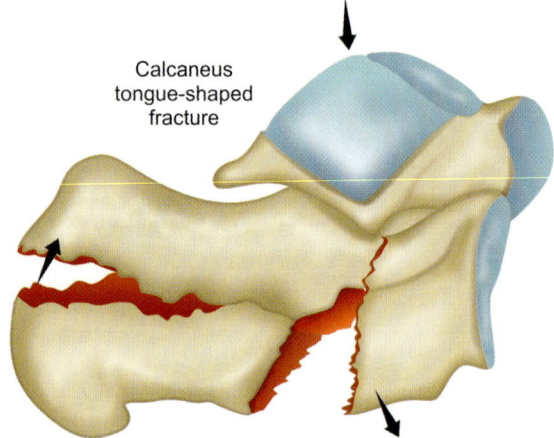

Fig. 63: Tongue fracture of calcaneum.

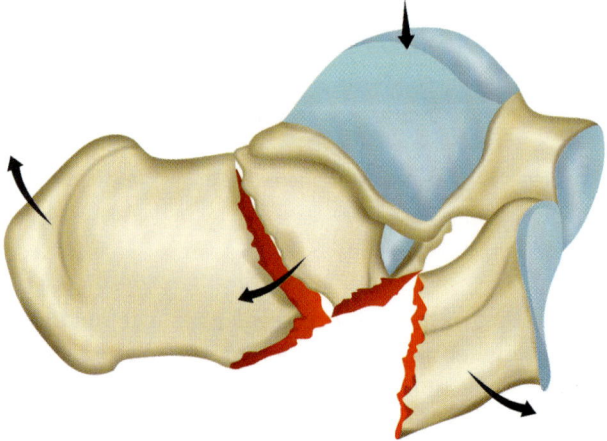

Fig. 64: Depressed fracture of calcaneum.

Infection is a major complication of calcaneus surgery. Compartment syndrome is also seen in calcaneum fractures.

The Bohler's angle and the Gissane's crucial angle are used to assess the status of the subtalar joint.

LISFRANC

The tarsometatarsal joint is known as the Lisfranc joint, whereas the mid tarsal joint (talonavicular and calcaneocuboid) is known as the Chopart's joint. The tarsometatarsal dislocation can produce compartment syndrome, ischemia of the forefoot and so is a significant injury. Open reduction using K-wires or screw fixation should be done.

FOOT

Crush injuries of the foot may lead to compartment syndrome and loss of vascularity. Metatarsal fractures may be managed using K-wire fixation of the shaft or neck injuries. Fasciotomy may be necessary in compartment syndromes.

TOES

Even though in common injuries, the management is cumbersome because to keep the toe immobilized till the fracture unites is time consuming. Even though circulatory impairment has to be watched for a simple protective dressing, metatarsal pad and shoe will suffice. Sometimes K-wire fixation may be needed.

CLAVICLE (FIG. 65)

It is the most commonly fractured bone accounting about 12% of the fractures. It is highly amenable to conservative management. The fracture of middle third accounts for 80% of the fractures. Subclavian vessels and brachial plexus are rarely injured. Surgery is usually by plating. Nonunion, neurovascular involvement, adult lateral end fracture near acromioclavicular joint, persistent separation with soft tissue interposition, and floating shoulder are indications for surgery. Although displaced fractures of the clavicle often cannot be reduced and maintained in perfect position, cosmesis is acceptable, functional results are uniformly excellent. Orthopedist should not be tempted to treat a fracture of the clavicle by open reduction. Scar produced can be more unsightly than a bony prominence. In 94% of 122 patients with clavicular fractures, Stanley et al. found the mechanism of injury to be consistent with a direct blow rather than a fall on the outstretched hand, which is widely believed to be the most common mechanism of injury. Floating shoulder is clavicle fracture neck of scapula.

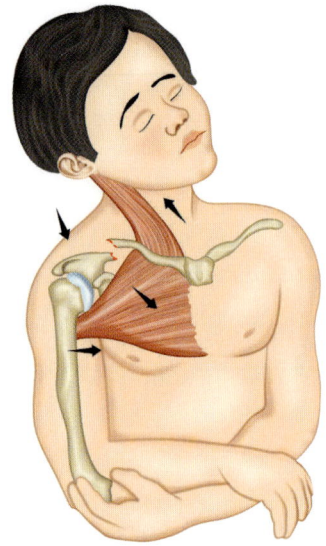

Fig. 65: Forces acting on fracture of the clavicle.

Acromion Scapula

Acromion fractures are managed conservatively. Neck of scapular fractures and body of scapular fractures are usually managed conservatively.

Acromioclavicular Dislocations

Even though previously managed by Robert Jone's strapping, now surgical management is more and more sought. Lateral end clavicle resection with coracoclavicular reconstruction using tendon grafts, nonabsorbable sutures, or Bosworth screws.

SHOULDER

Dislocation Types
- Anterior dislocation **(Fig. 66)**
- Posterior dislocation
- Inferior (Luxatio erecta) dislocation
- Superior (with rotator cuff tear) dislocation.

Dislocations (Figs. 67A to C)

Signs
- *Dugas' test*: Injured limb cannot touch the opposite shoulder.
- *Hamilton ruler test*: Acromion and lateral epicondyle can be approximated **(Fig. 68)**.
- *Callaway sign*: Circumference of the axilla is increased **(Fig. 69)**.

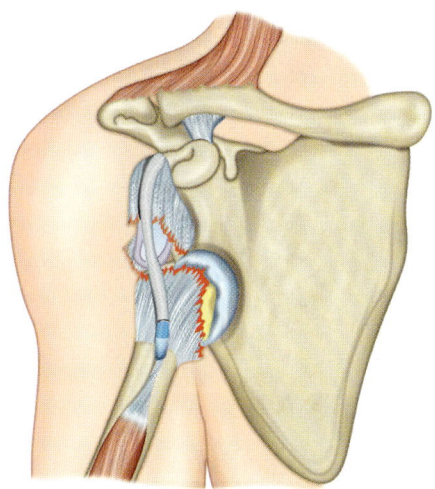

Fig. 66: Anterior dislocation of shoulder.

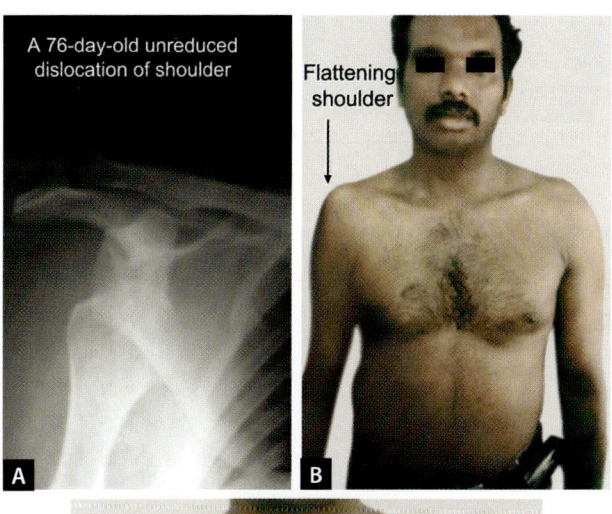

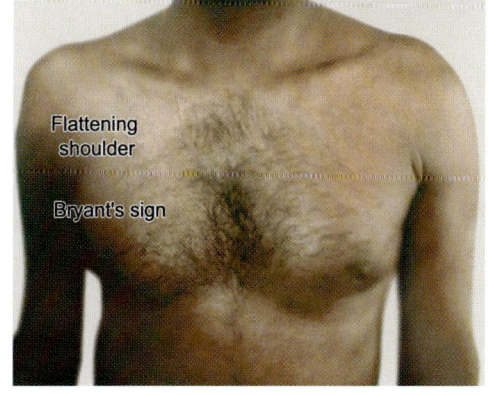

Figs. 67A to C: Chronic dislocation of shoulder.

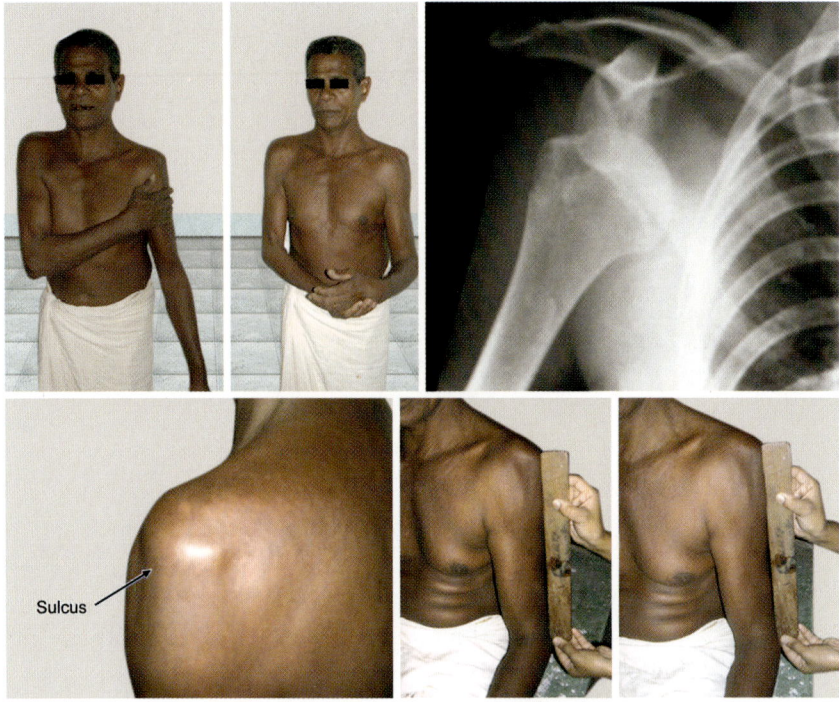

Fig. 68: Hamilton's ruler test.

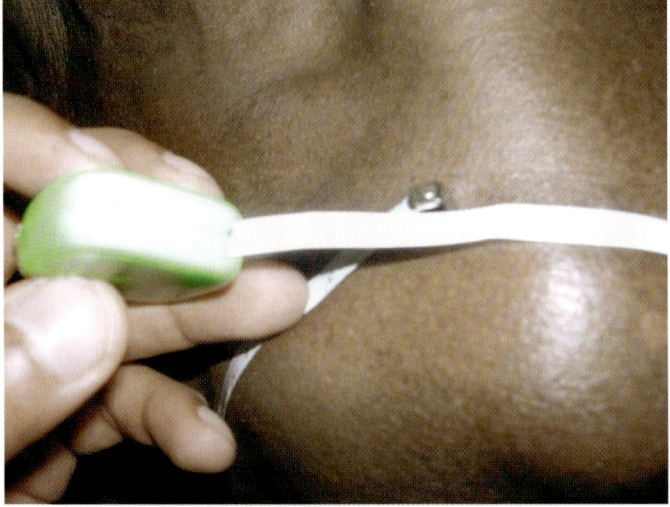

Fig. 69: Callaway's test.

- *Sulcus sign*: Sulcus below the acromion.
- *Drawers test*: For instability.
- *Bryant sign*: Anterior axillary fold is prominent.

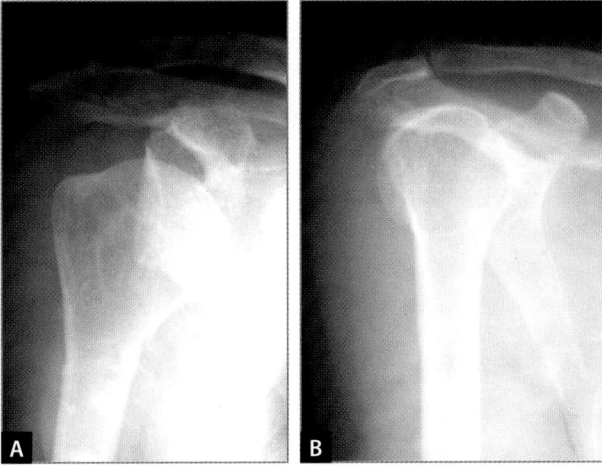

Figs. 70A and B: Radiographs of shoulder: (A) Prereduction; (B) Postreduction.

Methods of Reduction of Shoulder (Figs. 70A and B)

Stimson's Method

The patient is left prone with the arms hanging by the side. After 15–20 minutes, the shoulder may reduce.

Hippocratic Method

Gently increasing traction is applied to the arm with the shoulder in slight abduction, while the assistant applies firm counter.

Traction to the body (a towel slung around the patient's chest under axilla is helpful).

Kocher's Method

The elbow is bent to 90° close to the body; no traction is applied. The arm is rotated 75° laterally, then the point of the elbow is lifted forwards and finally the arm is rotated medially **(Fig. 71)**.

Fracture Neck of Humerus

This is seen in all ages and may be complicated by severe bruising. Manipulation under anesthesia of a displaced fracture may be done especially in a young adult. If unsuccessful, open reduction with internal fixation may be done. In an impacted fracture of elderly, early mobilization should be done to prevent severe post-traumatic stiffness of the shoulder.

Fracture Dislocation Shoulder (Figs. 72 and 73)

The shaft fragment, the head of the humerus, and the greater tuberosity may be three fragments and head may be dislocated. The head dislocation can

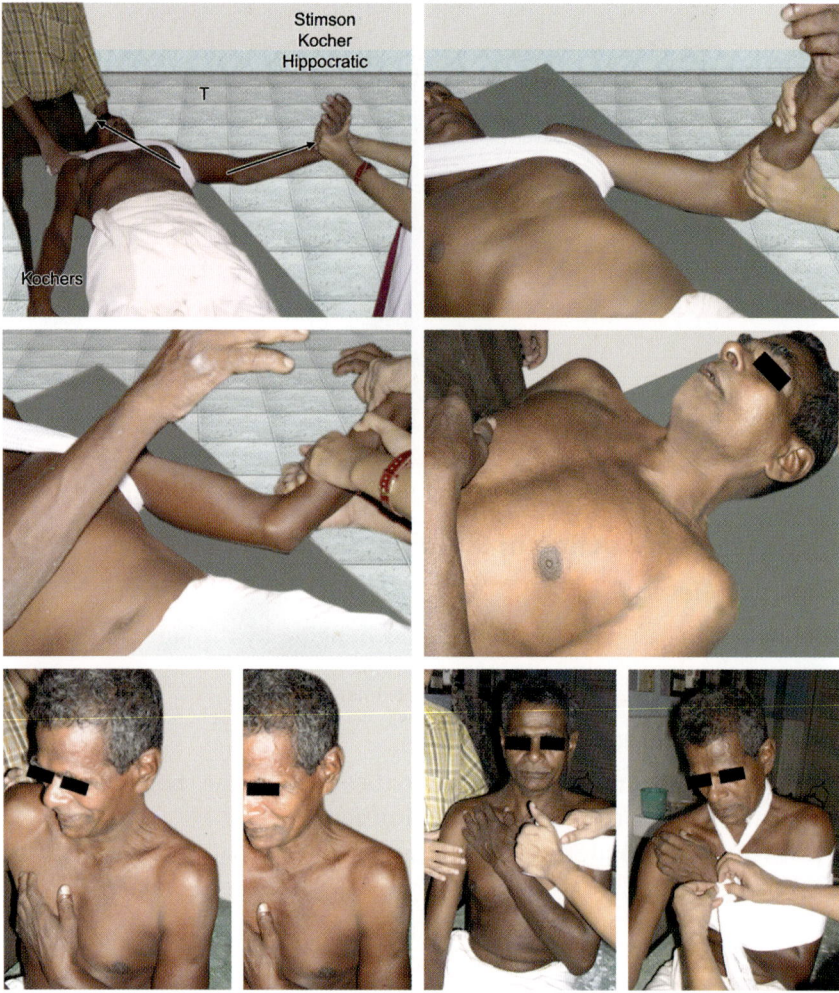

Fig. 71: Theodor Kocher's method of reduction of anterior dislocation shoulder.

be anterior and recent high-velocity injuries can be posterior. It is difficult to attain reduction even by open techniques. The greater tuberosity has to be brought back to its original position by suturing with nonabsorbable sutures such as ethibond.

Axillary Nerve

About 5 cm below the tip of the acromion, the axillary nerve winds around the neck of the humerus. So, this is injured in dislocations of the shoulder and fracture dislocation shoulder.

Fracture Shaft of Humerus

This is a common injury and may be due to a fall on the arm, or due to a direct trauma. Since the radial nerve winds around the distal third of the humerus

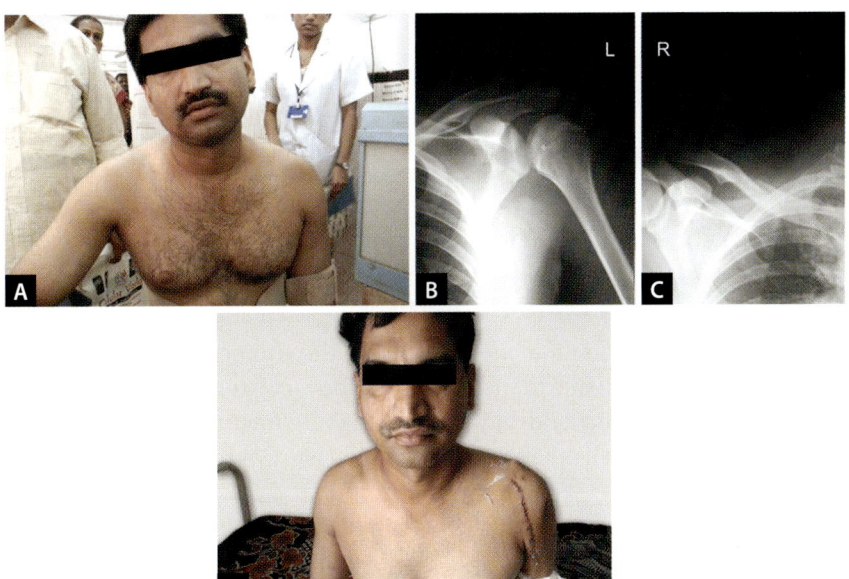

Figs. 72A to D: Posterior dislocation of shoulder, open reduction done.

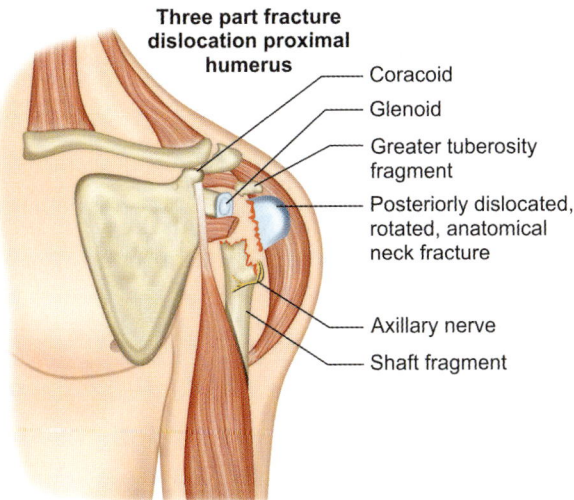

Fig. 73: Fracture–dislocation shoulder.

and is relatively fixed due to its penetration of the lateral intermuscular septum, this nerve is particularly vulnerable especially in spiral fractures. A postmanipulation radial nerve palsy is called Holstein–Lewis syndrome.

Management

In the past, closed manipulation and "U" slab and cast were given. Even shoulder spica was used to treat this condition. But, this is cumbersome and is becoming obsolete. Internal fixation usually by plating and rarely by interlocking nail is the common modality of the management. Since there is a good blood supply and plenty of muscle attachment, the union is usually achieved in 12 weeks.

OPEN FRACTURES

External fixator application is not comfortable due to the heavy muscles around the humerus. The same is applicable to Ilizarov method also.

Supracondylar Fracture Humerus

This fracture is common in children because the supracondylar area is thin in children and the hyperextension of the elbow concentrates the forces to pivot at the weak supracondylar area causing it to fracture. The mechanism of injury is usually a fall on outstretched hand **(Figs. 74 to 76)**.

Management

Type I fractures need only posterior slab. Type II fractures are managed by flexion and posterior slab. Type III fractures are managed by:
- CMR and plastering **(Figs. 77 and 78)**
- CMR and pinning (the best method)
- ORIF
- Traction—either skin traction (Dunlop traction) or olecranon skeletal traction.

Vessels

The rich vascular anastomosis is there around the elbow. Even though the collateral arteries and the recurrent arteries form a rich anastomosis, the

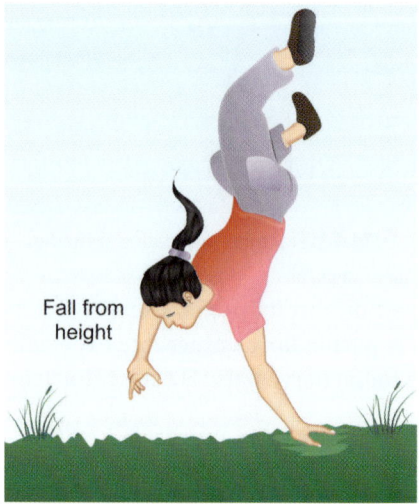

Fig. 74: Fall on outstretched hand.

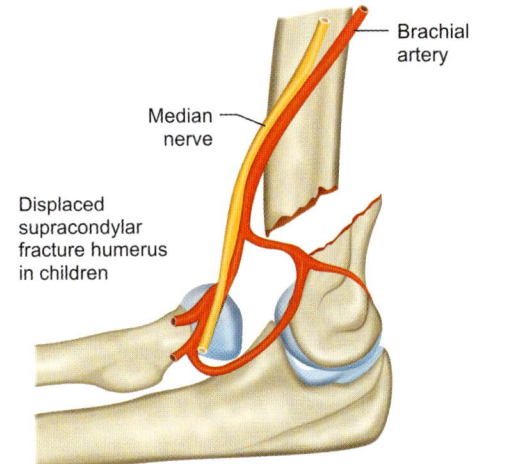

Fig. 75: The neurovascular anatomy of supracondylar fracture.

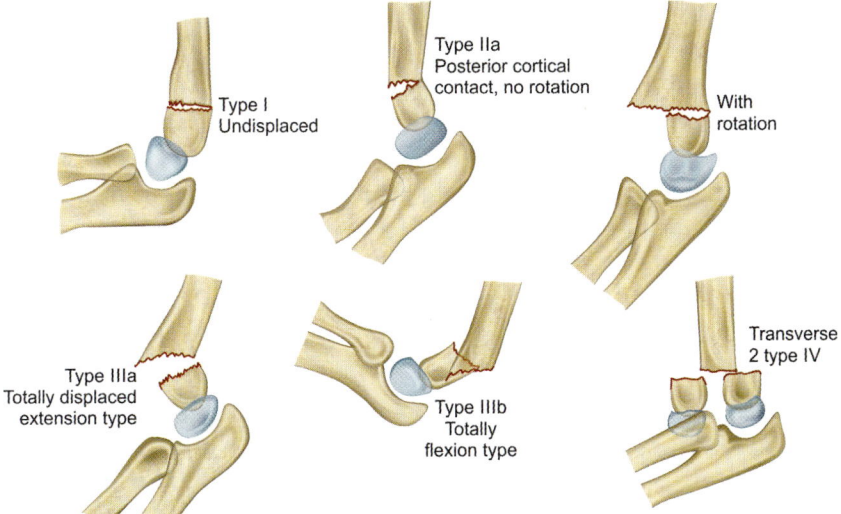

Fig. 76: Gartland classification of supracondylar fracture humerus in children.

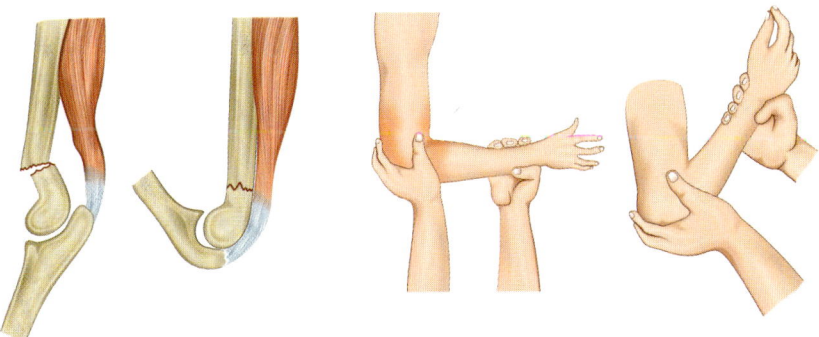

Fig. 77: The close manipulative reduction of supracondylar fracture.

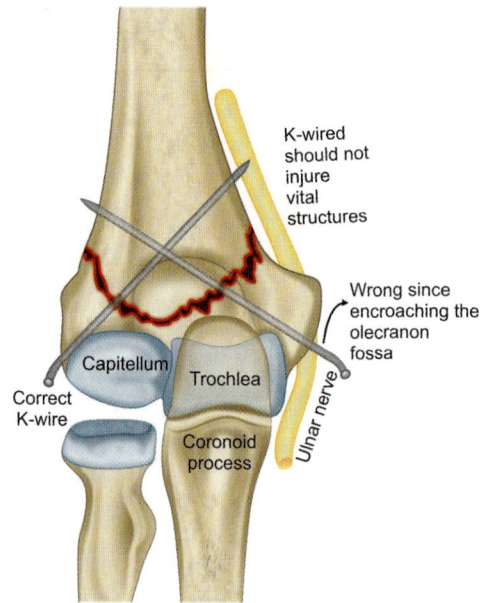

Fig. 78: K-wire fixation of supracondylar fractures either by closed or open method.

anterior interosseous artery, which supplies the deep muscles of the forearm namely flexor digitorum profundus and flexor pollicis longus, is an end artery impeded in compartment syndrome and leads to Volkmann's ischemia and contracture **(Fig. 79)**.

Complications

Complications of supracondylar fractures are malunion leading onto Gunstock deformity or cubitus varus, VIC following compartment syndrome, myositis ossificans, post-traumatic stiffness, and neurological involvement.

Gunstock Deformity

Gunstock deformity is cubitus varus due to extension, medial tilt, and internal rotation of the distal fragment. This is treated by lateral closing wedge osteotomy called French osteotomy **(Figs. 80A and B)**.

Lateral Condyle Fracture

Usually, lateral condyle fracture is a type IV or sometimes type II Salter–Harris epiphyseal injury. The common extensor origin attachment causes the fragment to rotate and the articular surface comes into contact with the fracture crater causing nonunion and cubitus valgus and tardy (late) ulnar nerve palsy. A malunited lateral condyle fracture produces cubitus varus and

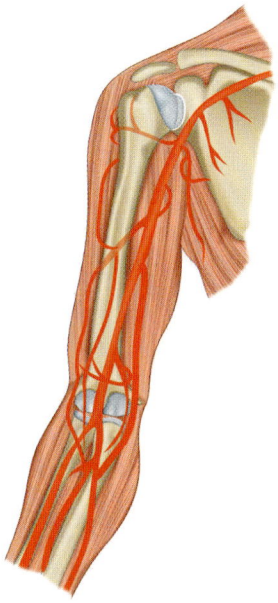

Fig. 79: The rich vascular anastomosis around elbow.

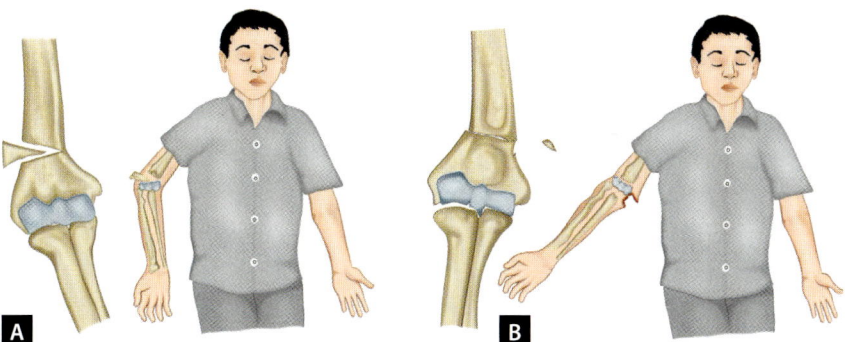

Figs. 80A and B: French osteotomy—lateral closing wedge.

a nonunion of lateral condyle fracture produces cubitus valgus. Since this is an inherently unstable fracture of necessity, conservative management by plastering is used only if the fracture line is less than 2 mm in all the three views. Usually K-wire fixation is done but care must be taken to avoid Kirschner wire to encroach into the olecranon fossa **(Figs. 81 and 82)**.

ELBOW DISLOCATIONS

This is an occasional injury and usually occurs by falling on the hand when the elbow is flexed. The radius and the ulnar dislocate posteriorly on the distal end of the humerus **(Fig. 83)**. The three bony landmarks of the elbow are mainly the olecranon and the medial and lateral epicondyle, which form scalene

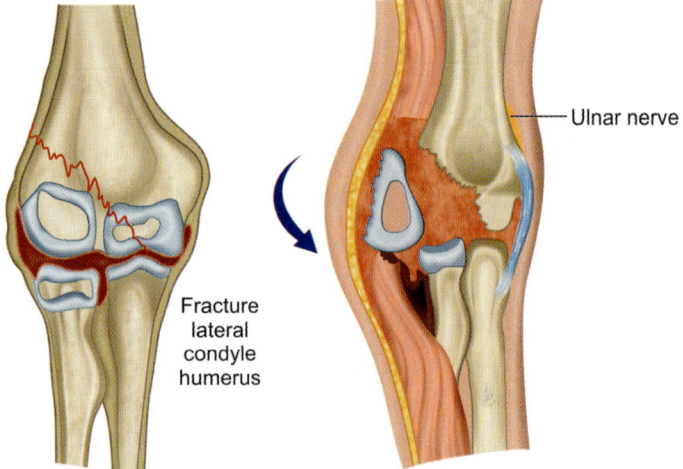

Fig. 81: Lateral condyle fractures of humerus.

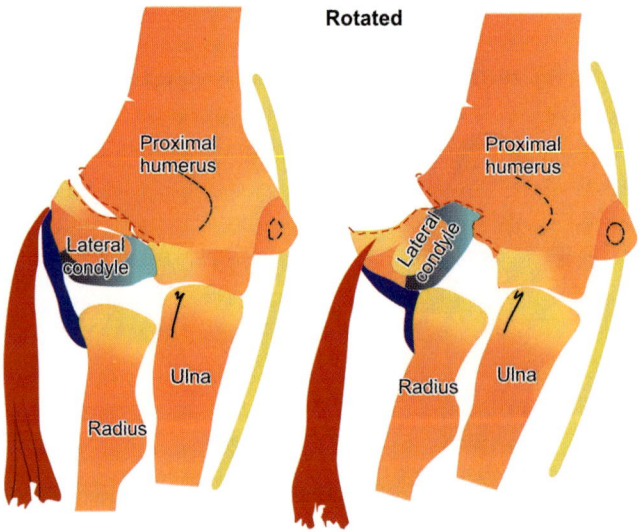

Fig. 82: Displacement of lateral condyle fractures.

triangle with the medial epicondyle olecranon, the smallest and between the epicondyle largest dimensions will be disrupted. Usually, a CMR can be achieved and a plaster is worn for 3 weeks. The median nerve and the brachial artery may be injured.

Fracture Dislocation Elbow

It is a very common injury now in an era of increasing road traffic accidents. The sideswipe injuries are a cause contributing to intercondylar and supracondylar fracture of the distal humerus. Anatomical osteosynthesis will be necessary. An olecranon osteotomy will aid in better exposure.

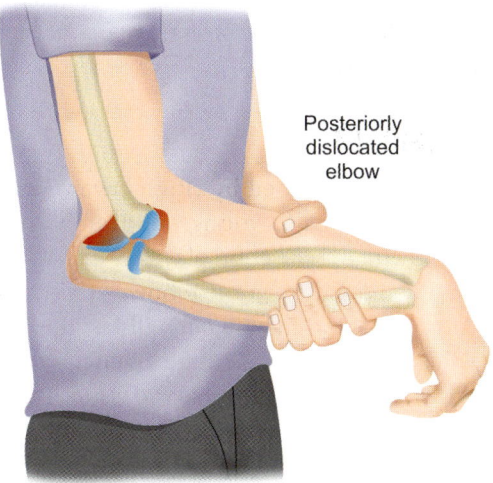

Fig. 83: Posterior dislocation elbow.

EPICONDYLE FRACTURE

Medial epicondyle fractures are common and lateral epicondyle fractures are uncommon. Types of medial epicondyle fractures are:
- *Type I*: Medial epicondyle at the level of the fracture (undisplaced)
- *Type II*: Medial epicondyle displaced
- *Type III*: Medial epicondyle at the level of the joint
- *Type IV*: Medial epicondyle incarcerated inside the joint.

Indications for Surgery
- Ulnar nerve injury
- Type IV epicondyle fracture
- Profound instability of the elbow.
  Fixation is usually done using cancellous screws.

OLECRANON FRACTURE

The fractures of the olecranon are usually displaced due to the pull of the triceps. A tension band wire fixation is the commonly used implant. Olecranon plates are recently available. An excision of the olecranon is done in small fragments. A fracture extending onto the coronoid is a contraindication for olecranon excision.

RADIAL HEAD FRACTURE

Radial head fracture can be an undisplaced fracture or comminuted and displaced one. For an undisplaced stable fracture, only a slab immobilization is necessary. But for a displaced fracture, either a fixation using screws or radial head excision may need to be done. Radial head excision is usually done at a later stage. Posterior interosseous nerve palsy has to be avoided when embarking on the surgery.

PULLED ELBOW (FIG. 84)

Pulled elbow, originally described by Hugh Owen Thomas, the father of modern orthopedics, is seen in young children who have been pulled forcibly by the arm. Swinging the child playfully can also lead to this injury. After the injury, the child will keep the elbow extended and pronated and will not use it. Any attempted movement will be resisted by the child and will cry. X-rays will be normal and accurate diagnosis and simple treatment by supination in a flexed elbow will solve the issue. The radiographer may actually reduce the elbow on attempting supination to take a proper AP view **(Fig. 85)**.

FRACTURE BOTH BONE FOREARM

It is a very common injury nowadays and may be open, if the injury is sufficiently severe. Previously CMR and plaster immobilization were done. Supination in an upper third BB fracture, mid prone position in a middle third BB fracture, and pronation in distal fractures were given during plastering. All the conservative management has given way to operative intervention. Dynamic compression plating and locked compression plating have taken over. Interlocking nailing is rarely done, especially in a segmental fracture.

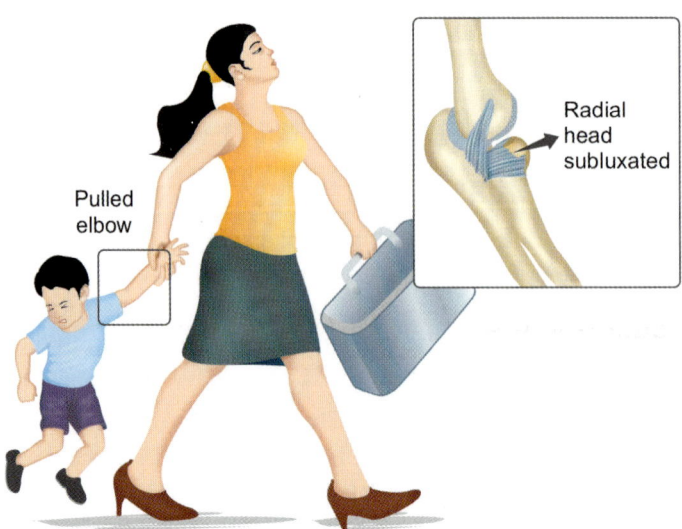

Fig. 84: Mechanism of injury in pulled elbow.

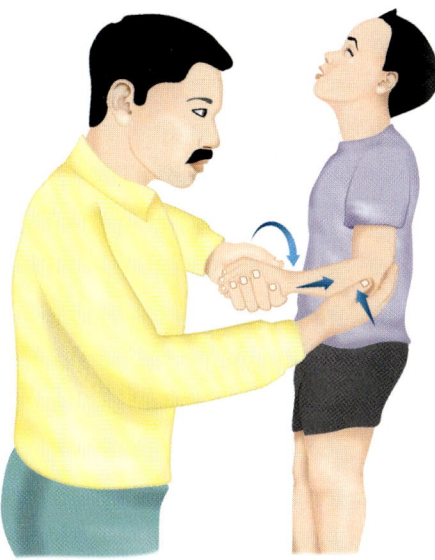

Fig. 85: Closed manipulative reduction of pulled elbow. Supination forearm, flex elbow over 90°, examiner's thump over radial head feels the snap of reduction.

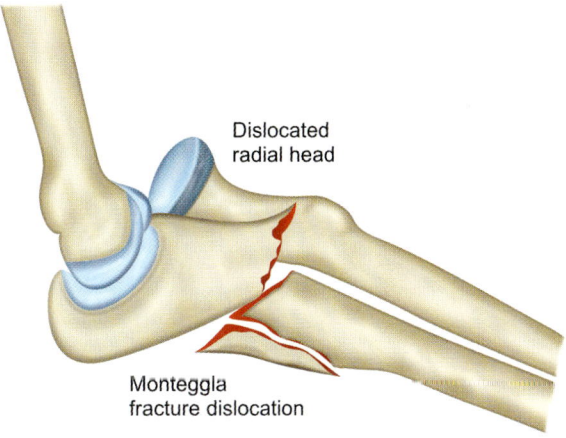

Fig. 86: Monteggia fracture.

Monteggia Fracture

Giovanni Battista Monteggia described this fracture 200 years ago in the Italian city of Milan in 1814 as the fracture of the upper third of the ulna with a dislocation of the superior radioulnar joint **(Fig. 86)**.

Bado has divided Monteggia fracture into:
- *Type I*—extension Monteggia with anterior dislocation of radial head.
- *Type II*—flexion Monteggia with posterior dislocation of radial head.

- *Type III*—lateral Monteggia with lateral dislocation of radial head.
- *Type IV*—fracture BBs forearm with dislocation of radial head.

Monteggia equivalents are:
- Isolated anterior radial head dislocation
- Fracture ulnar with radial neck fracture
- BBs forearm upper third with radial head dislocation.

Management

Conservative management by plastering can be attempted in this hyperpronation injury only in children. Rigid fixation of the ulnar, open reduction of the radial head is the management in adults.

Galeazzi Fracture

Riccardo Galeazzi described this fracture from Milan. This is a fracture of the lower end of the radius with inferior radioulnar dislocation **(Fig. 87)**.

Deforming forces are:
- Brachioradialis
- Pronator quadratus
- Abductor pollicis longus
- Gravity.

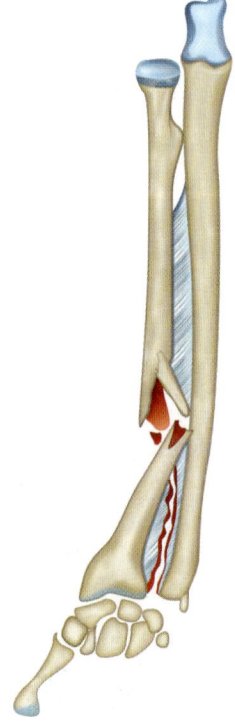

Fig. 87: Galeazzi fracture dislocation.

Types:
- Sprain of the inferior radioulnar joint
- Subluxation of the inferior radioulnar joint
- Dislocation of inferior radioulnar joint.
  Treatment: Rigid plating of distal radius. Nerve injured is ulnar nerve.

ESSEX-LOPRESTI FRACTURE

Acute longitudinal radioulnar disruption is seen in radial head fractures, where the whole interosseous membrane is torn and the distal radioulnar joint is injured.

COLLES' FRACTURE

Colles, who was working in Ireland, is often credited in the English literature as having first described the most common fracture pattern affecting the distal radius **(Fig. 88)**.

However, Pouteau, a French surgeon, may have described the same fracture earlier.

Definition

Colles' fracture can be defined as a fracture of the distal end of radius at the corticocancellous junction, 1 inch above the wrist joint in postmenopausal elderly ladies who fall on the outstretched hand producing dorsal displacement/step, dorsal tilt/volar angulation, lateral displacement/step, lateral tilt/medial angulation, impaction, and supination.

Six Displacements

1. Dorsal displacement/step
2. Dorsal tilt/volar angulation
3. Lateral displacement/step
4. Lateral tilt/medial angulation
5. Impaction
6. Supination.

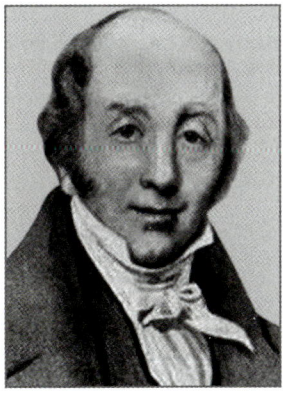

Fig. 88: Abraham Colles (1814).

Differential Diagnosis

- Smith's fracture
- Barton's fracture
- Bennett's fracture
- Chauffer's fracture
- Scaphoid fracture
- Lunate dislocation.
  Comminuted intra-articular distal end radius fracture.

Complications

- Malunion
- Stiffness
- Inferior radioulnar dislocation
- Carpal tunnel syndrome

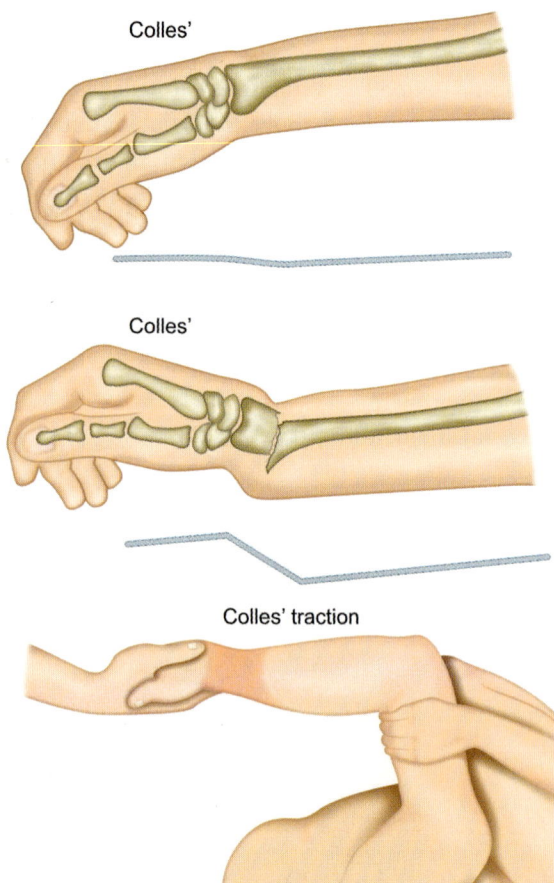

Fig. 89: Traction in Colles' fracture to disimpact.

- Extensor pollicis longus rupture
- Complex regional pain syndrome.

Management

Closed manipulative reduction may be done. Using general anesthesia/Bier's block/sedation, the assistants give traction countertraction and the surgeon reduces by disimpacting and reducing by giving a palmar flexion and ulnar deviation **(Fig. 89)**. Colles used to give a below elbow slab called the Colles' plaster which we follow even now, although as a fracture involving inferior radioulnar joint scientifically an above elbow slab should have been given as in Smith fracture. Time has proven that a below elbow plaster is ideal.

This should be applied for 5–6 weeks. A plaster check at day 3 and a repeat X-ray at day 10 are ideal **(Figs. 90 and 91)**.

For a malunited fracture, excision of the lower 1 inch of ulna retaining the ulnar styloid for ulnar collateral ligament is done commonly. A definitive management is osteotomy and plate fixation of the radius with Darrach's procedure.

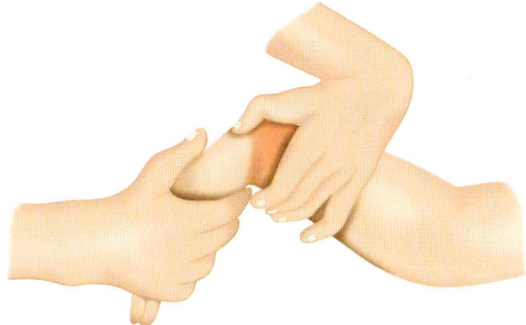

Fig. 90: Palmar flexion.

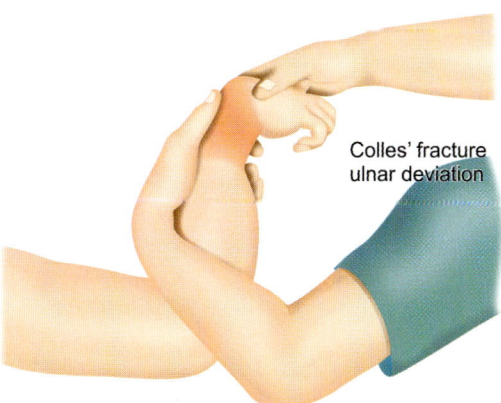

Fig. 91: Ulnar deviation.

SCAPHOID FRACTURE

Scaphoid fractures are complicated by the distally based blood supply. The fractures can be waist fracture, proximal and distal pole fractures, and the tuberosity fracture. The proximal pole fracture has a high incidence of avascular necrosis and nonunion. An attempt of CMR and conservative management can be done, and, if the fracture stays displaced, an ORIF and screw fixation can be done. Nonunion can be managed by bone grafting along with Herbert screw fixation. If there is coexisting arthritis, arthrodesis of the involved joint can be done.

BENNETT'S FRACTURE

Bennett's fracture is fracture dislocation of the base of the first metacarpal. The deforming force is the tendon of abductor pollicis longus. The differential diagnosis is a "T"-shaped fracture of the base of the first metacarpal called Rolando fracture. CMR and casting can be attempted. If the displacement persists, a K-wire fixation can be done.

Index

Page numbers followed by *f* refer to figure, *fc* refer to flowchart, and *t* refer to table.

A

Abdomen 345*f*
    butterfly strapping of 342, 343*f*
    closure of 92
    distension of 258
    magnetic resonance imaging of 132
Abdominal binder 341, 342*f*
Abductor pollicis longus 416
Abscess
    acute pilonidal 121
    deep 119
    drainage of 119, 121*f*
    perianal 121
    pulp space 120
    superficial 119
Absorbable sutures 101
Academia 322
Access, peripheral venous 66
Accidental damage 58
Acetic acid 328
Acid-base
    disorders 322
    imbalance 159
Acidosis 299, 329, 330
Acromioclavicular dislocations 402
Acromion scapula 402
Activated partial thromboplastin time 131
Acute respiratory distress syndrome 236
Adrenaline 75
    use of 76
Adult bradycardia, management of 301*f*
Adult cardiac arrest, management of 300*fc*
Adult tachycardia, management of 302*f*
Advanced trauma life support 276
Aggressive resuscitation 283
Airway 276, 304
    assessment 124
    control 276
    obstruction 280
Albumin, serum 131
Alcohol intoxication 312
Alkaline phosphatase 131
Alkalosis, hypochloremic 131
Allergy, history of 122
Allis maneuver 382
Ambu bag 279*f*
American Society of Anesthesiologists 34, 35
    Physical Status Classification System 34
Amnesia
    post-traumatic 309
    retrograde 309
Ampicillin 140
Amputation stump 340
    bandage 341*f*
Analgesia 322
Anastomosis
    techniques of 177
    types of 166
Anchor technique 178*f*
Anemia 321
Anesthesia 119, 254
Aneurysm, ruptured 319*f*
Ankle
    foot 395
    fractures 396
Anterior abdominal wall 227*f*
Anterior dislocation 402
    shoulder, Theodor Kocher's method of reduction of 406*f*
Anterior tibiofibular syndesmotic ligament 397, 398
Antibacterial ointments 330
Antibacterial sutures 139
Antibiotics 139-141
    five day rule for 4
    prophylaxis 132, 140, 140*f*
    concept of 138
Anticoagulants 285
    history of 312
Antiplatelet therapy 312
Antiseptics 328
    use of 328
Aortic aneurysm 259
Apnea 299, 302
Appendicectomy 133
Arrhythmias 123, 129
Arterial blood gas 281
Arterial pressure 285
Arterial transection 74
Arteriotomy, closure of 176
Artery forceps 92, 292*f*
    enlarging incision 291*f*
    inserting 291*f*
Arthritis 382
Ascites 124
Aspiration pneumonia 235, 260
Asthma 122
Atelectasis 233
Austin Moore's prosthetic replacement 389*f*
Automated external defibrillation 305
Avascular necrosis 382, 386, 386*f*
Avulsion fracture 355
Axillary nerve 406

B

Bacitracin 330
Bacteria, endogenous 137
Bandage, recurrent 334, 334*f*, 335
Bandaging 338*f*
   technique 332, 338*f*
Barbiturate coma 326
Barrel bandage 339, 339*f*
Barton's bandage 335
Barton's fracture 418
Basal metabolic rate 199*f*
Basal skull fracture 312
Basic life support 302
Basilic vein 72
Battered baby 360*f*
Battle's sign 312
Bennett's fracture 418, 420
Bigelow's method 382
Biliary stents 132
Bilirubin 131
Bimalleolar fracture 397
Biocides 328
Bipolar diathermy unit 40*f*
Blanket sutures 88
Bleeding 272
   diathesis 122, 312
   intra-abdominal 286
   time 125
Blenderized food 208
Blocked tube 260
Blood
   flashback of 57*f*
   grouping 128
   pressure 123
   sugar 126, 322
      estimation 128
   transfusion 126, 284
Bloody vicious cycle 285
Body mass index 123
Bogota bag 250, 250*f*
Bone
   marrow suppression 330
   wax 31
Bovie's device 36
Bovie's electrosurgical generator 38*f*
Bowel preparation 171
Bowel wall, anatomy of 161*f*
Brachioradialis 416
Bradyphrenia 309
Brain
   death 309
   herniation, types of 311*f*
Brainstem failure 309
Breast
   abscess 120
   bandage 339, 340*f*
   biopsy, incision for 98
   incisions 84, 85*f*, 98, 99*f*
Breath sounds 124
Breathing 276, 279, 304
Bruits 123
Bryant sign 404
Bupivacaine 75, 76
Burns, severe 331
Burst abdomen 248, 248

C

Calcaneum 400
   depressed fracture of 400*f*
   tongue fracture of 400*f*
Callaway's test 402, 404*f*
Cancellous bone 367
Cannula
   device information and choice of 55
   factors influencing choice of 55
   specifications for 56*f*
Capeline bandage 335, 335*f*
Caprini scoring system 243
Carbohydrate 210
   metabolism 188*fc*
Carbuncle 120
Cardiac arrest 299
   causes of 299
   types of 299
Cardiac evaluation, electrocardiography for 128
Cardiac tamponade 280
Cardiopulmonary collapse 51
Cardiorespiratory complications 251
Cardiovascular diseases 122
Carotid pulsation 302
Carpal tunnel syndrome 418
Cartilage damage 382
Castroviejo needle holder 183*f*
Castroviejo scissors 181*f*
Catabolism, overview of 187*fc*
Catheter
   block 272
   flow 60
   management of 272
   material 60, 262
   removal of 272
   sizes of 60, 266
   tip position 70
   types of 263, 263*f*
Cavitron ultrasonic surgical aspirator 47, 48*f*
   handpiece of 48*f*
Cefazolin 140, 141
Cefoxitin 140, 141
Cefuroxime 140
Cellulitis 74
Central fracture dislocation 382*f*

Central nervous system 373
Central vein 65*t*
    cannulation 65
Central venous access devices 60, 71
Central venous catheter 60, 61
    parts of 62*f*
Central venous pressure 64, 285
Cerebrospinal fluid 312
    rhinorrhea 326
Cerebrovascular accident, history of 122
Cervical
    injuries 380
    spinal cord injury 310
    spine 311, 315, 378
        fracture dislocation of 380*f*
        injury 379
        protection 276
    vertebrae 379
Chauffer's fracture 418
Cheatle cut on antimesenteric border 167*f*
Chemotherapy 248
Chest
    expansion 123
    pain 122
    tube 293, 294*f*
    X-ray of 128
Chlorhexidine 61, 328
Cholangitis, acute 132
Chromic catgut 101
    suture 102*f*
Chronic obstructive pulmonary disease 122
Ciprofloxacin 140
Circular bandage 333
Cirrhosis 132
Civil and criminal negligence 345
Clavicular fracture 339
Cleaning genitalia 268*f*
Clearing oral cavity, finger sweep method of 277*f*
Clindamycin 140
Closed antegrade intramedullary interlocking nail, method of 391*f*
Closed injuries, management of 395
Clostridium difficile-associated disease 139
Clotted blood 260
Clotting time 125
Clubbing 123
Coagulation 30, 39
Coagulopathy, management of 285
Coexisting cervical spine trauma 308
Collard anastomosis, modified 170*f*
Collecting bag 267*f*
    polyurimeter 267*f*
    system 266
Colles' fracture 373, 417, 418*f*
    dinner fork 362

Colloids 155
    controversy 156
    debate 282
    osmotic pressure 158
Colocolic anastomosis 171
Colostomy 248*f*
    consent for 133
Combitube 306
Comminuted fracture 354, 355*f*
Compartment syndrome 371*f*
Complex regional pain syndrome 419
Compound fracture 354
Compression 303*f*, 304
    fracture 355
    secondary 385
Condom catheter 264, 265*f*
Connell suture 168, 168*f*
Consciousness, loss of 299, 309, 312
Contusion 320*f*
    parenchymal 317*f*
Conventional tension 250
Cooley pediatric clamp 184*f*
Coronary artery disease 123
Corrosive poisoning, acute 259
Corticosteroids 248
Cosmetic impairment 365
Cotton's fractures 397
Coudé catheter 264
Cough 122
Cribriform plate, fracture of 259
Cricothyrotomy 306
Criminal negligence 346
Critical care 287
    management 322
Cruciate incision 120
Cruciate injuries 392
Crush syndrome 373
Cryoablation 50, 50*f*
Cryoshock 51
Crystalloid 156, 282
Cyanosis 123
Cyst
    inflamed sebaceous 116
    site of 114
Cystic swellings 114
    differential diagnosis of 114
    excision of 113
Cystostomy 258

D

Dakin solution 328
Damage control resuscitation 284
Danis-Weber classification 397, 398*f*
Debakey tissue forceps 182*f*
Debakey-Bahnson aortic aneurysm clamp 183*f*
Decompression 258

Deep incisional surgical site infections 143
Deep vein thrombosis 241
    prophylaxis of 240, 325
    treatment of 240, 245
Dentinogenesis imperfecta 360*f*
Depressed fracture 312, 327, 357*f*
Depression 350
Diabetes mellitus 129, 248
    history of 122
Diaphragmatic rupture 281
Diathermy 27, 30
    machines 37
Diffuse axonal injury 326
Digestive tract health 223
Digital nerve block 78, 79*f*
    techniques for 79
Dislocation 353, 402
    types 402
Displacement
    degree of 363
    direction of 363
Dorsal and palmar digital nerves 78*f*
Dorsolumbar spine fracture, Moss-Miami posterior stabilization of 381*f*
Drainage tube 270*f*, 288
    tip of 289*f*
Drawer's test 392*f*, 404
Dressing pad application 294*f*
Dugas' test 402
Dupuytren's fracture 397
Dyslipidemia 122
Dyspnea 12, 122

E

Ear 336, 339
Ecchymosis, periorbital 312
Edema 123
    bilateral periorbital 308
    lower limb 123
    pulmonary 235, 281, 373
Either propylthiouracil 128
Elbow
    dislocations 411
    fracture dislocation of 412
    profound instability of 413
Electrocardiography 123
Electrolyte 281
    disturbances 299
    replacement 151
Electrosurgery 39
    types of 38
Electrosurgical diathermy machine 39*f*
Elephant foot nonunion 376
Elevated intra-abdominal pressure 248
Emergency surgery 248
Endocrinology 128
Endotracheal tubes 278*f*, 306

End-to-end anastomosis 167, 179*f*
Enteral feeding 127
    complications of 210
    formulas, types of 208
Enteral nutrition 207
    rationale for 207
Enterococcus faecalis 138
Enterotomy 228
Enzymatic products 328
Epicondyle fracture 413
Epilepsy, history of 122
Erythrocyte sedimentation rate 374
Escherichia coli 138
Esophageal perforation 260
Esophageal varices 259, 260
Esophagogastric anastomosis 169
Esophagus, anatomic peculiarity of 160
Essex-Lopresti fracture 417
Eusol and Dakin solution 329
Extensor pollicis longus rupture 419
External jugular vein 68, 326
Extrahepatic biliary system, obstruction of 132
Extraperitoneal fat 92
Eye
    bandage 336
    opening response 308

F

Face mask 305
Fascia of Camper 95
Fascia of Scarpa 95
Fascial closure 248
Fasting blood sugar 129
Fat 210
    embolism 373, 373*f*
        syndrome, diagnosis of 373
    globules 374
    in urine 374
    metabolism 191*fc*
Fatigue 309
Feed, types of 210, 212
Feeding
    enteral routes for 210
    jejunostomy 226
        location of 227*f*
        tube 231*f*
Female catheterization 270
Femoral fractures 390*f*
Femoral head
    distally based blood supply of 385*f*
    Pipkin fracture of 383*f*
Femoral vein 69, 69*f*, 282
Femur
    fracture
        neck of 383
        shaft of 388
        interlocking nail of 391*f*

Fever 322
Fibular fracture 398*f*
Figure of eight bandage 334, 334*f*
Fistulas, arteriovenous 72
Fixing tube 294*f*
Flail chest 280
    severe 280
Flexion monteggia 415
Fluid 158
    adequacy of 151
    and electrolytes 220, 323
    controlled infusion of 283
    drinking lots of 273
    intravenous 154*f*
        replacement 156
        resuscitation 153
    therapy, indications for 147
Focal neurological deficits 310, 312, 314
Foley's catheter 263, 264*f*, 265, 281, 282
    parts of 266*f*
Four-tailed bandage 335
Fracture 353
    dislocation of hip, reduction of 385*f*
    neck of femur
        causes of nonunion of 388*f*
        Garden's staging of 387*f*
        osteosynthesis of 389*f*
    of clavicle, forces acting on 402*f*
    of proximal femur, types of 386*f*
    open depressed 312
    pathological 357*f*
    position of 373
    sacrum coccyx 378
    types of 354
French nasogastric tube 259
French osteotomy 411*f*
Fulguration 39
Full-length midline incision 93

G

Galea aponeurotica 315*f*
Galeazzi fracture dislocation 416*f*
Gallbladder wall thickness 132
Garden's spade deformity 361*f*
Garden's staging 387*f*
Gartland classification 409*f*
Gastric anastomosis 170
Gastroesophageal junction 257*f*
Gastrointestinal suturing 166
Gastrointestinal tract 137
General anesthesia 119
Gentamicin 140
Germinal matrix after total nail bed excision, removal of 256*f*
Gibbon catheter 264, 264*f*
Glasgow coma scale 281, 308

Gloving
    closed method of 15, 16*f*
    open method of 15, 17*f*
    steps of closed method of 16*f*
    techniques 15
Glucose 281
Glycemic control 325
Gram-positive cocci and bacilli 330
Granny knot 106, 107*f*
Gravity 416
Great saphenous vein 71, 282
Greenstick fracture 356, 356*f*
Gridiron incision 95
    problems of 96
Gunstock deformity 410
Gurd's criteria 373

H

Hamilton's ruler test 402, 404*f*
Hands
    hygiene, five moments for 11
    sanitization of 57*f*
Hand-sewn anastomosis, techniques of 167
Handwashing 6
    practice 10
    steps 14*f*
Harmonic focus 45, 46*f*
Harmonic scalpel 27, 45*f*
Harmonic wave 45, 46*f*
Hartmann's operation 137
Hartmann's solution 154
Head bandage 335
    types of 337*f*
Head injury 307
Headache 309, 312
Heart sounds 123
Hematologic syndromes 241
Hematoma 59, 74, 248, 375
    acute subdural 318*f*
    epidural 318*f*
    parenchymal 320*f*
    subacute subdural 319*f*
Hemiparesis 314
Hemiplegia 314
Hemodialysis 66
    catheters 65
Hemodynamic support 323
Hemoglobin-based oxygen carriers 284
Hemorrhage 281, 367
    conjunctival petechial 373*f*
    control 276
    intraventricular 320*f*
    subarachnoid 319*f*
    subconjunctival 312
    thoracic 281
Hemostasis 30

Hemothorax, massive 280
Hepatitis
    B virus 125
    C virus 125
Hilton's method 121
Hip
    dislocation, close manipulatory reduction of 384*f*
    fracture dislocation of 381, 383*f*
Hippocratic method 405
Holding needle, method of 86*f*
Horner's syndrome 311
Horse hoof nonunion 376
Hospital surgical surveillance program 146
Human body, composition of 186
Human immunodeficiency virus 32, 125
Humerus
    fracture
        neck of 405
        shaft of 406
        lateral condyle fracture of 412*f*
Hutchinson's pupil 310
Hydration, adequate preoperative 132
Hydrocolloids 328
Hydrogels 328
Hydrogen
    ion 299
    peroxide 328, 329, 331
Hypercapnia 321
Hypercoagulable states 241
Hyperglycemia 322
Hyperkalemia 299
Hyperosmolar therapy 324
Hypertension 122, 123, 248, 321
    abdominal 251
    portal 124
Hypertonic saline 283, 284
Hypervascular nonunions, types of 376*f*
Hypocapnia 321
Hypoglycemia 129, 322
Hypokalemia 299
Hyponatremia 321
Hypoosmolality 322
Hypoproteinemia 248
Hypotension 299, 321
Hypothermia 284, 285, 299, 309, 322
Hypothyroidism 129
Hypovascular nonunions, types of 376*f*
Hypovolemia 280
Hypoxemia 321, 373
Hypoxia 299

I

Icterus 123
Ileocolic anastomosis 170
Iliac crest bone grafting 377*f*
Immunonutrition 221
Immunosuppression 248
Impaired nutritional status 206
Incision 97, 116, 119, 121*f*, 291*f*
    abdominal 91, 91*f*
Index-finger hitch 109
    steps of 109*f*
Infected wounds, management of 328
Infection 272, 366, 372, 375
    catheter related 139
    intra-abdominal 248
Inferior radioulnar joint
    dislocation of 417
    sprain of 417
    subluxation of 417
Inflating balloon 270*f*
Infrasyndesmotic fibula fracture 397
Ingrowing toe nail 254
Injury
    abdominal 282
    dangerous mechanisms of 287
    mechanism of 414*f*
Internal fixation, failure of 377*f*
Internal jugular vein 64*f*, 65, 67, 68, 326
Intestinal anastomosis 160, 258
Intra-abdominal pressure 326
Intracranial air 327*f*
Intraoperative flow-directed fluid therapy 158
Intrathoracic esophagogastric anastomosis 139*f*
Intravenous cannula, parts of 55*f*
Intravenous drug abusers 66
Intravenous therapy 54
Iodophores 328
Ischemia 369
    mesenteric vascular arcades and critical points of 163*f*
Ivor Lewis operation 169*f*

J

Jaw thrust maneuver 277*f*
    modified 276
Jejunal mobilization 228
Joint stiffness 378

K

Kangaroo tendon 101
Kerosene poisoning 259
Kidney exposure, incision for 97
Kinked tube 260
Kirschner wires 367
Knee
    dislocation 393
    ligaments of 392
    tibia, fracture of 394

Kocher's forceps 92, 93
Kocher's method 405
Kocher's subcostal incision 96

L

Lachman's test 392*f*
Lanz incision 95
Laparostomy 249
Large bowel
  anastomosis 171
  operations 132
Large cyst under local anesthesia, excision of 116
Large intestine, anatomical peculiarity of 163
Large left parietal extradural hematoma 318*f*
Larger gauge catheter 272
Laryngeal mask airway 306
Lateral condyle fracture 410
  displacement of 412*f*
Lauge-Hansen's classification 396, 396*f*
Lefort-Wagstaffe fracture 398
Lembert sutures 168
Ligament strains 395
Ligasure 51
  tip 52*f*
  unit with probes 52*f*
Lignocaine 75, 259, 266, 269*f*, 270
Linea alba 92
Lipoma 113, 116
  excision of 118
  finger dissection 117*f*, 118*f*
  lobule, dissection of 118*f*
Liquefies necrotic tissue 331
Lithotomy position 270
Liver 131
  diseases 124
  function tests 131
  metastasis 132
  parenchyma 48*f*
  secondaries, palliative ablation of 49
Lloyd-Davies position 28*f*
Local anesthesia 113
  infiltration of 73*f*, 76*f*
Looser's zone 360*f*
Lumbar injury 378
Lunate dislocation 418
Lung injury, acute 236
Lymph node biopsy 113
Lymphadenopathy 123
Lymphoma 357*f*

M

Mafenide acetate 330
Magnetic resonance cholangiopancreatography 132

Male catheterization procedure 266, 267
Malnutrition 248
Malunion 365, 374, 418
Malunited fracture 374*f*, 375*f*
Masogastric tube, parts of 257, 257*f*
Mastectomy, incision for 99*f*
Mastoid bandage 336, 339*f*
Mastoid ecchymosis 312
Mayo-Hegar needle holder 182*f*
McBurney's point 95
McKeown operation 170*f*
Mechanical ventilation 322
Medial cubital vein 72*f*
Medical literature, evidence-based classification of 7*t*
Memory
  deficits 312
  short-term 309
Meniscal injuries 393, 394*f*
Menisci of knee 392
Meniscus 393*f*
Mental state 285
Metformin 130
Methicillin-resistant staphylococcus aureus 139, 252
Methimazole 128
Metronidazole 140
Middle-finger hitch 109, 110
  steps of 111*f*
Midline incision, advantages of 92
Minocycline 61
Mobility, abnormal 362
Monopolar diathermy lead 40*f*
Monteggia fracture 415, 415*f*
Mount Fuji sign 327*f*
Multidrug resistant pathogens, emergence of 139
Multisystem trauma 281
Murmurs 123
Muscle splitting incision 95
Myocardial contusion 310

N

Nail
  avulsion of 254
  bed, excision of 255, 255*f*
Nasal intubation 277
Nasogastric feeding 258
Nasogastric intubation 257
Nasogastric tube 131, 257, 281, 282
  contraindications for 282
  dislodged 260, 261
  insertion 259*f*
  problems of 260
  removal of 261
Nasopharyngeal airway 276, 306

Nasopharynx 259
Neck
    bandage 340
    computed tomography of 128
    lymph node biopsy of 113
    ultrasound of 128
    X-ray of 128
Necrotic tissue 329, 331
Needle 105
    catheter jejunostomy 232
    insertion of 57*f*
Negative pressure wound therapy 250
Neomycin 330
Nephrectomy 27*f*, 258
Neuropathy 329
Neurovascular injury 368
Nipple areola complex 99*f*
Nonabsorbable sutures 103
Nonunions, types of 376
No-touch technique 266, 269*f*
Novus actus interveniens 345
Nutrient 220
    absorption 219
Nutrition pyramid 214*f*
    concept of 211
Nutritional therapy, decision-making for 206

O

Obesity 66, 122, 248
Oblique incisions 95
Ofloxacin 140
Olecranon fracture 413
Oligomeric formulas 208
Oligotrophic nonunion 376
Open fractures 408
Open injuries, management of 395
Opening parotid abscess, Blair method of 121
Oral contraceptives 125
Oral hypoglycemic agents 124, 129
Oral intubation 277
Organ space surgical site infection 144
Orogastric tube 131
Oropharyngeal airway 278*f*, 306
Osteoarthritis 382
Osteomalacia 358*f*, 359*f*
Osteomyelitis 331
Otorrhea 312, 314
Oxygen 127
    saturation 285

P

Packed red cells 285
Pain 359
Pallor 123
Palmar flexion 419*f*
Palpitation 122

Pancreas, diagnose pseudocyst of 258
Pancreatic operations 131
Papain-based products 331
Parachute technique 178*f*
Paralysis 322
Paralyzed limb 282
Paramedian incision 93
    closure of 93
    problems of 93
Paraphimosis 272
Paraplegia, traumatic 380
Parenteral nutrition 216
    complications of 218
Partial thromboplastin time 125
Pass bladder neck 272
Patella 391
    dislocation 391
Pauwels' classification 386*f*
Pelvic
    fractures, control of 280
    injuries 282
Pelvis, fracture of 381
Peripherally inserted central catheters 64
Peritoneum 92
    parietal 230*f*
Pfannenstiel incision 94
Philadelphia collar 315*f*
Phlebitis 58, 74
Phonophobia 309
Photophobia 309
Physical fitness, ASI classification of 33
Planned enterotomy, site of 228*f*
Plasma-derived colloids 157
Plastic catheter 264, 265*f*
Platelet
    aggregation 283
    count 125
    derived growth 331
    values 374
Pleura, gloved finger separating adhesions of 292*f*
Pneumatic antishock garment 280
Pneumocephalus 327
    large 327*f*
Pneumonia 139, 234
Pneumothorax 69
    open 280
Poliglecaprone 102
Polyamide 104
    sutures 104*f*
Polydioxanone 102
    sutures 103*f*
Polyester 104
    suture 104*f*
Polyethylene
    glycol 133
    sutures 104*f*

Index

Polyglactin 102
    sutures 102f
Polyglycolic acid 102
    sutures 102f
Polymeric formula 208
Polymyxin 330
Polypropylene 104
    sutures 180
Polysporin 330
Polytetrafluoroethylene sutures 180
Polytrauma 367
Postcardiac arrest care 300fc
Postcompartment syndrome sequelae 370f
Posterior auricular artery 312
Posterior dislocation 402
    elbow 413f
Posterior tibial artery 383f
Postoperative fluid management 147
Potts's fractures 397
Potts's scissors 181f
Povidone iodine 266, 328, 329, 331
Pressure sore 371
Prilocaine 75
Prolene 180
Promotes granulation tissue 331
Pronation abduction injury 396
Pronation external rotation injury 396, 397, 398f
Pronator quadratus 416
Prophylactic mesh, use of 250
Prostatic disease 264
Protein 210
    metabolism 193f
Prothrombin time 125, 131
Proximal femur 385
    trabecular pattern of 386f
Pseudofracture 357
Pseudomonas infection 328
Pulled elbow 414
    closed manipulative reduction of 415f
Pulmonary embolism 237, 240
    diagnosis of 243
    prophylaxis of 243
    treatment of 247
Pulsations, peripheral 123
Pulse 123
    pressure 281
    rate 281, 284
Pulseless electrical activity 299
Pulseless ventricular tachycardia 299
Pupils 310
Purse string suture 228f
Pyrexia 373

Q

Q mechanism 391
Quadriceps mechanism 356f

R

Raccoon eyes 312
Radial head dislocation 416
Radial head
    anterior dislocation of 415, 416
    dislocation of 416
    fracture 413, 416
    posterior dislocation of 415
Radiation therapy 248
Radical mastectomy, modified 99f
Radiofrequency 49f
    ablation 48
    energy 44
Raised intracranial pressure 311f
Raised jugular venous pressure 123
Red rubber catheter 263, 263f
Reef knot 107, 107f
Refeeding syndrome 211, 214, 215, 216f
Reflux esophagitis 260
Rehabilitation 364, 366, 367
Rehydration formula 208
Removing nail segment 255f
Res iudicata 347
Respiration, cessation of 302
Respiratory complications after surgery 233
Respiratory diseases 259
Respiratory rate 281
Resuscitation 274, 284, 287
    cardiopulmonary 299, 302, 304
    conventional aggressive 281
Retroperitoneal approach 97
Reverse spiral bandage 333, 333f
Rhinorrhea 312
Rib fractures 280
Rifampin 61
Right frontal hemorrhagic contusion 320f
Right frontoparietal intracerebral hematoma 321f
Ringer's lactate 154
Rooftop incision 97
Rotator cuff tear 402
Routine knot tying 111f
    steps of 112f
Rush nails 367
Rutherford-Morrison incision 97
Ryle's tube 257
    inserting 259

S

Sacral injury 378
Safe surgery, ten essential objectives for 136
Satinsky clamp 184f
Scalp
    infiltration of 76f
    layers of 315f

suturing 315
swellings in 115
Scandinavian guidelines 313
Scaphoid fracture 418, 420
Sciatic nerve palsy 383
Scissors 181
Screw fixation 389*f*
Sealing suture 293
Sebaceous cyst 116, 117*f*
  excision of 114, 115*f*, 117*f*
Sedation 322
Segmental fracture 354, 355*f*
Segmental nail bed excision 256*f*
Seizure 312
  prophylaxis 325
  recurrent 314
Seldinger technique, modified 62
Seroma 248
Shock therapy 281
Shoulder 402
  anterior dislocation of 403*f*
  chronic dislocation of 403*f*
  dislocated 353*f*
  fracture dislocation of 405, 407*f*
  posterior dislocation of 407*f*
  pull-down view 380
  radiographs of 405*f*
  reduction of 405
Silicone catheter 271
Silk suture 103*f*
Silver
  alloy 262
  fork deformity 362
  nitrate 329, 330
  sulfadiazine 61, 329, 330
Simple fracture 354, 354*f*
Simple interrupted suture 85
Simple running suture 87*f*
Sinusitis 260
Skin 92
  adhesive strips 88
  clips 89
  damage 368
  incisions 81, 82, 135
  loss 368
  necrosis 251, 369*f*
Skull
  open fractures of 314
  X-ray 316
Sleep disturbances 309
Slip knot 107, 108*f*
Small bowel, vascularity of 162*f*
Small intestine, anatomical peculiarity of 161
Small sebaceous cyst simple incision over dome, excision of 115*f*
Smith's fracture 418
  garden spade deformity 362

Soft-tissue
  interposition of 365, 375
  necrosis 369*f*
Sono-guided fine needle aspiration cytology 128
Spatulate needles 105
Spinal injury, emergency management of 379
Spine
  dislocation of 378
  fracture of 378
  three-column concept of 379
  trauma 315
Spiral bandage 333, 333*f*
Staphylococcus aureus 137
Staphylococcus epidermidis 137
Sterile cotton balls 266
Sterile drapes 266
Sterile gloves 259, 266
Sterile precautions 67
Sterilization 105
Sternocleidomastoid muscle 67, 68
Steroids 325
Stiffness 418
Stimson's method 405
Stomach
  anatomical peculiarity of 160
  vascular anatomy of 162*f*
Streptococcus pyogenes 119
Stress 196
  hypermetabolic 200
  starvation 196
  ulcer prophylaxis 325
Subclavian vein 68
Subconjunctival petechiae 373
Subcutaneous swellings, minor surgical procedures of 113
Subcutaneous tissue 92
Suction apparatus 259
Sudeck's osteodystrophy 378
Sulbactam 140
Sulcus
  below acromion 404
  sign 404
Superficial surgical site infection 142
Superior dislocation 402
Superior vena cava 61
Supination adduction injury 396, 397*f*
Supination external rotation injury 396, 397*f*
Supination forearm 415*f*
Supracondylar fracture
  close manipulative reduction of 409*f*
  deformity in 362
  humerus 408
  Gartland classification of 409*f*
  K-wire fixation of 410*f*
  neurovascular anatomy of 409*f*
Suprapubic transverse incision 95

Suprasyndesmotic fibula fracture 397
Surgeon's knots 106, 108, 108f
Surgical blades, types of 81f
Surgical scrub team 29
Surgical site infection 137, 142
    organisms for 138
    three different types of 142f
Surgical sterile instruments 26
Suture 101
    materials 101
    removal 89, 89f
    techniques 85
    types 163
Swan-Ganz catheter 285
Swelling 362
Swirl sign 317
Syncope 59
    history of 122

T

Tachycardia 373
Tachypnea 279
Talar neck fractures, Hawkins classifications of 399f
Talus 398
Tamponade cardiac 299
T-bandage 340, 341f
Teacher-student model 8
Tenderness 362
Tensile strength 102
Tension
    pneumocephalus 327f
    pneumothorax 280, 299, 310
    secondary 385
    sutures 248
Theodor Kocher's method 406f
Thomas splint, open fracture on 354f
Thoracic injuries 380
Thoracolumbar injury 378, 380
Thrombophlebitis, superficial 247
Thrombosis prophylaxis 245
Thrombus, physical properties of 283
Thyroid
    function tests 128
    stimulating hormone 128
Thyroidectomy 128
Tibia fracture 394
Tibial condyle, split fracture of 357f
Tiemann neoplex catheter 264, 265f
Tight cervical collar 326
Tight tape fixation 326
Tillaux-Chaput fractures 397
Tissue
    ablation 49f
    forceps 181
    glue 89

Tobramycin 140
Torsion wedge nonunions 376
Total nail bed excision 255f
Total parenteral nutrition 66
Toxicity 300
Trace minerals 221
Trachea bronchial tree injury 280
Tracheoesophageal fistula 258
Tracheostomy 306
Tranexamic acid 285
Transient ischemic attacks, history of 122
Transient neutropenia 330
Trans-syndesmotic fibula fracture 397
Transtracheal jet ventilation 306
Transvenous cardiac pacing 66
Transverse elliptical incision 99f
Transverse incision 94
Trauma, abdominal 280
Traumatic brain injury, clinical classification of 307
Traumatic circulatory arrest 280
Trendelenburg position 27
Triangular bandage 336, 338f
Trimalleolar fracture 397
Triple throw knot 107, 108f
Trochanteric fractures, proximal femoral nail fixation for 389f
Trunk, least skin tension of 84f
Tube drain 31
Tube tip, intraluminal position of 229f

U

Ugly wound 251
Ulnar deviation 419f
Ulnar nerve injury 413
Ultrasonic activated scalpel 45f
Ultrasonic devices 44
Ultrasonography machine 27
Unicameral bone cyst 357
Upper abdominal transverse incision 94
Upper gastrointestinal
    endoscopy 131, 132
    surgery 130
Upper limb
    hemorrhage 281
    venous anatomy of 72f
Upper midline incision 91
Urethra, prostatic 271
Urethral catheterization 262, 266
    technique of 266
Urethral meatus 282
Urethral strictures 272
Urinary catheter 27
Urine
    outflow 270f
    output 281

V

Vacuum pack closure 250
Valvular heart disease 123
Vancomycin 140
Varicose veins, ablation of 49
Vascular anastomosis, complications of 184
Vascular reconstruction, basics of 173
Vascular sutures 180
Vasovagal faint 59
Vein, perforation of posterior wall of 74
Venous air embolism 69
Venous cutdown insertion, complications of 74
Venous thrombosis 74
Ventilation 276, 279
Ventricular fibrillation 299
Vertical compression injury 396
Vertical mattress suture 87, 87f
Vessels 408
Visual infusion phlebitis score 59f
Vital signs 309
Vitamins 220, 222
Volkmann's ischemic contracture 371f
Volkmann's sign 372f
Vomiting 312

W

Wheeze 122
World Health Organization 6, 25, 124, 134
    surgical safety checklist 134
Wound 331
    breakdown 372
    care of 328
    closure 81, 85
    dehiscence 248
    epithelialization of 331
    full-thickness 331
    infection 248
        risk of 144
    management, ointments for 328

X

Xylocaine 76

Z

Zadik's operation 254
Zollinger-Ellison syndrome 258